Farm Animal Medicine and Surgery

For Small Animal Veterinarians

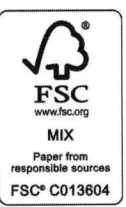

FSC
www.fsc.org
MIX
Paper from
responsible sources
FSC® C013604

I would like to dedicate this book to all the veterinary students that I have had the privilege of helping with their learning, starting with Shartry and Ramazan in Mombasa in 1967 and continuing through to my daughter Amelia in 2013. They have all helped me and taught me so much about life in general. I hope they will enjoy their veterinary careers as much as I have and find this book useful.

Farm Animal Medicine and Surgery

For Small Animal Veterinarians

Dr Graham R. Duncanson BVSc, MSc (VetGP), DProf, FRCVS

Equine and Farm Animal Practitioner,
Westover Veterinary Practice, UK

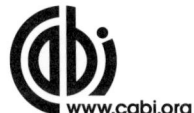

www.cabi.org

CABI is a trading name of CAB International

CABI	CABI
Nosworthy Way	38 Chauncey Street
Wallingford	Suite 1002
Oxfordshire OX10 8DE	Boston, MA 02111
UK	USA
Tel: +44 (0)1491 832111	Tel: +1 800 552 3083 (toll free)
Fax: +44 (0)1491 833508	Tel: +1 (0)617 395 4051
E-mail: info@cabi.org	E-mail: cabi-nao@cabi.org
Website: www.cabi.org	

A catalogue record for this book is available from the British Library, London, UK.

Library of Congress Cataloging-in-Publication Data

Duncanson, Graham R.
  Farm animal medicine and surgery : for small animal veterinarians / Graham R. Duncanson.
    p. ; cm.
  Includes bibliographical references and index.
  ISBN 978-1-84593-882-6 (hb) -- ISBN 978-1-84593-883-3 (pb)
  1. Veterinary medicine--Handbooks, manuals, etc. 2. Animal health--Handbooks, manuals, etc. I. C.A.B. International. II. Title.
    [DNLM: 1. Animal Diseases--therapy. 2. Animal Diseases--diagnosis.
3. Livestock. 4. Poultry. 5. Surgical Procedures, Operative--veterinary. SF 745]

  SF745.D86 2013
  636.089--dc23
                          2012025557

ISBN-13: 978 1 84593 882 6 (hbk)
ISBN-13: 978 1 84593 883 3 (pbk)

Commissioning editor: Sarah Hulbert
Editorial assistant: Emma McCann
Production editor: Shankari Wilford

Typeset by SPi, Pondicherry, India.
Printed and bound in the UK by MPG Printgroup.

Contents

Foreword   vii

Abbreviations   ix

Introduction   xiii

 1 Veterinary Equipment   1

 2 Veterinary Medicines   8

 3 Cattle Medicine   27

 4 Cattle Surgery   54

 5 Sheep and Goat Medicine   82

 6 Sheep and Goat Surgery   122

 7 South American Camelid (SAC) Medicine   143

 8 South American Camelid (SAC) Surgery   166

 9 Pig Medicine   182

10 Pig Surgery   198

11 Domestic Poultry Medicine and Surgery   207

12 Notifiable Diseases   223

13 Zoonotic Diseases   228

Glossary   237

References   243

Index   245

The colour plates can be found following p. 146

Foreword

What constitutes a large animal emergency?

Is it every farm call for the mixed practice vet with the 5% farm animal caseload? Is it the dreaded phone call to see a farrowing sow while being the duty vet on call? What about the new graduate vets panicking over the large animal out of hours rota with thoughts of caesareans, uterine prolapses, unpackings, chokes, embryotomies, fractures and ditch rescues racing through their minds? Or is it simply the 5 a.m. call to the experienced veterinarian at 10 degrees below freezing with snow expected and farmer Giles informing you that 'The heifer in the field down yonder is off colour' and you get there to find a blown, recumbent heifer that has been attempting to calve a dead rotten calf for the past 6 hours!

These are among some of the unbelievably impossible and truly unimaginable situations we commonly find ourselves presented with when working as veterinarians. We often feel inexperienced and ill prepared to deal with the daunting tasks that we are presented with in both a correct and effective manner, especially if 90% of our caseload is small animal biased!

This book is intended as a quick reference (to keep in your car!) guide to those common large animal emergencies that we can be faced with as practising veterinarians. The author uses his vast knowledge and lifelong experiences in both the UK and abroad to summarize some of the most common, and indeed uncommon, medical and surgical situations encountered in large animal practice. In a simple yet comprehensive way, the author aims to both inform and settle the reader with the goal of providing the veterinarian with the essential information required to become better equipped and prepared when dealing with an emergency – while at all times keeping the animal's well-being at the forefront.

As a new graduate veterinarian myself, I feel we are often overwhelmed and underprepared for the harsh realities that face us in large animal practice. We are thrown in at the deep end upon graduation, and the reality of this in my experience is often vastly different from college textbooks and theory! This book is practically minded, focusing more on the 'how tos' as opposed to the 'whys?', and provides a logical and rational approach to large animal cases with the author's wealth of experience to back it up.

As my guide and mentor as a newly qualified veterinarian, the author of this book, Graham Duncanson, can only be described as a true inspiration. His enthusiasm for life and work is exceptional, along with his desire to continue to develop himself professionally. He is a very 'hands on' teacher and is happy to share his wealth of experience with others. His positive 'can do' attitude and kind-hearted, encouraging nature towards veterinary students and younger members of the profession is admirable and something we should all aspire to achieve.

Katie Rosslee
BSc (Hons) BVetMed MRCVS

Abbreviations (excluding disease and virus names)

ad lib	As much as desired
AGID	Agar gel immunodiffusion
AI	Artificial insemination
ASF	African swine fever
AST	Aspartate aminotransferase
BCS	Body condition score
BHC	Benzene hexachloride
bid	Twice daily
BUN	Blood urea nitrogen
C	Celsius
CAE	Caprine arthritis and encephalitis
cal	Calorie
CCN	Cerebrocortical-necrosis
CFT	Complement fixation test
CK	Creatine kinase
CLA	Caseous lymphadenitis
cm	Centimetre
CNS	Central nervous system
C-NS	Coagulase-negative staphylococci
CSF	Cerebrospinal fluid (also used for 'classical swine fever')
CT	Controlled test
cu.	Cubic
Cu	Copper
DEET	Diethyl-meta-toluamide
DIC	Disseminated intravascular coagulation
DM	Dry matter
DMSO	Dimethyl sulfoxide
DNA	Deoxyribonucleic acid
EAE	Enzootic abortion of ewes
ECG	Electrocardiogram
EDTA	Ethylenediaminetetraacetic acid
e.g.	For example

EHA	Egg hatch assay
EHV	Equine herpes virus
ELISA	Enzyme-linked immunosorbent assay
EPG	Eggs per gram
EU	European Union
F	Fahrenheit
FAT	Fluorescent antibody test
FCE	Feed conversion efficiency
FCR	Feed conversion ratio
FEC	Faecal egg count
FECRT	Faecal egg count reduction test
FMD	Foot-and-mouth disease
FPT	Failure of passive transfer
ft	Feet (measurement)
g	Gram
G	Gauge
GA	General anaesthetic
GGT	Gamma glutamyltransferase
GI	Gastrointestinal
GLDH	Glutamate dehydrogenase
GnRH	Gonadotrophin-releasing hormone
GVS	Goat Veterinary Society in the UK
h	Hour
Hb	Haemoglobin
IgE	Immunoglobulin E
IgG	Immunoglobulin G
i.e.	That is
im	Intramuscularly
in.	Inch
ip	Intraperitoneally
IU	International units
iv	Intravenously
kg	Kilogram
l	Litre
LAT	Latex agglutination test
LDT	Larval development test
LN	Lymph node
m	Metre
MCF	Malignant catarrhal fever
mcg	Microgram
MCH	Mean corpuscular haemoglobin
MCHC	Mean corpuscular haemoglobin concentration
MCV	Mean corpuscular volume
ME	Metabolizable energy
mg	Milligram
MIU	Million international units
min	Minute
ml	Millilitre
MOET	Multiple ovulation and embryo transfer
MRCT	Malignant round cell tumours
MRI	Magnetic resonance imaging
MV	Maedi-Visna (virus)

NSAID	Nonsteroidal anti-inflammatory drug
OIE	World Organisation for Animal Health (formerly Office International des Epizooties)
PAGE	Polyacrylamide gel electrophoresis
PCR	Polymerase chain reaction
PCV	Packed cell volume
pH	Negative logarithm of hydrogen ion activity
PI	Persistently infected
PLR	Papillary light reflex
PM	Post-mortem
PRA	Progressive retinal atrophy
PrP	Prion protein
PUBH	Polymerized ultrapurified bovine haemoglobin
pme	Post-mortem examination
PMN	Polymorphic nuclear cell
PMSG	Pregnant mare serum gonadotrophin
PO	Per os, orally
pp.	Pages
ppm	Part(s) per million
PPR	Peste des petits ruminants
PUPD	Polyuria–polydipsia
qid	Four times daily
RBC	Red blood cell
RFI	Residual feed intake
RNA	Ribonucleic acid
RPM	Revolutions per minute
RT-PCR	Reverse transcriptase polymerase chain reaction
s	Second
SAC	South American camelid
SCV	Small cell variant
SG	Specific gravity
sid	Once a day
SNT	Serum neutralization test
sub cut	Subcutaneously
TAT	Tetanus antitoxin
TDN	Total digestible nutrients
tid	Three times daily
TMS	Trimethoprim–sulfadoxine
TPR	Temperature, pulse and respiration
UK	United Kingdom
USA	United States of America
VDS	Veterinary Defence Society
VLA	Veterinary Laboratory Agency
VNT	Virus neutralization test
vol.	Volume
WBC	White blood cell
WCC	White cell count
wt	Weight
ZN	Ziehl–Neelsen

Introduction

The book aims to provide an easily accessible reference to the information required by practising veterinarians confronted by the emergency care of farm animals. Although information on the provision of emergency care is the prime aim of the book, information is also provided on likely surgical procedures (in the broadest possible sense) that will need to be carried out by clinicians in farm animal practice. Each chapter follows a similar format in consisting of a series of sections, often with subsections, generally with either a brief summary of or introduction to the subject concerned, and with or without accompanying lists of the information relevant to that topic, be it equipment, medicines, disease signs, diagnosis and treatment, or surgical conditions and procedures.

First, there are two general chapters on veterinary equipment and medicines, mostly consisting of practical checklists for use in an emergency. The rest of the book presents information on the medicine and surgery of farm animal species. Cattle, camelids and pigs are addressed in separate chapters, while sheep and goats are linked together in a single chapter, though highlighting the differences between the two. The chapter on domestic poultry is centred on chickens, but waterfowl, guinea fowl, peafowl and quails are referenced when relevant. The chapter on notifiable diseases near the end of the book is mainly for the UK and Europe, but other areas are included if thought to be of note.

The author hopes this book will be useful for veterinary practitioners throughout the world who are treating farm animals. However, it has mainly been written for small animal practitioners who are asked to treat pet farm animals or who are asked by smallholders to treat their animals. The author also hopes that the book will be particularly useful for veterinary students and younger graduates.

Veterinary science is evolving at an ever increasing rate and so some of the information presented here may be out of date before publication. The author apologizes for this and any inaccuracies. He hopes that these can be corrected in future editions and would be really grateful for any contact from readers via email to vetdunc@btinternet.com

Dr Graham R. Duncanson,
BVSc, MSc (VetGP), DProf, FRCVS

1

Veterinary Equipment

Introduction

Equipping an ambulatory veterinary surgeon to carry out emergency farm animal practice may appear expensive. However, the author feels that having the correct equipment is vital, and that anything substandard will create unnecessary stress for the veterinarian and be open to criticism by the client. The items in the lists below need not all be carried by the veterinarian but, on the whole, they represent the minimum equipment that should be readily available. Veterinary practices should consider very carefully their position in undertaking emergency work with farm animals if they are not properly equipped to do so.

Equipment for Handling

The items that are listed below for handling animals might not seem to be essential equipment because, except for rubber boots and waterproofs, it is reasonable to expect that the other items will be provided by the farmer. Indeed, established farmers will provide all of these items, particularly as they are well aware of the danger of spreading disease. Hobby farmers and pet farm animal owners will not be so helpful, and so I suggest that the items listed below are carried by the ambulatory practitioner. Compared with

so much modern imaging equipment, they are very inexpensive:

- A bucket, brush, farmyard disinfectant, rubber boots and waterproofs.
- Small halter. This is required for calves, sheep, goats and South American camelids (SACs).
- Large halter. This should be strong enough for bulls.
- Lung line. This is for herding SACs.
- Strong rope. A 10 m length of rope is required for casting cattle.
- 4 × 1 m lengths of thin rope are required to help with restraint of sheep, goats and SACs during Caesarean section.
- Bulldog clip.
- A pig snare. A suitable type is shown in Figure 1.1.

Equipment for Diagnosis

These items are very small and inexpensive, except for the centrifuge, McMaster slide and microscope, which it is not necessary to carry. However, the author considers the other items in the list to be essential:

- Arm-length sleeves are required for internal examinations but are probably not used for actual parturition procedures.
- Blood slides and coverslips are essential items.

- Blood tubes are required with different anticoagulants:
  - Red top – serum – routine serology and biochemistry
  - Green top – heparin – glutathione peroxidase (selenium)-BVD (bovine virus diarrhoea) antigen
  - Lilac top – EDTA – haematology
  - Grey top – oxidase/fluoride – glucose
  - Blue top – acid wash – special ions e.g. Zn (must be non-rubber top for Zn).
- Biopsy punches of the small 8 mm disposable type are useful for skin biopsies. There are sophisticated biopsy gadgets available, which are vital for certain biopsies, e.g. liver biopsies. These need not be taken as a routine in the vehicle by an ambulatory clinician.
- A digital camera is important so that the clinician has the ability to download the photographs, label them, store them and send them as attachments to emails.
- Faeces sample bottles of sufficient size are required. Clinicians should be aware that quite large amounts of faeces are required for certain examinations. At least 70 g should be collected.
- Haematocrit centrifuge tubes can be used without a centrifuge to get a quick idea of packed cell volume (PCV). However, a mini centrifuge is useful and relatively inexpensive. A hand-driven centrifuge for larger tubes is very cheap and can give adequate results. This need not be taken in the vehicle as a routine by an ambulatory clinician.
- Labels, notebook and a pen are all required for recording cases and sample taking.
- A magnifying glass is useful in skin examination.
- A 'McMaster' slide is required for carrying out faecal worm egg counts. Great care should be taken when handling the coverslip (with the squares), as they are delicate and expensive. These need not be taken as a routine in the vehicle by an ambulatory clinician.
- A microscope is a delicate piece of equipment. It is not recommend that it is routinely carried in the vehicle. However, the use of a microscope at the base is vital. It needs to be equipped for oil immersion. 'Diff-Quik'-stained slides are also useful. Gram stain, Giemsa and methylene blue are important.
- Sample bottles containing formalin are required for preserving biopsy material. They should be stored separately from swabs required for bacteriological sampling.
- Small strong polythene bags are useful for skin samples and for double sealing various other samples, e.g. faeces sample bottles.
- A stethoscope is a vital piece of diagnostic equipment. Ideally it needs to be slim so that auscultation is possible under the muscles caudal to the shoulder, and both a bell and a diaphragm should be present. Obviously, there are sophisticated stethoscopes available, e.g. 'Litmans', but the inexpensive models are quite adequate.
- A thin stomach tube is required with a rectangular piece of wood to act as a gag with a hole to pass the tube through. This is useful for relieving bloat in calves, sheep and goats. It can also be used for obtaining samples of the rumen contents.
- Various types of swab are required. Some should have transport media and some should be plain. Sometimes a very narrow swab will be required.
- A clinical thermometer is vital. The traditional glass thermometers will last for years if kept carefully in a plastic case, but they are hard to acquire in the UK because of their mercury content. However, there are digital thermometers available. The clinician needs to choose whether the thermometer reads Celsius (Centigrade) or Fahrenheit – this is just a matter of which the clinician is happy with.
- Urine dipsticks are useful occasionally.

Equipment for Treatment

Practitioners might consider a force pump (an 'Agger's pump' is recommended) to be too expensive to be supplied to all ambulatory veterinary surgeons. Indeed large volumes of

liquid can be administered to cows with a funnel, but this very time-consuming and does
not look very professional. In these days,
when farmers are charged by the minute, the
author considers that most of them will not be
impressed with such old-fashioned methods
of treatment. The other items listed are essential and very inexpensive:

- force pump for administering large volumes of fluid to cows (e.g. an Agger's pump)
- calf rehydration bag
- non-disposable 30 ml syringes
- hypodermic needles (Luer fitting)
- disposable syringes (Luer mount)
- spinal needles 15 cm
- 25 cm Seaton needle with uterine tape
- 6 inch curved cutting edged suturing
  needle

Equipment for the Feet

Cattle hoof trimmers are not cheap, but there
is no realistic alternative and so the author
considers them to be essential equipment,
together with the other inexpensive items
that are described below.

Hoof knife

The type of knife is a very individual choice.
Obviously, there are knives for left and right
hands. Equally, there are double-sided knives
which can be used in either hand. Looped
knives are useful for removing the softer parts
of the hoof.

Hoof trimmers

The large size is required for adult cattle.

Gutter tape

A roll of this tape is very useful for making
bandages waterproof in the hoof area. The
tape is also useful for covering poultices.

Small sheep-size hoof clippers

These should be kept well oiled.

Equipment for the Limbs

Fractured limbs not only require immediate
immobilization but also, in the eyes of both
farmers and the public, need immediate
stabilization. Splints and bandages are, therefore, essential; they should be kept in a sturdy
case to avoid damage from pressure and
liquid contamination.

Oscillating saw

This might be considered not to be essential as
a hand-held plaster saw can be used. However,
with modern plastering materials it is seriously
hard work. An oscillating saw is quick and
accurate. These need not be routinely taken in
the vehicle by an ambulatory clinician.

Splints

Where funds are tight there is no need for
sophisticated splints. Smooth lengths of wood
and plastic guttering are quite adequate. Any
sharp ends can be rasped smooth and covered
with gutter tape.

Bandages and dressings

Sufficient materials should be included to
cover a very large leg wound on a cow. An
adequate amount of hydroponic gel is required.
There should be enough bandaging to put a
'Robert Jones' splint on a cow.

Equipment for the Eyes

There is no doubt that eyes will need urgent
attention and consequently the two items
described below are essential for the ambulatory clinician.

Fluorescein strips

These are inexpensive and vital not only for revealing the presence of deep corneal ulcers but also for testing the patency of the tear ducts. It should be remembered that it takes up to 30 min for the fluorescein to reach the nasal end of the tear ducts in ruminants after instillation in the eye.

Ophthalmoscope

This is an expensive piece of equipment but is important to the clinician. Much can be found out by examining the eyes carefully with a bright small torch and a magnifying glass. Sadly, however, without a good ophthalmoscope some pathological conditions will be missed. Although a slit lamp is very useful for examining dog's eyes, it is not required for farm animals.

Equipment for Dentistry

Unlike eyes, the teeth of farm animals do not need very urgent attention. In fact, there is much to recommend a more structured approach to their treatment. As a result, the items noted below may be kept at the practice rather than carried. The only exception is the drinkwater gag which will be required urgently to enable the removal of potatoes in the oesophagus of cows.

Dental elevators

Dental elevators as used for removing wolf teeth in horses are helpful.

Dental picks

These should be strong to allow the practitioner to pick out the food matter compacted between the teeth in diastemata.

Dental rasps

A small diamond-covered rasp is required.

Drinkwater gag

These are available for both the left and the right jaws of adult cattle. Only one is required. Normally the gag for the right jaw is required for a right-handed operator.

Headlight

There are some seriously bright torches available with heavy battery packs, but these are not really required, and a headlight which is easily taken on and off is preferable.

Molar extraction forceps

Two pairs are required. They should be 20 cm long, one should be straight and the other should have the extracting jaws at right angles.

Molar spreaders

A small pair 20 cm long is required.

Mouthwashing syringe

A catheter tip 60 ml syringe is adequate for this purpose.

Small ruminant gag

These are hard to obtain. A suitable type is shown in Fig. 6.2. on page 124.

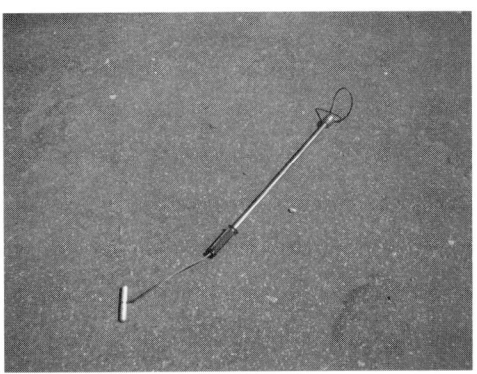

Fig. 1.1. Pig snare.

Equipment for Stitching

These items are self-explanatory. They are listed below for completeness. The clinician can manage with very few.

Artery forceps

These can be straight or curved. Several pairs are required.

Clippers

These are a luxury. However, they make stitching and wound management so much cleaner and easier, particularly in rough-haired animals. The ideal is the rechargeable battery type.

Drapes

A single sterile drape is required as a tray cloth by the ambulatory clinician, although drapes will be required for other surgery.

Dressing forceps

The ends of dressing forceps are important: they can be flat or 'rat toothed'. A pair of each would be required.

Dressing scissors

A pair of curved, blunt-ended scissors needs to be readily available for trimming hair. However, a straight pair with pointed ends is required for a stitch-up kit. There are various different sizes.

Needle holders

There are various types. The most convenient for stitching up wounds are the combination of cutting and holding type called 'Gillies'.

Scalpel blades

These come in different sizes and shapes for different procedures.

Scalpel handle

It is important that the scalpel handle is the same size as the blades.

Stitch-cutting scissors

These small scissors need to be available for removing sutures.

Suture material

This may be absorbable or non-absorbable. It may also be either monofilament or braided. On the whole, monofilament nylon is the non-absorbable material recommended for suturing the skin. Polyglactin is the ideal absorbable suture material.

Suture needles

These come in various shapes. They are also either cutting or non-cutting. Generally, cutting needles will be required for the skin and non-cutting needles for soft tissue.

Tissue forceps

These forceps are for lifting tissue. A minimum of two pairs is required.

Towel clips

These are not normally required by the ambulatory clinician unless surgery is going to be performed under a general anaesthetic (GA).

Swabs

Sets of sterile swabs are required for a variety of tasks.

Equipment for the Reproductive System

Parturition is an urgent event and therefore the items listed below are vital to the ambulatory practitioner.

Calving jack

This should include a set of two short calving ropes of different colours.

Calving and lambing equipment

This should include:

- long strong calving ropes
- thin lambing ropes
- three 20 cm lengths of alkathene pipe
- a calf resuscitator pump
- calving lubricant and J lube
- doxapram hydrochloride drops
- a heavy introducer
- a thin long flexible introducer
- two small eye hooks

- an embryotomy knife
- a calf feeder bag
- resuscitation equipment
- a 5 l container, containing 0.5 l sterile water containing 20 g of sodium citrate
- a small trocar and cannula
- a large plastic bloodline
- a McLean's knife

Embryotome

This should have a threader, a long length of embryotomy wire, a pair of small wire cutters and a set of two handles for the wire.

Vaginal speculum

These can be disposable and used with a head torch or a small hand torch. The small duck-billed type affords the very best visibility for ewes, does, sows and SACs. The large duck-billed type affords the best visibility for cows.

A dedicated box for Caesarean section

This should contain:

- Sterile instruments, including several 4 inch non-cutting and cutting curved suturing needles, one pair of needle holders, one pair of 'Gillies', one pair of rat-toothed dressing forceps, one pair of flat-ended dressing forceps, one scalpel blade holder, one large pair of straight scissors, four large pairs of artery forceps, two small pairs of artery forceps, and two pairs of uterus-holding forceps.
- Scalpel blades which must fit the scalpel blade holder in the sterile instrument pack.
- Polyglactin suture material.
- Monofilament nylon suture material.
- A sterile tray cloth.
- Two sterile calving ropes.
- A navel clip.
- Hair clippers (or razors).
- A sterile scrubbing brush.
- Two packets of large sterile swabs.

- A sterile embryotomy knife or a disposable embryotomy knife.
- Disposable syringes (10, 20 and 30 ml).
- Disposable needles (4 cm × 18 G).
- Pieces of cotton wool in a bag for cleaning the skin.
- Bottle of surgical spirit.
- Bottle of chlorhexidine.
- 1 × 25 ml oxytocin injection containing 10 IU/ml.
- 1 × 100 ml water for injection.
- 1 × 50 ml solution of clenbuterol hydrochloride containing 30 micrograms/ml.
- 3 × 5 mega crystalline penicillin.
- 3 × 100 ml local anaesthetic.
- 100 ml aqueous suspension of a mixture of procaine penicillin and dihydrostreptomycin.
- Dopram drops.
- 50 ml solution of clenbuterol hydrochloride containing 30 micrograms/ml.
- A 100 ml bottle of an injectable nonsteroidal anti-inflammatory drug (NSAID) licensed for ruminants.
- An antibiotic aerosol.
- A 5 m length of rope to be tied around the right hind leg and brought under the cow's body so that it can be pulled if the cow is appearing to go down. This will make sure the cow falls with her left flank uppermost.

Other reproductive equipment

- a Burdizzo, for castration
- a McLean's teat knife

Equipment for Post-mortem (PM)

These articles are not normally carried by an ambulatory clinician:

- large plastic bucket with disinfectant, warm water, soap and towel

- butcher's knife and flaying knife
- scalpel and blades that fit
- rat-toothed forceps (15 cm)
- fine forceps (15 cm)
- blunt-nosed straight scissors (20 cm)
- bowel scissors
- bone cutters, saw and hedge loppers

Sampling materials

These include the following:

- plastic trays (50 × 30 × 5 cm)
- plastic bags or various sizes
- sterile universal bottles
- plastic jars (1 l)
- bottles of formalin (kept separate)
- pots containing 50% glycerol for virus isolation
- swabs (plain, transport media and specialized for respiratory pathogens)
- red Vacutainers® for collecting blood, aqueous humour, body fluids
- Pasteur pipettes and rubber sucker
- clipboard
- PM report form, lab submission form

Specialist Equipment

The pieces of equipment listed below are included for completeness. It would be very useful to have the use these items, although within the scope of this book a full description would not be worthwhile. Throughout the text a feasible alternative will be suggested wherever possible to save on financial investment. The list is as follows:

- blood analyser
- centrifuge
- gaseous anaesthetic machine
- operating table
- refractometer
- ultrasound scanner
- X-ray machine

2

Veterinary Medicines

Introduction

In the UK, veterinary medicines are licensed for use in a particular species. They may only be used in a different species if there is no licensed product for that species available. There are very few medicines licensed for goats and no medicines licensed for camelids, although all products licensed for sheep and cattle can be used in goats and camelids (excepting those that contain the antibiotic tilmicosin). Only products required for emergency veterinary cases (i.e. no mastitis prevention antibiotics, no vaccines and no products for disease prevention) are included in the drug lists below, which are arranged first by animal species (cattle, sheep, pigs and poultry) and then by medicine type; proprietary names are used throughout.

The lists that are presented cover the majority of licensed medicines available for cattle, sheep, pigs and poultry in the UK; these are included as a guide only. Practitioners from other countries will have other products available which are similar or are actually generic replicas. Such generic products may well be not only suitable but also legal in other countries; however, they are not legal in the UK.

General advice on products that need to be carried and/or used by the emergency practitioner is given at the head of each main category of medicines.

Cattle Medicines

Anti-inflammatory preparations

Practitioners need to be very selective with these preparations. Only a single NSAID (non-steroidal anti-inflammatory drug – indicated at the end of the drug description) is essential so, on balance, the author would choose a preparation containing flunixin meglumine. This drug will be useful for its analgesic, anti-inflammatory and antitoxic properties. A preparation containing dexamethasone which can be given iv is also required. A solution containing butylscopolamine 4 mg/ml and metamizole 500 mg/ml should be included as well. The complete list follows:

- Binixin: flunixin meglumine 50 mg/ml; 2 ml/45 kg iv daily for up to 5 days. Meat withhold 8 days. Milk withhold 12 h. NSAID.
- Buscopan: hyoscine butylbromide 20 mg/ml; 2 ml/100 kg im as a single injection. Meat withhold 2 days. Not to be used in lactating animals.
- Buscopan Compositium: butylscopolamine 4 mg/ml and metamizole 500 mg/ml; 5 ml/100 kg iv or im as a single injection. Meat withhold 9 days after iv and 28 days after im. Not to be used in lactating animals. NSAID.

- Carprieve Solution for Injection for Cattle: carprofen 50 mg/ml; 1 ml/35 kg as a single injection sub cut. Meat withhold 21 days. Zero milk withhold. NSAID.
- Colvasone: dexamethazone 2 mg/ml; 1 ml/25 kg iv or im as a single injection. Milk withhold 84 h. Meat withhold 21 days.
- Comforion vet 100 mg/ml Solution for Injection for Horse, Cattle and Swine: ketoprofen 100 mg/ml; 1 ml/33 kg iv or im daily. Meat withhold 4 days. Zero milk withhold. NSAID.
- Dexadreson: dexamethasone 2 mg/ml; 1.5 ml/50 kg iv or im once and repeated in 48 h. Meat withhold 7 days. Milk withhold 60 h.
- Dexafort: dexamethazone sodium phosphate 1.38 mg/ml and dexamethazone phenylpropionate 2.67 mg/ml; 1 ml/50 kg im. Meat withhold 63 days. Milk withhold 6 days.
- Duphacort Q: dexamethasone 2 mg/ml; 1 ml/25 kg iv or im. Meat withhold 21 days. Milk withhold 84 h.
- Finadyne Solution: flunixin meglumine 50 mg/ml; 2 ml/45 kg im. Meat withhold 5 days. Milk withhold 24 h. NSAID.
- Flunixin Injection: flunixin meglumine 50 mg/ml; 2 ml/45 kg im. Meat withhold 7 days. Milk withhold 36 h. NSAID.
- Ketodale 100 mg/ml Solution for Injection for Horses, Cattle and Swine: ketoprofen 100 mg/ml; 3 ml/100 kg im. Meat withhold 4 days. Zero milk withhold. NSAID.
- Ketofen 10%: ketoprofen 100 mg/ml; 3 ml/100 kg im. Meat withhold 4 days. NSAID.
- Melovem 5 mg/ml Solution for Injection for Cattle and Pigs: meloxicam 5 mg/ml; 2 ml/25 kg im daily for two injections. Meat withhold 5 days. Zero milk withhold. NSAID.
- Meloxidyl 20 mg/ml Solution for Injection for Cattle, Pigs and Horses: meloxicam 20 mg/ml; 2 ml/100 kg im daily for two injections. Meat withhold 5 days. Milk withhold 120 h. NSAID.
- Metacam 20 mg/ml Solution for Injection for Cattle, Pigs and Horses: meloxicam 20 mg/ml; 2 ml/100 kg im daily for two injections. Meat withhold 5 days. Milk withhold 120 h. NSAID.
- Norocarp Injection for Cattle and Horses: carprofen 50 mg/ml; 1 ml/35 kg iv or sub cut as a single injection. Meat withhold 21 days. Not licensed for lactating cattle. NSAID.
- Rapidexon: dexamethasone 2 mg/ml; 1.5 ml/50 kg iv or im once and repeated in 48 h. Meat withhold 2 days. Milk withhold 72 h.
- Rheumocam 20 mg/ml Injection for Cattle, Pigs and Horses: meloxicam 20 mg/ml; 2.5 ml/100 kg sub cut or iv. Meat withhold 15 days. Milk withhold 5 days. NSAID.
- Rimadyl Cattle: carprofen 50 mg/ml; 1 ml/35 kg iv or sub cut as a single injection. Meat withhold 21 days. Zero milk withhold. NSAID.
- Solacyl 100%, Powder for Oral Solution for Calves and Pigs: sodium salicylate 1000 mg/g; 35 mg/kg orally in drinking water for 3–5 days. Zero meat withhold. Not for use in cows producing milk for human consumption. NSAID.
- Tolfine: tolfenamic acid 4 mg/ml; 1 ml/20 kg im as a single injection. Meat withhold 3 days. Milk withhold 24 h, discard the first milking after treatment. NSAID.
- Voren Suspension for Injection, 1 mg/ml: dexamethazone 1 mg/ml; 2 ml/100 kg im. Meat withhold 55 days. Milk withhold 60 h.

Mixed anti-inflammatory and antimicrobial preparations

These are suitable for farmers' use but are not essential for practitioners. Preparations containing NSAIDs are indicated at the end of the drug description:

- Hexasol LA Injection: oxytetracycline 300 mg/ml and flunixin meglumine 20 mg/ml; 1 ml/10 kg im as a single injection. Meat withhold 35 days. Not to be used in lactating animals. NSAID.

- Resflor Injectable Solution: florfenicol 300 mg/ml and flunixin meglumine: 16.5 mg/ml; 2 ml/15 kg as a single sub cut injection. Meat withhold 46 days. Not to be used in lactating animals. NSAID.

Antimicrobials

There are a very wide range of antimicrobials available to the modern practitioner, not only with different ingredients but also with different durations of action. It could be argued that the emergency clinician does not actually require any long-acting preparations as the task required is urgent antimicrobial therapy which, if not effective in 24 h, requires adjustment in either drug type or dosage. This may certainly be the case when cattle are being treated by experienced farmers, but when treating cattle for smallholders with poor handling facilities, or when treating cattle kept in extensive conditions, e.g. when they are out on open land (range) or on marshland, a different approach will be required that entails the use of longer acting antimicrobials. Another factor to be considered is the stress induced by handling yarded cattle on a daily basis, particularly beef cattle with pneumonia. In these cases too long-acting preparations will be required. The author would, therefore, advise that ambulatory practitioners carry a minimum of a selection of five different types of injectable antibiotics with at least two potentially long-acting preparations. At least one oral and one topical antimicrobial will also be required.

In the following lists, drugs containing tilmicosin are marked as not recommended for use in goats and camelids at the end of the drug description:

Injectables

- Advocin 2.5% Solution for Injection: danofloxacin 25 mg/ml; 1 ml/20 kg im or iv daily. Meat withhold 5 days. Milk withhold 2 days.
- Advocin 180: danofloxacin 180 mg/ml; 1 ml/30 kg subcutaneously or iv as a single injection. Meat withhold 8 days. Milk withhold 4 days.

- Alamycin 10: oxytetracycline 100 mg/ml; 1 ml/11–50 kg im daily. Meat withhold 20 days. Milk withhold 86 h.
- Alamycin LA: oxytetracycline 200 mg/ml; 1 ml/10 kg im as a single injection. Meat withhold 31 days. Milk withhold 10 days.
- Alamycin LA 300: oxytetracycline 300 mg/ml; 1 ml/10–15 kg im as a single injection. Meat withhold 14–35 days depending on dosage. Milk withhold 10 days.
- Amfipen LA: ampicillin 100 mg/ml; 1.5 ml/10 kg im every 2 days. Meat withhold 60 days. Not to be used in animals producing milk for human consumption.
- Amoxycare Injection: amoxicillin 150 mg/ml; 1 ml/22.5 kg im daily. Meat withhold 18 days. Milk withhold 24 h.
- Amoxycare LA Injection: amoxicillin 150 mg/ml; 1 ml/10 kg im every 2 days. Meat withhold 23 days. Milk withhold 84 h.
- Amoxypen Injection: amoxicillin 150 mg/ml; 1 ml/20 kg im daily. Meat withhold 18 days. Milk withhold 24 h.
- Amoxypen LA: amoxicillin 150 mg/ml; 1 ml/10 kg im daily. Meat withhold 23 days. Milk withhold 79 h.
- Baytril 5% Solution for Injection: enrofloxacin 50 mg/ml; 1 ml/20 kg im daily. This dose rate may be doubled for treating salmonellosis and complicated respiratory disease. Meat withhold 14 days. Not to be used in animals producing milk for human consumption.
- Baytril 10% Solution for Injection: enrofloxacin 100 mg/ml; 2.5 ml/100 kg daily sub cut (dose rate may be doubled for treating salmonellosis and complicated respiratory disease; this double dose may be given slowly intravenously to treat toxic mastitis). Meat withhold 10 days, milk withhold 84 h after sub cut injection. Meat withhold 4 days, milk withhold 72 h after iv injection.
- Betamox Injection: amoxicillin 150 mg/ml; 1 ml/22.5 kg im daily. Meat withhold 18 days. Milk withhold 24 h.
- Betamox LA: amoxicillin 150 mg/ml; 1 ml/10 kg im every 2 days. Meat withhold 23 days. Milk withhold 79 h.

- Cefenil 50 mg/ml Powder and Solvent Solution for Injection for Cattle and Pigs: ceftiofur 1 g/20 ml; 1 ml/50 kg im daily. Meat withhold 2 days. Milk withhold zero.
- Ceftiocyl 50 mg/ml: ceftiofur 50 mg/ml; 1 ml/50 kg sub cut daily. Meat withhold 8 days. Milk withhold zero.
- Cevaxel-RTU: ceftiofur 50 mg/ml; 1 ml/50 kg sub cut daily. Meat withhold 8 days. Milk withhold zero.
- Clamoxyl Ready-to-use Injection: amoxicillin 150 mg/ml; 1 ml/21 kg im daily. Meat withhold 54 days. Milk withhold 60 h.
- Cobactan 2.5%: cefquinome 25 mg/ml; 2 ml/50 kg im daily. Meat withhold 5 days. Milk withhold 24 h.
- Cobactan 4.5%: cefquinome 45 mg/ml; 1 ml/45 kg im daily. Meat withhold 2 days. Milk withhold 36 h.
- Combiclav Injection: amoxicillin 140 mg/ml and clavulanic acid 35 mg/ml; 1 ml/20 kg im daily. Meat withhold 42 days. Milk withhold 60 h.
- Cyclosol LA: oxytetracycline 200 mg/ml; 1 ml/10 kg im every 3 days. Meat withhold 35 days. Milk withhold 192 h.
- Depocillin: procaine benzylpenicillin 300 mg/ml; 1 ml/25 kg im daily. Meat withhold 5 days. Milk withhold 11 days.
- Devomycin 250 mg/ml Solution for Injection: streptomycin 250 mg/ml; 1 ml/25 kg im daily. Meat withhold 16 days. Milk withhold 48 h.
- Devomycin D: streptomycin 150 mg/ml and dihydrostreptomycin 150 mg/ml; 1 ml/12 kg im daily. Meat withhold 14 days. Milk withhold 48 h.
- Draxxin 100 mg/ml Solution for Injection for Cattle and Pigs: tulathromycin 100 mg/ml; 1 ml/40 kg im as a single injection. Meat withhold 49 days. Not for use in lactating cattle producing milk for human consumption. Not to be used in pregnant cows or heifers intended to produce milk for human consumption within 2 months of expected parturition.
- Duphacillin: ampicillin 150 mg/ml; 1 ml/20 kg im daily. Meat withhold 18 days. Milk withhold 24 h.
- Duphacycline 10%: oxytetracycline 100 mg/ml; 1 ml/13–40 kg im daily. Meat withhold 20 days. Milk withhold 84 h.
- Duphacycline LA 20% Solution for Injection: oxytetracycline 200 mg/ml; 3 ml/50 kg im as a single injection. Meat withhold 31 days. Milk withhold 240 h.
- Duphamox: amoxicillin 150 mg/ml; 1 ml/21 kg im daily. Meat withhold 18 days. Milk withhold 24 h.
- Duphamox LA: amoxicillin 150 mg/ml; 1 ml/10 kg im as a single injection. Meat withhold 21 days. Milk withhold 60 h.
- Duphapen: procaine penicillin 300 mg/ml; 1 ml/30 kg im daily. Meat withhold 7 days. Milk withhold 84 h.
- Duphapen Fort: procaine benzylpenicillin 300 mg/ml; 1 ml/15 kg im every 72 h. Meat withhold 13 days. Milk withhold 132 h.
- Duphapen+Strep: procaine benzylpenicillin 200 mg/ml + dihydrostreptomycin 250 mg/ml; 1 ml/25 kg im daily. Meat withhold 23 days. Milk withhold 60 h.
- Duphatrim IS Injectable Solution: trimethoprim 40 mg/ml + sulfadiazine 200 mg/ml; 1 ml/16 kg im or iv daily. Meat withhold 12 days. Milk withhold 24 h.
- Eficur: ceftiofur 50 mg/ml; 1 ml/50 kg im daily. Meat withhold 8 days. Milk withhold zero.
- Engemycin 10% (DD): oxytetracycline 100 mg/ml; 1 ml/12.5 kg im or iv daily or 1 ml/5 kg im every 60 h. Meat withhold 36 days with daily dose and 21 days with 60 h dose; milk withhold for both dosages 6 days.
- Engemycin 10% Farm Pack: oxytetracycline 100 mg/ml; 3 ml/100 kg im daily or 1 ml/10 kg im every 60 h. Meat withhold 35 days with daily dose and 21 days with 60 h dose; milk withhold for both dosages 6 days.
- Engemycin LA: oxytetracycline 200 mg/ml; 1 ml/10 kg im as a single injection. Meat withhold 31 days. Milk withhold 10 days.
- Enrocare 5%: enrofloxacin 50 mg/ml; 1 ml/20 kg sub cut daily; this dose may be doubled when treating salmonellosis and complicated respiratory disease. Meat withhold 14 days. Not permitted

for animals producing milk for human consumption.

- Enrocare 10%: enrofloxacin 100 mg/ml; 1 ml/40 kg sub cut or iv daily (dose may be doubled when treating salmonellosis and complicated respiratory disease). Meat withhold 10 days for sub cut injection and 4 days for iv injection. Milk withhold 84 h for sub cut injection and 72 h for iv injection.
- Enroxil Solution for Injection 50 mg/ml for Calves, Pigs and Dogs: enrofloxacin 50 mg/ml; 1 ml/20 kg im daily (dose may be doubled when treating complicated respiratory disease). Meat withhold 10 days. Not permitted for animals producing milk for human consumption.
- Enroxil Solution for Injection 100 mg/ml for Calves and Pigs: enrofloxacin 100 mg/ml; 1 ml/20 kg sub cut daily (dose may be doubled when treating salmonellosis and complicated respiratory disease). Meat withhold 14 days, milk withhold 120 h.
- Excenel RTU 50 mg/ml Suspension for Injection for Pigs and Cattle: ceftiofur 50 mg/ml; 1 ml/50 kg im daily. Meat withhold 8 days. Milk withhold zero.
- Excenel Sterile Powder for Solution for Injection: ceftiofur 50 mg/ml; 1 ml/50 kg sub cut daily. Meat withhold 1 day. Milk withhold zero.
- Fenflor 300 mg/ml Solution for Injection for Cattle: florfenicol 300 mg/ml; 1 ml/15 kg im every 48 h. Meat withhold 30 days. Not permitted for animals producing milk for human consumption.
- Fenoflox 50 mg/ml Injection for Cattle, Pigs, Dogs and Cats: enrofloxacin 50 mg/ml; 1 ml/20 kg sub cut daily (dose may be doubled when treating complicated respiratory disease). No withhold periods stated.
- Fenoflox 100 mg/ml Injection for Cattle and Pigs: enrofloxacin 100 mg/ml; 1 ml/40 kg sub cut daily (dose may be doubled when treating complicated respiratory disease). No withhold periods stated.
- Florkem: florfenicol 300 mg/ml; 1 ml/20 kg im every 48 h. Meat withhold 37 days. Not permitted for animals producing milk for human consumption.

- Forcyl: marbofloxacin 160 mg/ml; 1 ml/16 kg im. Meat withhold 5 days. Milk withhold 48 h.
- Intradine: sulfadimidine 308.9 mg/ml; 1 ml/1.5 kg sub cut initially followed by 1 ml/3 kg daily. Meat withhold 18 days. Milk withhold 156 h.
- Kefloril 300 mg/ml: florfenicol 300 mg/ml; 1 ml/15 kg im every 48 h or 2 ml/15 kg sub cut every 4 days. Meat withhold 30 days for im injection and 44 days for sub cut injection. Not permitted for animals producing milk for human consumption.
- Mamyzin 333.3 mg/ml powder and solvent: available as 5 g and 15 ml diluent, and as 10 g and 30 ml diluent. 3.5–5 ml/100 kg im. Meat withhold 7 days. Milk withhold 108 h.
- Marbiflox 100 mg/ml Solution for Cattle and Pigs: marbofloxacin 100 mg/ml; 2 ml/25 kg im for respiratory disease; 1 ml/50 kg im, sub cut and iv for acute mastitis. Meat withhold 3 days for respiratory disease dose, 6 days for the mastitis dose. Milk withhold 72 h for respiratory disease dose and 36 h for the mastitis dose.
- Marbocyl 2% Solution for Injection: marbofloxacin 2 mg/ml; 1 ml/10 kg sub cut daily. To be used in pre-ruminant calves. Meat withhold 6 days.
- Marbocyl 10% Solution for Injection: marbofloxacin 10 mg/ml; 1 ml/50 kg im, sub cut or iv daily. Meat withhold 6 days. Milk withhold 36 h.
- Marbocyl solo 10% Solution for Injection for Cattle: marbofloxacin 100 mg/ml; 2 ml/25 kg im as a single injection. Meat and milk withhold 3 days.
- Micotil: tilmicosin 300 mg/ml; 1 ml/30 kg for pneumonia and 1 ml/60 kg for interdigital necrobacillosis sub cut as a single injection. Meat withhold 60 days. Milk withhold 864 h. *This medicine can only be injected by a veterinary surgeon. Not recommended for use in goats or camelids.*
- Milbotyl: tilmicosin 300 mg/ml; 1 ml/30 kg for pneumonia and 1 ml/60 kg for interdigital necrobacillosis sub cut as a single injection. Meat withhold 60 days. Not to be used in lactating animals. *This medicine can only be injected by a veterinary*

surgeon. Not recommended for use in goats or camelids.

- Naxcel 200 mg/ml Suspension for Injection for Cattle: 200 mg ceftiofur per ml. 1 ml/30 kg sub cut as a single injection. Meat withhold 9 days. Milk withhold zero.
- Nisamox Suspension for Injection: amoxicillin 140 mg/ml + clavulanic acid 35 mg/ml; 1 ml/20 kg im daily. Meat withhold 42 days. Milk withhold 60 h.
- Norobrittin 15%: ampicillin 150 mg/ml; 1 ml/20 kg im daily. Meat withhold 18 days. Milk withhold 24 h.
- Norocillin 30%: procaine penicillin 300 mg/ml; 1 ml/30 kg im daily. Meat withhold 7 days. Milk withhold 84 h.
- Noroclav Injection: amoxicillin 140 mg/ml and clavulanic acid 35 mg/ml; 1 ml/20 kg im daily. Meat withhold 42 days. Milk withhold 80 h.
- Norodine 24: sulfadiazine 200 mg/ml + trimethoprim 40 mg/ml; 1 ml/16 kg im or iv daily. Meat withhold 12 days. Milk withhold 48 h.
- Norotril Max 100 mg/ml Solution for Injection for Cattle: enrofloxacin 100 mg/ml; 7.5 ml/100 kg sub cut as a single injection. Meat withhold 14 days. Milk withhold 84 h.
- Nuflor 300 mg/ml Solution for Injection for Cattle: florfenicol 300 mg/ml; 1 ml/15 kg im every 48 h or 2 ml/15 kg sub cut every 4 days. Meat withhold with im injection 30 days, with sub cut injection 44 days. Not permitted for use in animals producing milk for human consumption.
- Nuflor Minidose 450 mg/ml Solution for Injection for Cattle: florfenicol 450 mg/ml; 4 ml/45 kg sub cut as a single dose. Meat withhold 64 days. Not permitted for use in lactating animals producing milk for human consumption.
- Oxycare 10%: oxytetracycline 100 mg/ml; 1.5 ml/30–100 kg im daily. Meat withhold 20 days. Milk withhold 84 h.
- Oxycare 20% LA: oxytetracycline 200 mg/ml; 1 ml/10 kg im as a single injection. Meat withhold 31 days. Milk withhold 10 days.
- Oxytetrin 20 LA: oxytetracycline 200 mg/ml; 1 ml/10 kg im as a single injection. Meat withhold 39 days. Not be used in animals producing milk for human consumption.
- Pen & Strep: procaine penicillin 200 mg/ml + dihydrostreptomycin 250 mg/ml; 1 ml/25 kg im daily. Meat withhold 23 days. Milk withhold 60 h.
- Penacare: procaine benzylpenicillin 300 mg/ml; 1 ml/30 kg im daily. Meat withhold 7 days. Milk withhold 84 h.
- Powerflox 50 mg/ml Injection: enrofloxacin 50 mg/ml; 1 ml/20 kg sub cut daily (dose may be doubled when treating complicated respiratory disease). Meat withhold 14 days. Not permitted for use in lactating animals producing milk for human consumption.
- Powerflox 100 mg/ml Injection: enrofloxacin 100 mg/ml; 1 ml/40 kg sub cut or iv daily (dose may be doubled when treating complicated respiratory disease). Meat withhold for sub cut usage 14 days, for iv usage 4 days. Milk withhold for sub cut usage 96 h, for iv usage 72 h.
- Readycef Injection: ceftiofur 50 mg/ml; 1 ml/50 kg sub cut daily. Meat withhold 8 days. Milk withhold zero.
- Selectan: florfenicol 300 mg/ml; 1 ml/15 kg im every 48 h. Meat withhold 30 days. Not to be used in cattle producing milk for human consumption.
- Shotaflor 300 mg/ml Solution for Cattle: florfenicol 300 mg/ml; 1 ml/15 kg im every 48 h; 2 ml/15 kg sub cut as a single injection. Meat withhold 30 days for im dose, 44 days for sub cut dose. Not to be used in cattle producing milk for human consumption.
- Streptacare: procaine penicillin 200 mg/ml + dihydrostreptomycin 250 mg/ml; 1 ml/25 kg im daily. Meat withhold 23 days. Milk withhold 60 h.
- Synulox Ready-To-Use Suspension for Injection: clavulanic acid 35 mg/ml + amoxicillin 140 mg/ml; 1 ml/20 kg im daily. Meat withhold 42 days. Milk withhold 60 h.
- Terramycin/LA 200 mg/ml Solution for Injection: oxytetracycline 200 mg/ml; 1 ml/10 kg im as a single injection. Meat withhold 36 days. Milk withhold 7 days.

- Tilmodil 300 mg/ml solution: tilmicosin 300 mg/ml; 1 ml/30 kg for pneumonia and 1 ml/60 kg for interdigital necrobacillosis sub cut as a single injection. Meat withhold 60 days. Not to be used in cows producing milk for human consumption. *This medicine can only be injected by a veterinary surgeon. Not recommended for use in goats or camelids.*
- Tribrissen Injection 48%: trimethoprim 80 mg/ml + sulfadiazine 80 mg/ml; 1 ml/32 kg im daily. Meat withhold 34 days. Milk withhold 156 h.
- Trimacare 24% Injection: trimethoprim 40 mg/ml + sulfadiazine 200 mg/ml; 1 ml/16 kg im or iv daily. Meat withhold 12 days. Milk withhold 48 h.
- Trinacol Solution for Injection: trimethoprim 40 mg/ml + sulfadiazine 200 mg/ml; 1 ml/16 kg im daily. Meat withhold 12 days. Milk withhold 48 h.
- Tylan 200: tylosin 200 mg/ml; 1 ml/20–50 kg im daily. Meat withhold 28 days. Milk withhold 108 h.
- Ultrapen LA: procaine benzylpenicillin 300 mg/ml; 1 ml/15 kg im or sub cut as a single injection. Meat withhold 13 days after sub cut injection, 23 days after im injection. Milk withhold 132 h.
- Zactran: gamithromycin 150 mg/ml; 1 ml/25 kg sub cut as a single injection. Meat withhold 64 days. Not permitted for use in lactating animals producing milk for human consumption. Not to be used in pregnant cows or heifers intended to produce milk for human consumption within 2 months of expected parturition.
- Zuprevo: tildipirosin 180 mg/ml; 1 ml/45 kg sub cut as a single injection. Meat withhold 47 days. Not licensed for lactating animals.

Oral products to be given as bolus/tablet to calves

- Duphatrim Bolus: trimethoprim 200 mg/bolus and sulfadiazine 1 g/bolus; 1 bolus/40 kg daily for calves only. Meat withhold 15 days.
- Marbocyl Bolus: marbofloxacin 50 mg/bolus; 1 bolus/50 kg daily for calves only. Meat withhold 6 days.

- Norodine Bolus Tablets: trimethoprim 200 mg/bolus and sulfadiazine 1 g/bolus; 1 bolus/40 kg daily for calves only. Meat withhold 15 days.
- Occrycetin Bolus 500 mg tablet: oxytetracycline 500 mg/bolus; 1 bolus/50 kg twice daily for non-ruminating calves only. Meat withhold 14 days.
- Strinacin 11 Tablets: sulfadiazine 1.0 g/tablet + trimethoprim 200 mg/tablet; 1 tablet per 40 kg daily. Meat withhold 15 days.
- Synulox Bolus 500 mg Film-Coated Tablet: clavulanic acid 100 mg/bolus + amoxicillin 400 mg/bolus; 0.5 bolus/40 kg twice daily. Meat withhold 9 days.
- Trimacare Bolus: 1.0 g sulfadiazine + 200 mg trimethoprim per bolus; 1 bolus/40 kg daily. Meat withhold 15 days.

Oral products for calves to be used in the drinking water, milk or milk replacer

- Apralan Soluble Powder: apramycin sulfate 1 g/sachet; 1–2 sachets/50 kg daily. Meat withhold 28 days.
- Baycox 50 mg/ml Oral Suspension for Piglets, Calves and Lambs: toltrazuril 50 mg/ml; 0.4 ml/kg once orally. Meat withhold 63 days. Not for use in milking cows.
- Halocur: halofuginone lactate 0.5 mg/ml; 2 ml/kg daily. Meat withhold 13 days.
- Pulmotil AC: tilmicosin 250 mg/ml; 1 ml/20 kg twice daily. Meat withhold 42 days. Not to be used in lactating animals. *Not recommended for use in goats or camelids.*
- Terramycin Soluble Powder 5%: oxytetracycline 50 g/kg in a water-soluble base; 9–18 mg/kg daily for calves, 2–4 mg/kg daily for ruminating cattle. Meat withhold 10 days. Milk withhold zero.
- Terramycin Soluble Powder Concentrated 20%: oxytetracycline 200 g/kg in a water soluble base; 9–18 mg/kg daily for calves, 2–4 mg/kg daily for ruminating cattle. Meat withhold 10 days. Milk withhold zero.
- Tilmovet 250 mg/ml Concentrate for Oral Solution: tilmicosin 250 mg/ml; 1 ml/20 kg per os twice daily. For calves

only. Meat withhold 42 days. *Not recommended for use in goats or camelids.*

- Tylan Soluble: tylosin 100 g/bottle; 1 g/calf twice daily. Meat withhold 14 days.

Topical products

- Alamycin Aerosol: active substance oxytetracycline. Zero meat and milk withhold.
- Cyclo Spray: active substance chlortetracycline. Zero meat and milk withhold.
- Engemycin Spray 3.84% w/w: active substance oxytetracycline. Zero meat and milk withhold.
- Oxycare Spray: active substance oxytetracycline. Zero meat and milk withhold.
- Tetcin Aerosol: active substance oxytetracycline. Zero meat and milk withhold.

Antiprotozoals

Antiprotozoal injectable preparations will be required by the ambulatory clinician in tropical and subtropical areas where blood-borne protozoan parasites cause massive problems in cattle. Specific treatments are given in Chapter 3 in the section dealing with the circulatory system (which also describes treatments for tropical diseases caused by other types of organisms). There is only one licensed product for the protozoal disease of babesiosis in the UK:

- Imizol Injection: imidocarb 85 mg/ml sub cut. Meat withhold 213 days. Milk withhold 21 days.

Cardiovascular and respiratory preparations

The preparation described here is not required to be carried as a routine if a NSAID is available:

- Bisolvon Injection: bromhexine hydrochloride 3 mg/ml; 17 ml/100 kg im daily for 5 days. Meat withhold 28 days. Not to be used in lactating animals.

Dietary supplements and fluid metabolites

Metabolic diseases need to be treated urgently and therefore clinicians will require sources of injectable calcium, magnesium, phosphorus and dextrose. Thiamine by injection will also be needed urgently for the treatment of Cerebrocortical necrosis (CCN). Oral electrolytes will be an urgent requirement not only for adult cattle but also for calves. The list follows:

- Anivit 4BC Injection: thiamine 35 mg/ml, riboflavin 0.5 mg/ml, pyridoxine 7 mg/ml, nicotinamide 23 mg/ml and ascorbic acid 70 mg/ml; 20–30 ml/adult cow im, iv or sub cut (5–10 ml/calf) daily. Zero meat and milk withhold.
- Anivit B12: vitamin B_{12} 250 mcg/ml; 2–4 ml/calf im or sub cut; repeat in 7 days. Zero meat withhold.
- Anivit B12 1000 Micrograms/ml Injection: vitamin B_{12} 1000 mcg/ml; 1–3 ml/adult cow im or sub cut (0.5–1 ml/calf) every 7 days. Zero meat and milk withhold.
- Calciject 20 CM: calcium 5.92 g and magnesium 1.85 g in 400 ml; 400–800 ml/adult cow iv or sub cut. Zero meat and milk withhold.
- Calciject 40: calcium 11.88 g/400 ml; 150–500 ml/adult cow iv or sub cut. Zero meat and milk withhold.
- Calciject 40 CM: calcium 400 mg/ml and magnesium 50 mg/ml; 200–400 ml/adult cow. Zero meat and meat withhold.
- Calciject LV: calcium 4.2 g and magnesium 0.78 g in 100 ml; 100–200 ml/adult cow sub cut. Zero meat and milk withhold.
- Combivit: thiamine 35 mg/ml, riboflavin 0.5 mg/ml, pyridoxine 7 mg/ml, nicotinamide 23 mg/ml and ascorbic acid 70 mg/ml; 20–30 ml/adult cow and 5–10 ml/calf im, iv or sub cut. Zero meat and milk withhold.
- Duphafral Extravite Solution: thiamine 35 mg/ml, riboflavin 0.5 mg/ml, pyridoxine 7.0 mg/ml, nicotinamide 23 mg/ml and ascorbic acid 70 mg/ml; 20–30 ml/cow sub cut, im or iv daily (calves 5–10 ml). Zero meat and milk withhold.
- Duphafral Multivitamin 9: retinol 15,000 IU/ml, cholecalciferol 25 mcg/ml,

alpha-tocopheryl acetate 20 mg/ml, thiamine 10 mg/ml, riboflavin 5 mg/ml, pyridoxine 3 mg/ml, nicotinamide 35 mg/ml, dexpanthenol 25 mg/ml and cyanocobalamin 25 mcg/ml; 20–30 ml/ cow im or sub cut (5–10 ml/calf). Meat withhold 28 days. Zero milk withhold.

• Duphalyte: combination of B-complex vitamins, electrolytes, amino acids and dextrose; 100 ml/50 kg iv for adults; 30 ml/5 kg for calves. May be followed up by sub cut injections. Zero meat and milk withhold.

• Effydral Effervescent Tablet: sodium chloride 2.34 g, potassium chloride 1.12 g, sodium bicarbonate 6.72 g, citric acid 3.84 g, lactose 32.44 g and glycine 2.25 g per tablet; 1 tablet/l water 2–3 times daily for calves. Zero meat and milk withhold.

• Forketos Oral Solution for Cattle and Sheep: propylene glycol 80% v/v and cobalt sulfate heptahydrate 0.1 % w/v; 2 ml/kg (maximum dose 120 ml) orally, repeat in 8 h. Zero meat and milk withhold.

• Glucose 40%: glucose 40% w/v; 1 mg/kg iv repeat in 6 h. Zero meat and milk withhold.

• Intravit 12: cyanobalamin 0.5 g/ml; 2–5 ml/adult cow im or sub cut, 1–3 ml/ calf. Zero meat and milk withhold.

• Ketol: propylene glycol 0.8 ml/ml + mineral glycerophosphates, choline, cobalt, iodine; adult cows 225 ml orally twice daily for 1 day, then 115 ml twice daily for 3 days. Zero meat and milk withhold.

• Lectade Powder for Oral Solution: glycine 6.18 g, citric acid 0.48 g, potassium citrate 0.12 g, potassium dihydrogen phosphate 4.08 g and sodium chloride 8.58 g in sachet A; glucose 44.61 g in sachet B; add both sachets to 2 l water; calves 2 l orally twice daily for 2 days. Zero meat withhold.

• Lectade Plus Powder for Oral Solution: glycine 3.01 g, sodium chloride 4.59 g, sodium citrate 0.66 g, potassium citrate 3.24 g, potassium dihydrogen phosphate 1.36 g and sodium acid citrate 1.80 g in sachet A; glucose 62.69 g in sachet B; add

both sachets to 2 l water; calves 2 l orally twice daily for 2 days. Zero meat withhold.

• Life Aid Xtra: electrolyte powder 83.74 g/sachet; calves 1 sachet/l warm water fed orally twice daily for 2 days. Zero meat withhold.

• Liquid Life-Aid: concentrated aqueous solution for dilution with 11.5 times its own volume of water; calves 2 l orally twice daily for 2 days. Zero meat withhold.

• Magniject Injection: magnesium sulfate 25% w/v; 400 ml/cow as a single injection sub cut. Zero meat and milk withhold.

• Multivitamin Injection: vitamin A 15,000 IU/ml, vitamin D 25 mcg/ml, vitamin E 20 mg/ml, vitamin B_1 10 mg/ml, vitamin B_2 5 mg/ml, vitamin B_6 3 mg/ml, nicotinamide 35 mg/ml, dexpanthenol 25 mg/ml and vitamin B_{12} 25 mcg/ml; 20–30 ml/ adult (5–10 ml/calf) im or sub cut, repeated in 10–14 days. Meat withhold 28 days. Zero milk withhold.

• Vitbee 250: vitamin B_{12} 0.025% w/v; 2–4 ml/calf im or sub cut. Zero meat and milk withhold.

• Vitesel Emulsion for Injection: alpha-tocopheryl acetate 68 mg/ml and potassium selenate 1.5 mg/ml; calves 1–2 ml/ 45 kg im repeated in 2–4 weeks. Zero meat withhold.

Other medicines

The four medicines (five products) listed below are all required, mainly for parturition cases:

• Adrenacaine Solution for Injection for Cattle: procaine hydrochloride 50 mg/ml and adrenaline 0.02 mg/ml. Zero meat and milk withhold.

• Dopram-V Drops: doxapram hydrochloride 20 mg/ml; 2–5 ml/calf sublingually. Newborn calves meat withhold 28 days.

• Dopram-V Injection: doxapram hydrochloride 20 mg/ml; calves 2–5 ml iv, im, sub cut or sublingually. Newborn calves meat withhold 28 days.

- Oxytocin S: oxytocin 10 IU/ml; 0.2–1 ml/ cow im. Zero meat and milk withhold.
- Planipart Solution for Injection 30 micrograms/ml: clenbuterol 30 mcg/ml; 10 ml per cow iv. Meat withhold 14 days. Milk withhold 60 h.

Sheep Medicines

Anti-inflammatory preparations

There are no licensed products for sheep in the UK. Anti-inflammatory preparations licensed for cattle should be used in sheep, goats and South American camelids (SACs) under the cascade principle. Clinicians who do not intend to carry out cattle practice will need to be aware that they will have to carry – selected from the cattle medicines that are available (see Cattle Medicines, Anti-inflammatory preparations) – at least one NSAID, a solution containing dexamethazone (Colvasone, Dexafort or Voren Suspension for Injection) and a solution containing butylscopolamine 4 mg/ml and metamizole 500 mg/ml (Buscopan Compositium).

Antimicrobials

The requirements for antimicrobials in sheep practice are not as large as in cattle practice, but if the requirements for goats and SACs are included, then the range will need to be as large as for the treatment of cattle. Oral and topical antimicrobial preparations will also be required. (Note that in the list that follows, drugs containing tilmicosin are marked as not recommended for use in goats and camelids at the end of the drug description.)

Injectables

- Alamycin LA: oxytetracycline 200 mg/ml; 1 ml/10 kg im as a single injection. Meat withhold 9 days. Milk withhold 7 days.
- Alamycin LA 300: oxytetracycline 300 mg/ml; 1 ml/10–15 kg im as a single injection. Meat withhold 28 days. Milk withhold 8 days.

- Amfipen LA: ampicillin 100 mg/ml; 7.5 ml/50 kg im every 2 days. Meat withhold 60 days. Not to be used for animals producing milk for human consumption.
- Amoxycare Injection: amoxicillin 150 mg/ml; 3 ml/65 kg im daily. Meat withhold 10 days. Not to be used in sheep producing milk for human consumption.
- Amoxycare LA Injection: amoxicillin 150 mg/ml; 1 ml/10 kg im every 2 days. Meat withhold 16 days. Not to be used in sheep producing milk for human consumption.
- Amoxypen Injection: amoxicillin 150 mg/ml; 1 ml/20 kg im daily. Meat withhold 10 days. Not to be used in sheep producing milk for human consumption.
- Amoxypen LA: amoxicillin 150 mg/ml; 1 ml/10 kg im daily. Meat withhold 16 days. Not to be used in sheep producing milk for human consumption.
- Betamox Injection: amoxicillin 150 mg/ml; 3 ml/65 kg im daily. Meat withhold 10 days. Not to be used in sheep producing milk for human consumption.
- Betamox LA: amoxicillin 150 mg/ml; 1 ml/10 kg im every 2 days. Meat withhold 16 days. Not to be used in sheep producing milk for human consumption.
- Clamoxyl LA: amoxicillin 150 mg/ml; 1 ml/ 10 kg im every 48 h. Meat withhold 45 days. Not to be used in sheep producing milk for human consumption.
- Clamoxyl Ready-to-use Injection: amoxicillin 150 mg/ml; 1 ml/20 kg im daily. Meat withhold 47 days. Not to be used in sheep producing milk for human consumption.
- Depocillin: procaine benzylpenicillin 300 mg/ml; 1 ml/20 kg im daily. Meat withhold 5 days. Not to be used in sheep producing milk for human consumption.
- Devomycin 250 mg/ml Solution for Injection: streptomycin sulfate 250 mg/ml; 1 ml/25 kg im daily. Meat withhold 18 days. Not to be used in sheep producing milk for human consumption.
- Devomycin D solution for injection: streptomycin sulfate 150 mg/ml + dihydrostreptomycin sulfate 150 mg/ml; 1 ml/30 kg daily. Meat withhold 14 days. Not to be used in sheep producing milk for human consumption.

- Duphacillin: ampicillin 150 mg/ml; 1 ml/20 kg im daily. Meat withhold 18 days. Not to be used in sheep producing milk for human consumption.
- Duphacycline LA 20% Solution for Injection: oxytetracycline 200 mg/ml; 1 ml/10 kg im as a single injection. Meat withhold 9 days. Milk withhold 168 h.
- Duphamox: amoxicillin 150 mg/ml; 3 ml/65 kg im daily. Meat withhold 10 days. Not to be used in sheep producing milk for human consumption.
- Duphamox LA: amoxicillin 150 mg/ml; 1 ml/10 kg im as a single injection. Meat withhold 21 days. Not to be used in sheep producing milk for human consumption.
- Duphapen: procaine penicillin 300 mg/ml; 1 ml/30 kg im daily. Meat withhold 7 days. Not to be used in sheep producing milk for human consumption.
- Duphapen+Strep: procaine benzylpenicillin 200 mg/ml + dihydrostreptomycin 250 mg/ml; 1 ml/25 kg im daily. Meat withhold 31 days. Not to be used in sheep producing milk for human consumption.
- Engemycin 10% (DD): oxytetracycline 100 mg/ml; 1 ml/12.5 kg im daily or 1 ml/5 kg im every 60 h. Meat withhold 14 days. Not to be used in sheep producing milk for human consumption.
- Engemycin 10% Farm Pack: oxytetracycline 100 mg/ml; 1 ml/12.5 kg im daily or 1 ml/5 kg im every 60 h. Meat withhold 14 days. Not to be used in sheep producing milk for human consumption.
- Engemycin LA: oxytetracycline 200 mg/ml; 1 ml/10 kg im as a single injection. Meat withhold 9 days. Milk withhold 7 days.
- Intradine: sulfadimidine 308.9 mg/ml; 1 ml/1.5 kg sub cut initially followed by 1 ml/3 kg daily. Meat withhold 18 days. Not to be used in sheep producing milk for human consumption.
- Micotil: tilmicosin 300 mg/ml; 1 ml/30 kg for pneumonia and mastitis; and 1 ml/60 kg for foot rot sub cut as a single injection. Meat withhold 42 days. Milk withhold 360 h. *This medicine can only be injected by a veterinary surgeon. Not recommended for use in goats or camelids.*
- Milbotyl: tilmicosin 300 mg/ml; 1 ml/30 kg sub cut as a single injection. Meat withhold 42 days, milk withhold 15 days. *This medicine can only be injected by a veterinary surgeon. Not recommended for use in goats or camelids.*
- Neopen: neomycin 100 mg/ml + procaine benzylpenicillin 200 mg/ml; 1 ml/20 kg im daily. Meat withhold 70 days. Not to be used in sheep producing milk for human consumption.
- Norobrittin 15%: ampicillin 150 mg/ml; 1 ml/20 kg im daily. Meat withhold 18 days. Not to be used in sheep producing milk for human consumption.
- Norocillin 30%: procaine penicillin 300 mg/ml; 1 ml/30 kg im daily. Meat withhold 7 days. Not to be used in sheep producing milk for human consumption.
- Oxycare 20% LA: oxytetracycline 200 mg/ml; 1 ml/10 kg im as a single injection. Meat withhold 9 days. Milk withhold 7 days.
- Oxytetrin 20 LA: oxytetracycline 200 mg/ml; 1 ml/10 kg im as a single injection. Meat withhold 28 days. Not to be used in sheep producing milk for human consumption.
- Pen & Strep: procaine penicillin 200 mg/ml + dihydrostreptomycin 250 mg/ml; 1 ml/25 kg im daily. Meat withhold 31 days. Not to be used in sheep producing milk for human consumption.
- Penacare: procaine benzylpenicillin 300 mg/ml; 1 ml/30 kg im daily. Meat withhold 7 days. Not to be used in sheep producing milk for human consumption.
- Streptacare: procaine penicillin 200 mg/ml + dihydrostreptomycin 250 mg/ml; 1 ml/25 kg im daily. Meat withhold 31 days. Not to be used in sheep producing milk for human consumption.
- Terramycin Q-100 mg/ml Solution for Injection: oxytetracycline 100 mg/ml; 1 ml/10 kg im daily. Meat withhold 28 days. Not to be used in sheep producing milk for human consumption.
- Terramycin/LA 200 mg/ml Solution for Injection: oxytetracycline 200 mg/ml; 1 ml/10 kg im as a single injection. Meat withhold 24 days. Not to be used in sheep producing milk for human consumption.

- Tilmodil 300 mg/ml injection: tilmicosin 300 mg/ml; 1 ml/30 kg sub cut as a single injection. Do not inject lambs under 15 kg. Meat withhold 42 days. Milk withhold 360 h. *This medicine can only be injected by a veterinary surgeon. Not recommended for use in goats or camelids.*

Oral products to be given directly by mouth

- Baycox 50 mg/ml Oral Suspension for Piglets, Calves and Lambs: toltrazuril 50 mg/ml; 0.4 ml/kg once orally. Meat withhold 42 days. Not for use in sheep producing milk for human consumption.
- Spectam Scour Halt Oral Solution 50 mg/ml: spectinomycin 50 mg/ml; 1 ml once by mouth for lambs soon after birth. Meat withhold 10 days.

Topical products

- Alamycin Aerosol: active substance oxytetracycline. Zero meat and milk withhold.
- Cyclo Spray: active substance chlortetracycline. Zero meat and milk withhold.
- Engemycin Spray 3.84% w/w: active substance oxytetracycline. Zero meat and milk withhold.
- Oxycare Spray: active substance oxytetracycline. Zero meat and milk withhold.
- Tetcin Aerosol: active substance oxytetracycline. Zero meat and milk withhold.

Dietary supplements and fluid metabolites

These preparations will be required urgently, and although the amounts per animal will be much less than those required in cattle, it is likely that several animals will be affected. Therefore, the author advises that a similar range and quantity as for cattle are carried, as follows:

- Anivit 4BC Injection: thiamine 35 mg/ml, riboflavin 0.5 mg/ml, pyridoxine 7 mg/ml, nicotinamide 23 mg/ml and ascorbic acid 70 mg/ml; 5–10 ml/sheep im, iv or sub cut daily. Zero meat and milk withhold.

- Anivit B12: vitamin B_{12} 250 mcg/ml; 1–3 ml/adult im or sub cut. Repeat in 7 days. Zero meat and milk withhold.
- Calciject 20 CMD: calcium 5.92 g/ml, magnesium 1.84 g/ml and glucose 80 g/ml; 50–80 ml/sheep sub cut. Zero meat and milk withhold.
- Duphafral Extravite: thiamine 35 mg/ml, riboflavin 0.5 mg/ml, pyridoxine 7.0 mg/ml, nicotinamide 23 mg/ml and ascorbic acid 70 mg/ml; 5–10 ml/sheep im, iv or sub cut. Zero meat and milk withhold.
- Duphafral Multivitamin 9: retinol 15,000 IU/ml, cholecalciferol 25 mcg/ml, alpha-tocopheryl acetate 20 mg/ml, thiamine 10 mg/ml, riboflavin 5 mg/ml, pyridoxine 3 mg/ml, nicotinamide 35 mg/ml, dexpanthenol 25 mg/ml and cyanocobalamin 25 mcg/ml; 5–10 ml per adult (lambs 2–5 ml) im or sub cut repeated in 10–14 days. Meat withhold 28 days. Milk withhold zero.
- Forketos Oral Solution for Cattle and Sheep: propylene glycol 80% v/v and cobalt sulfate heptahydrate 0.1 % w/v; 2 ml/kg (maximum dose 120 ml) orally, repeated in 8 h. Zero meat and milk withhold.
- Glucose 40%: glucose 40% w/v; 1 mg/kg iv repeat in 6 h. Zero meat and milk withhold.
- Intravit 12: cyanobalamin 0.5 g/ml; 0.5–1.5 ml/sheep im or sub cut. Zero meat and milk withhold.
- Ketol: propylene glycol 0.8 ml + mineral glycerophosphates, choline, cobalt, iodine; 115 ml orally daily for several days. Zero meat and milk withhold.
- Lectade Powder for Oral Solution: glycine 6.18 g, citric acid 0.48 g, potassium citrate 0.12 g, potassium dihydrogen phosphate 4.08 g and sodium chloride 8.58 g in sachet A; glucose 44.61 g in sachet B; add both sachets to 2 l water; lambs 150–200 ml orally 2–4 times daily. Zero meat withhold.
- Liquid Life-Aid: concentrated aqueous solution for dilution with 11.5 times its own volume of water; 160 ml to be given orally 3–6 times a day. Zero meat withhold.

- Magniject Injection: magnesium sulfate 25% w/v; 75 ml/sheep as a single injection sub cut. Zero meat withhold.
- Multivitamin Injection: vitamin A 15,000 IU/ml, vitamin D 25 mcg/ml, vitamin E 20 mg/ml, vitamin B_1 10 mg/ml, vitamin B_2 5 mg/ml, vitamin B_6 3 mg/ml, nicotinamide 35 mg/ml, dexpanthenol 25 mg/ml and vitamin B_{12} 25 mcg/ml; 5–10 ml per adult (2–5 ml per lamb) im or sub cut, repeated in 10–14 days. Meat withhold 28 days. Zero milk withhold.
- Vitbee 250: vitamin B_{12} 0.025% w/v; 1–3 ml/sheep im or sub cut. Zero meat and milk withhold.
- Vitesel: alpha-tocopheryl acetate 68 mg/ml and potassium selenate 1.5 mg/ml; 2 ml/ 45 kg sub cut as a single injection to ewes, 0.5 ml to newborn lambs and 1 ml to older lambs either im or sub cut to be repeated in 2–4 weeks. Zero meat withhold for lambs but 28 days for ewes.

Other medicines

All the preparations listed below, together with a solution for injection of clenbuterol 30 mcg/ml (Planipart Solution for Injection 30 micrograms/ml; see Cattle Medicines, Other medicines) will be required for sheep, goats and SACs:

- Dopram-V Drops: doxapram hydrochloride 20 mg/ml; 0.25–0.5 ml sublingually per lamb. Newborn lambs meat withhold 28 days.
- Dopram-V Injection: doxapram hydrochloride 20 mg/ml, 0.25–0.5 ml/lamb iv, im, sub cut or sublingually. Newborn lambs meat withhold 28 days.
- Oxytocin S: oxytocin 10 IU/ml; 0.2–1 ml im. Zero meat and milk withhold.

Pig Medicines

Anti-inflammatory preparations

For clinicians undertaking emergency pig practice, only one injectable NSAID preparation

(NSAIDs are indicated at the end of the drug description below), together with an injectable preparation of dexamethazone (Voren Suspension for Injection in the UK) is required. A complete list of anti-inflammatory preparations for pigs is given below:

- Comforion vet 100 mg/ml Solution for Injection for Horse, Cattle and Swine: 100 mg ketoprofen per ml; 1 ml/33 kg im daily. Meat withhold 4 days. NSAID.
- Dexadreson: dexamethasone 2 mg/ml; 1.5 ml/50 kg iv or im once and repeated in 48 h. Meat withhold 2 days.
- Finadyne Solution: flunixin meglumine 50 mg/ml; 2 ml/45 kg im. Meat withhold 22 days. NSAID.
- Flunixin Injection: flunixin meglumine 50 mg/ml; 2 ml/45 kg im. Meat withhold 22 days. NSAID.
- Ketodale 100 mg/ml Solution for Injection for Horses, Cattle and Swine: ketoprofen 100 mg/ml; 3 ml/100 kg im. Meat withhold 4 days. NSAID.
- Ketofen 10%: ketoprofen 100 mg/ml; 3 ml/100 kg im. Meat withhold 4 days. NSAID.
- Melovem 5 mg/ml Solution for Injection for Cattle and Pigs: meloxicam 5 mg/ml; 2 ml/25 kg im daily for two injections. Meat withhold 5 days. NSAID.
- Meloxidyl 20 mg/ml Solution for Injection for Cattle, Pigs and Horses: meloxicam 20 mg/ml; 2 ml/100 kg im daily for two injections. Meat withhold 5 days. NSAID.
- Metacam 20 mg/ml Solution for Injection for Cattle, Pigs and Horses: meloxicam 20 mg/ml; 2 ml/100 kg im daily for two injections. Meat withhold 5 days. NSAID.
- Rapidexon: dexamethasone 2 mg/ml; 1.5 ml/50 kg iv or im once and repeated in 48 h. Meat withhold 2 days.
- Rheumocam 20 mg/ml Injection for Cattle, Pigs and Horses: meloxicam 20 mg/ml; 2 ml/100 kg im. Meat withhold 5 days. NSAID.
- Solacyl 100%, Powder for Oral Solution for Calves and Pigs: sodium salicylate 1000 mg/g; 35 mg/kg orally in drinking water for 3–5 days. Zero meat withhold. NSAID.

- Tolfine: tolfenamic acid 4 mg/ml; 1 ml/20 kg im as a single injection. Meat withhold 3 days. NSAID.
- Voren Suspension for Injection, 1 mg/ml: dexamethazone 1 mg/ml; 2 ml/100 kg im in growing pigs and adults; 1 ml/10 kg im in piglets. Meat withhold 55 days.

Antimicrobials

There are a large number of licensed and available antimicrobials for pigs in the UK, together with similar generic preparations in other parts of the world. The ambulatory clinician requires only as few as five injectable preparations, which should include two long-acting drugs. The latter are very useful for the busy pig farmer as well as for the busy practitioner treating pet pigs whose owners are unable to inject their stock. Clinicians would be well advised to carry one oral preparation for prolonged antimicrobial therapy. A spray of topical antimicrobial is also useful.

Injectables

- Advocin 2.5% Solution for Injection: danofloxacin 25 mg/ml; 1 ml/20 kg im daily. Meat withhold 3 days.
- Alamycin 10: oxytetracycline 100 mg/ml; 1 ml/11–50 kg im daily. Meat withhold 20 days.
- Alamycin LA: oxytetracycline 200 mg/ml; 1 ml/10 kg im as a single injection. Meat withhold 18 days.
- Alamycin LA 300: oxytetracycline 300 mg/ml; 1 ml/10–15 kg im as a single injection. Meat withhold 14–28 days depending on dosage.
- Amfipen LA: ampicillin 100 mg/ml; 1 ml/4 kg im every 2 days. Meat withhold 60 days.
- Amoxycare Injection: amoxicillin 150 mg/ml; 1 ml/21 kg im daily. Meat withhold 16 days.
- Amoxycare LA Injection: amoxicillin 150 mg/ml; 1 ml/10 kg im every 2 days. Meat withhold 16 days.
- Amoxypen Injection: amoxicillin 150 mg/ml; 1 ml/20 kg im daily. Meat withhold 16 days.
- Amoxypen LA: amoxicillin 150 mg/ml; 1 ml/10 kg im daily. Meat withhold 16 days.
- Baytril 5% Solution for Injection: enrofloxacin 50 mg/ml; 2.5 ml/100 kg im daily (dose rate may be doubled for treating salmonellosis and complicated respiratory disease). Meat withhold 10 days.
- Baytril 10% Solution for Injection: enrofloxacin 100 mg/ml; 0.5 ml/10 kg im daily (dose rate may be doubled for treating salmonellosis and complicated respiratory disease). Meat withhold 10 days.
- Baytril Max: enrofloxacin 100 mg/ml; 0.75 ml/10 kg as a single injection. Meat withhold 12 days.
- Betamox Injection: amoxicillin 150 mg/ml; 1 ml/21 kg im daily. Meat withhold 16 days.
- Betamox LA: amoxicillin 150 mg/ml; 1 ml/10 kg im every 2 days. Meat withhold 16 days.
- Cefenil 50 mg/ml Powder and Solvent Solution for Injection for Cattle and Pigs: ceftiofur 1 g/20 ml; 1 ml/50 kg im daily. Meat withhold 2 days.
- Ceftiocyl 50 mg/ml: ceftiofur 50 mg/ml; 1 ml/16 kg im daily. Meat withhold 6 days.
- Cevaxel: ceftiofur 50 mg/ml; 1 ml/16 kg im daily. Meat withhold 5 days.
- Clamoxyl Ready-to-use Injection: amoxicillin 150 mg/ml; 1 ml/20 kg im daily. Meat withhold 47 days.
- Cobactan 2.5%: cefquinome 25 mg/ml; 2 ml/25 kg im daily. Meat withhold 3 days.
- Cyclosol LA: oxytetracycline 200 mg/ml; 1 ml/10 kg im every 3 days. Meat withhold 28 days.
- Denagard 200 Solution for Injection: tiamulin 200 mg/ml; 3 ml/40 kg im daily. Meat withhold 14 days.
- Depocillin: procaine benzylpenicillin 300 mg/ml; 1 ml/20 kg im daily. Meat withhold 5 days.
- Draxxin 100 mg/ml Solution for Injection for Cattle and Pigs: tulathromycin 100 mg/ml; 1 ml/40 kg im as a single injection. Meat withhold 33 days.
- Duphacillin: ampicillin 150 mg/ml; 1 ml/20 kg im daily. Meat withhold 18 days.

- Duphacycline 10%: oxytetracycline 100 mg/ml; 1 ml/11–50 kg im daily. Meat withhold 20 days.
- Duphacycline LA 20% Solution for Injection: oxytetracycline 200 mg/ml; 1 ml/10 kg im as a single injection. Meat withhold 18 days.
- Duphamox: amoxicillin 150 mg/ml; 1 ml/21 kg im daily. Meat withhold 16 days.
- Duphamox LA: amoxicillin 150 mg/ml; 1 ml/10 kg im as a single injection. Meat withhold 21 days.
- Duphapen: procaine penicillin 300 mg/ml; 1 ml/30 kg im daily. Meat withhold 7 days.
- Duphapen Fort: procaine benzylpenicillin 300 mg/ml; 1 ml/15 kg im every 72 h. Meat withhold 10 days.
- Duphapen+Strep: procaine benzylpenicillin 200 mg/ml + dihydrostreptomycin 250 mg/ml; 1 ml/25 kg im daily. Meat withhold 18 days.
- Duphatrim IS Injectable Solution: trimethoprim 40 mg/ml + sulfadiazine 200 mg/ml; 1 ml/16 kg im daily. Meat withhold 20 days.
- Eficur: ceftiofur 50 mg/ml; 1 ml/16 kg im daily. Meat withhold 5 days.
- Engemycin 10% (DD): oxytetracycline 100 mg/ml; 1 ml/12.5 kg im daily or 1 ml/5 kg im every 60 h. Meat withhold 14 days with daily dose and 10 days with 60 h dose.
- Engemycin 10% Farm Pack: oxytetracycline 100 mg/ml; 1 ml/12.5 kg im daily or 1 ml/5 kg im every 60 h. Meat withhold 14 days with daily dose and 10 days with 60 h dose.
- Engemycin LA: oxytetracycline 200 mg/ml; 1 ml/10 kg im as a single injection. Meat withhold 18 days.
- Enrocare 5%: enrofloxacin 50 mg/ml; 1 ml/20 kg im daily (dose may be doubled when treating salmonellosis and complicated respiratory disease). Meat withhold 10 days.
- Enrocare 10%: enrofloxacin 100 mg/ml; 1 ml/40 kg im daily (dose may be doubled when treating salmonellosis and complicated respiratory disease). Meat withhold 10 days.
- Enroxil Solution for Injection 50 mg/ml for Calves, Pigs and Dogs: enrofloxacin 50 mg/ml; 1 ml/20 kg im daily (dose may be doubled when treating complicated respiratory disease). Meat withhold 10 days.
- Enroxil Solution for Injection 100 mg/ml for Calves and Pigs: enrofloxacin 100 mg/ml; 1 ml/40 kg im daily (dose may be doubled when treating salmonellosis and complicated respiratory disease). Meat withhold 10 days.
- Excenel RTU 50 mg/ml Suspension for Injection for Pigs and Cattle: ceftiofur 50 mg/ml; 1 ml/16 kg im daily. Meat withhold 5 days.
- Excenel Sterile Powder for Solution for Injection: ceftiofur 50 mg/ml; 1 ml/16 kg im daily. Meat withhold 2 days.
- Fenflor 300 mg/ml Solution for Injection for Pigs: florfenicol 300 mg/ml; 1 ml/20 kg im every 48 h. Meat withhold 18 days.
- Fenoflox 50 mg/ml Injection for Cattle, Pigs, Dogs and Cats: enrofloxacin 50 mg/ml; 1 ml/20 kg im daily (dose may be doubled when treating complicated respiratory disease). Meat withhold 10 days.
- Fenoflox 100 mg/ml Injection for Cattle and Pigs: enrofloxacin 100 mg/ml; 1 ml/40 kg im daily (dose may be doubled when treating complicated respiratory disease). Meat withhold 10 days.
- Florkem: florfenicol 300 mg/ml; 1 ml/20 kg im every 48 h. Meat withhold 18 days.
- Intradine: sulfadimidine 308.9 mg/ml; 1 ml/1.5 kg sub cut initially followed by 1 ml/3 kg daily. Meat withhold 42 days.
- Kefloril 300 mg/ml: florfenicol 300 mg/ml; 1 ml/20 kg im every 48 h. Meat withhold 18 days
- Lincocin Sterile Solution: lincomycin 100 mg/ml; 1 ml/9–22 kg im daily. Meat withhold 3 days.
- Lincojet 10%: lincomycin 100 mg/ml; 1 ml/9–22 kg im daily. Meat withhold 3 days.
- Marbiflox 100 mg/ml Solution for Cattle and Pigs: marbofloxacin 100 mg/ml; 1 ml/50 kg im daily for 3 days. Meat withhold 4 days.

- Marbocyl 2% Solution for Injection: marbofloxacin 2 mg/ml; 1 ml/10 kg im daily. Meat withhold 2 days.
- Marbocyl 10% Solution for Injection: marbofloxacin 10 mg/ml; 1 ml/50 kg im daily. Meat withhold 2 days.
- Naxcel 100 mg/ml Suspension for Injection for Pigs: ceftiofur 100 mg/ml; 1 ml/20 kg im as a single injection. Meat withhold 71 days.
- Neopen: neomycin 100 mg/ml + procaine benzylpenicillin 200 mg/ml; 1 ml/20 kg im daily. Meat withhold 60 days.
- Norobrittin 15%: ampicillin 150 mg/ml; 1 ml/20 kg im daily. Meat withhold 18 days.
- Norocillin 30%: procaine penicillin 300 mg/ml; 1 ml/30 kg im daily. Meat withhold 7 days.
- Norodine 24: sulfadiazine 200 mg/ml + trimethoprim 40 mg/ml; 1 ml/16 kg im daily. Meat withhold 20 days.
- Norotyl LA 15%: tylosin 150 mg/ml; 1 ml/7.5 kg im as a single injection. Meat withhold 7 days.
- Nuflor Swine 300 mg/ml Solution for Injection: florfenicol 300 mg/ml; 1 ml/20 kg im every 48 h. Meat withhold 18 days.
- Oxycare 10%: oxytetracycline 100 mg/ml; 1 ml/11–50 kg im daily. Meat withhold 20 days.
- Oxycare 20% LA: oxytetracycline 200 mg/ml; 1 ml/10 kg im as a single injection. Meat withhold 18 days.
- Oxytetrin 20 LA: oxytetracycline 200 mg/ml; 1 ml/10 kg im as a single injection. Meat withhold 70 days.
- Pen & Strep: procaine penicillin 200 mg/ml + dihydrostreptomycin 250 mg/ml; 1 ml/25 kg im daily. Meat withhold 18 days.
- Penacare: procaine benzylpenicillin 300 mg/ml; 1 ml/30 kg im daily. Meat withhold 7 days.
- Powerflox 50 mg/ml Injection: enrofloxacin 50 mg/ml; 1 ml/20 kg im daily (rate may be doubled when treating complicated respiratory disease). Meat withhold 10 days.
- Powerflox 100 mg/ml Injection: enrofloxacin 100 mg/ml; 1 ml/40 kg im daily (rate may be doubled when treating complicated respiratory disease). Meat withhold 10 days.
- Readycef Injection: ceftiofur 50 mg/ml; 1 ml/16 kg im daily. Meat withhold 5 days.
- Selectan: florfenicol 300 mg/ml; 1 ml/20 kg im every 48 h. Meat withhold 18 days.
- Streptacare: procaine penicillin 200 mg/ml + dihydrostreptomycin 250 mg/ml; 1 ml/25 kg im daily. Meat withhold 18 days.
- Synulox Ready-To-Use Suspension for Injection: clavulanic acid 35 mg/ml + amoxicillin 140 mg/ml; 1 ml/20 kg im daily. Meat withhold 31 days.
- Terramycin Q-100 mg/ml Solution for Injection: oxytetracycline 100 mg/ml; 1 ml/10 kg im daily. Meat withhold 21 days.
- Terramycin/LA 200 mg/ml Solution for Injection: oxytetracycline 200 mg/ml; 1 ml/10 kg im as a single injection. Meat withhold 36 days.
- Tiamutin 200 Injection: tiamulin 200 mg/ml; 3 ml/40 kg im daily. Meat withhold 14 days.
- Tribrissen Injection 48%: trimethoprim 80 mg/ml + sulfadiazine 80 mg/ml; 1 ml/32 kg im daily. Meat withhold 28 days.
- Trimacare 24% Injection: trimethoprim 40 mg/ml + sulfadiazine 200 mg/ml; 1 ml/16 kg im daily. Meat withhold 20 days.
- Trinacol Solution for Injection: trimethoprim 40 mg/ml + sulfadiazine 200 mg/ml; 1 ml/16 kg im daily. Meat withhold 20 days.
- Tylan 200: tylosin 200 mg/ml; 1 ml/20–100 kg im daily. Meat withhold 9 days.
- Tyluvet 20% w/v, Solution for Injection: tylosin 200 mg/ml; 1 ml/20 kg im daily. Meat withhold 46 days.
- Ultrapen LA: procaine benzylpenicillin 300 mg/ml; 1 ml/15 kg im as a single injection. Meat withhold 10 days.
- Vetmulin 162 mg/ml Solution for Injection for Pigs: tiamulin 162 mg/ml; 1 ml/20 kg im daily. Meat withhold 5 days.

Oral products to be used in the feed or drinking water

- Aivlosin 625 mg/g Granules for Use in Drinking Water: tylvalosin 8.5 mg/g; 2.125 mg/kg orally in feed for 7 days for treatment of enzootic pneumonia; 4.25 mg/kg orally in feed for 7 days for treatment of porcine proliferative enteropathy and swine dysentery. Meat withhold 2 days.
- Amoxinsol 50: amoxicillin trihydrate 50% w/w; 20 mg/kg in drinking water for 5 days. Meat withhold 2 days.
- Apralan Soluble Powder: apramycin 1 g/sachet or apramycin 50 g in 220 ml powder; 7.5–12.5 mg/kg in drinking water daily for 7 days. Meat withhold 14 days.
- Chlorsol: chlortetracycline 50%; 20 mg/kg in drinking water for 5 days. Meat withhold 6 days.
- Coliscour Solution: colistin 2 MIU/ml; 0.25 ml/10 kg orally direct into the mouth or in drinking water. Meat withhold 1 day.
- Denagard 12.5% Oral Solution: tiamulin 125 mg/ml; 8.8 mg/kg daily in drinking water for 3–5 days. Meat withhold 2 days.
- HydroDoxx: doxycycline 500 mg/g; 10 mg/kg doxycycline in drinking water for 5 days. Meat withhold 6 days.
- Linco-Spectin 100 Soluble Powder: lincomycin 33.3 g and spectinomycin 66.7 g in a pack; 10 mg/kg in drinking water for 7 days. Zero meat withhold.
- Lincocin Soluble Powder: lincomycin 400 mg/g; 4.5 mg/kg in drinking water for a minimum of 5 days. Zero meat withhold.
- Liquidox Oral Solution for use in Drinking Water for Chickens and Pigs: doxycycline 100 mg/ml; 10 mg /kg daily. Meat withhold 7 days.
- Nuflor Drinking Water Concentrate for Swine: florfenicol 23 mg/ml; 10 mg/kg in drinking water for 5 days. Meat withhold 20 days.
- Octacillin 697 mg/g Powder for use in Pigs: amoxicillin 697 mg/g; 14 mg/kg in drinking water for 3–5 days. Meat withhold 2 days.
- Pulmodox Granules for Oral Solution: doxycycline 500 mg/g; 12–15 mg/kg in drinking water for 4 days. Meat withhold 4 days.
- Soludox: doxycycline 500 mg/g; 20 mg/kg in drinking water for 5 days. Meat withhold 3 days.
- Stabox 50% Oral Soluble Powder Pig: amoxicillin 500 mg/g; 20 mg/kg in liquid feed for 5 days. Meat withhold 14 days.
- Terramycin Soluble Powder Concentrated 20%: oxytetracycline 200 g/kg; 10–30 mg/kg in drinking water daily for 3–5 days. Meat withhold 7 days.
- Tetsol 800: tetracycline hydrochloride 800 g/kg; 40 mg/kg in drinking water for 5 days. Meat withhold 6 days.
- Tiamutin 12.5% Solution: tiamulin 125 mg/ml; 8.8 mg/kg daily in drinking water for 3–5 days. Meat withhold 2 days.
- Tiamvet 12.5% Solution: tiamulin 125 mg/ml; 8.8 mg/kg daily in drinking water for 3–5 days. Meat withhold 2 days.
- Tylan Soluble: tylosin tartrate 100 g/bottle; 25 mg/kg in drinking water for 3–10 days. Zero meat withhold.
- Vetmulin 125 mg/ml Oral Solution: tiamulin 125 mg/ml; 7 ml/100 kg daily for 5 days for the treatment of swine dysentery; 12–16 ml/per 110 kg daily for 5 days for the treatment of enzootic pneumonia. Meat withhold 5 days.

Oral products to be given directly by mouth

- Baytril Piglet Doser 0.5% Oral Solution: 5 mg/ml enrofloxacin. 1 ml once daily per os to piglets under 3 kg daily. 3 ml once daily per os to piglets between 3 and 10 kg. Meat withhold 10 days.
- Baycox 50 mg/ml Oral Suspension for Piglets, Calves and Lambs: toltrazuril 50 mg/ml; 0.4 ml/kg once orally. Meat withhold 77 days.
- Cevazuril 50 mg/ml Oral Suspension for Piglets: toltrazuril 50 mg/ml; 0.4 ml/kg once orally. Meat withhold 77 days.
- Coliscour Solution: colistin 2 MIU/ml; 0.25 ml/10 kg orally direct into the mouth or in drinking water. Meat withhold 1 day.
- Spectam Scour Halt Oral Solution 50 mg/ml: spectinomycin 50 mg/ml; 1 ml orally twice daily for 3–5 days for piglets under 4.5 kg. The dose should be doubled for heavier piglets. Meat withhold 12 days.

Topical products

- Alamycin Aerosol: active substance oxytetracycline. Zero meat withhold.
- Cyclo Spray: active substance chlortetracycline. Zero meat withhold.
- Engemycin Spray 3.84% w/w: active substance oxytetracycline. Zero meat withhold.
- Oxycare Spray: active substance oxytetracycline. Zero meat withhold.
- Tetcin Aerosol: active substance oxytetracycline. Zero meat withhold.

Cardiovascular and respiratory preparations

These rather specialized medications are not normally required by the general practitioner:

- Bisolvon Injection: bromhexine 3 mg/ml; 7–17 ml/100 kg im daily. Meat withhold 28 days.
- Bisolvon Powder: bromohexine 10 mg/g; 2–5 g/100 kg in drinking water daily. Meat withhold zero.

Dietary supplements and fluid metabolites

Clinicians should carry a licensed injectable vitamin supplement together with a soluble powder for rehydration purposes:

- Anivit 4BC Injection: thiamine 35 mg/ml, riboflavin 0.5 mg/ml, pyridoxine 7 mg/ml, nicotinamide 23 mg/ml and ascorbic acid 70 mg/ml; 5–10 ml/pig im, iv or sub cut daily. Zero meat withhold.
- Duphafral Multivitamin 9: retinol 15,000 IU/ml, cholecalciferol 25 mcg/ml, alpha-tocopheryl acetate 20 mg/ml, thiamine 10 mg/ml, riboflavin 5 mg/ml, pyridoxine 3 mg/ml, nicotinamide 35 mg/ml, dexpanthenol 25 mg/ml and cyanocobalamin 25 mcg/ml; 5–10 ml/pig im or sub cut (2–5 ml per weaner). Meat withhold 28 days.
- Duphalyte: combination of B-complex vitamins, electrolytes, amino acids and dextrose; 100 ml/50 kg iv for adults; 30 ml/5 kg for younger pigs. May be followed up by sub cut injections. Zero meat withhold.
- Effydral Effervescent Tablet: sodium chloride 2.34 g, potassium chloride 1.12 g, sodium bicarbonate 6.72 g, citric acid 3.84 g, lactose 32.44 g and glycine 2.25 g in each tablet; 1 tablet/1 water. Give ad lib to pigs. Zero meat withhold.
- Forgastrin Oral Powder: attapulgite 73% and bone charcoal 27%; 6–10 g thrice daily for pigs as a drench with a little water or in a little food; for piglets, 10 g/60 ml water and 5 ml daily. Zero meat withhold.
- Intravit 12: cyanobalamin 0.5 g/ml; 0.5–1.5 ml/pig im or sub cut. Zero meat withhold.
- Lectade Powder for Oral Solution: glycine 6.18 g, citric acid 0.48 g, potassium citrate 0.12 g, potassium dihydrogen phosphate 4.08 g and sodium chloride 8.58 g in sachet A; glucose 44.61 g in sachet B; add both sachets to 2 l water; solution should be readily available to young pigs. Zero meat withhold.
- Liquid Life-Aid: concentrated aqueous solution for dilution with 11.5 times its own volume of water; 200–300 ml/piglet orally daily; 1 l/weaned pig daily. Zero meat withhold.
- Multivitamin Injection: vitamin A 15,000 IU/ml, vitamin D 25 mcg/ml, vitamin E 20 mg/ml, vitamin B_1 10 mg/ml, vitamin B_2 5 mg/ml, vitamin B_6 3 mg/ml, nicotinamide 35 mg/ml, dexpanthenol 25 mg/ml and vitamin B_{12} 25 mcg/ml; 5–10 ml/adult (2–5 ml/weaner, 0.5–2 ml/piglet) im or sub cut, repeated in 10–14 days. Meat withhold 28 days.
- Vitesel: alpha-tocopheryl acetate 68 mg/ml and potassium selenate 1.5 mg/ml; 1 ml/25 kg im to piglets to be repeated in 2–4 weeks. Zero meat withhold.

Other medicines

Vetrabutine (Monzaldon 100 mg/ml Solution for Injection below) is recommended by some practitioners for porcine parturition, but the evidence for its effectiveness is not strong. However, oxytocin and azaperone (listed below) are vital medicines to be carried by practitioners carrying out pig practice:

- Monzaldon 100 mg/ml Solution for Injection: vetrabutine hydrochloride 100 mg/ml; 2–4 ml/sow im as a single injection. Meat withhold 28 days.
- Oxytocin-S: oxytocin 10 IU/ml; 0.2–1 ml im. Zero meat withhold.
- Stresnil 40 mg/ml Solution for Injection for Pigs: azaperone 40 mg/ml; 0.5–1 ml/ 20 kg im. Meat withhold 10 days.

Poultry Medicines

In commercial situations, antimicrobials are initially supplied to poultry in the drinking water and then, if required, the same antimicrobial can be included in the food. In backyard flocks and individual birds, injectable antimicrobials licensed for other stock can be used under the cascade principle. Hence, the ambulatory practitioner does not normally need to carry specifically licensed poultry products.

Antimicrobials

- Aivlosin 625 mg/g granules: tylvalosin 25 mg/kg. Meat withhold 2 days for chickens and pheasants. Not to be used in laying hens.
- Amoxinsol: amoxicillin 20 mg/kg. Meat withhold 1 day for chickens, 5 days for turkeys, 9 days for ducks. Not to be used in laying hens.
- Apralan Soluble Powder: apraycin 40 mg/kg. Meat withhold 7 days for chickens. Not to be used in laying hens.
- Baytril 10% Oral Solution: enrofloxacin 10 mg/kg. Meat withhold 8 days for chickens and turkeys. Not to be used in laying hens.
- Chlorosol 50: chlortetracycline 20 mg/kg. Meat withhold 3 days. Not to be used in laying hens.
- Colibird: colistin 75,000 IU/kg. Meat withhold 1 day. Zero egg withhold in poultry.
- Denagard 12.5% Oral Solution: tiamulin 25 mg/kg. Meat withhold in chickens 2 days. Meat withhold in turkeys 5 days. Zero egg withhold.
- Dicural Oral Solution: difloxacin 10 mg/kg. Meat withhold 1 day. Not to be used in laying hens or turkeys.
- Enroxil Oral Solution: enrofloxacin 10 mg/kg. Meat withhold 10 days in chickens, 11 days in turkeys. Not to be used in laying hens.
- Erythrocin Soluble: erythromycin 25.5 mg/kg. Meat and egg withhold 6 days.
- Linco-Spectin 100 Soluble Powder: 33.3 g lincomycin and 66.7 g spectinomycin per pack; prevention, 50 mg/kg lincomycin and 100 mg/kg spectomycin (150 mg antibiotic) as fresh solution in drinking water for first 3–5 days of life; further prevention and treatment, 50 mg/kg antibiotic daily for 1–2 days during the fourth week or after vaccination, and at first signs of disease for 3–7 days. Meat withhold 5 days. Not to be used in laying hens.
- Octacillin WSP: amoxicillin 16 mg/kg. Meat withhold 1 day. Not to be used in laying hens.
- Pulmotil AC: tilmicosin 20 mg/kg. Meat withhold 12 days. Not to be used in laying hens.
- Soludox: doxycycline 10 mg/kg. Meat withhold 3 days. Not to be used in laying hens.
- Tetsol 800: tetracycline 60 mg/kg. Meat withhold 6 days. Not to be used in laying hens.
- Tilmovet 250 mg/ml Oral Solution: tilmicosin 20 mg/kg. Meat withhold 12 days. Not to be used in laying hens.
- Tylan Soluble: tylosin 200 mg/kg. Meat withhold 1 day in chickens. Nil meat withhold in turkeys. Zero egg withhold.
- Vetremox: amoxicillin 20 mg/kg. Meat withhold 2 days for chickens, 5 days for turkeys. Not to be used in laying hens.

Antiprotozoals

- Baycox 2.5% Oral Solution: toltrazuril 7 mg/kg. Meat withhold 18 days for chickens. Not to be used in laying hens.

3

Cattle Medicine

Introduction

The chapter starts with a brief discussion on carrying out a clinical examination and taking a case history in cattle practice. This is followed by an account of cattle medicine which is organized by system, with sections on diseases of the gastroenteric system, diseases of the neurological system, metabolic diseases (which can also be viewed as a category of neurological diseases), diseases of the respiratory system, diseases of the circulatory system, diseases of the urinary system, diseases of the reproductive system, diseases of the locomotory system and diseases of the integument. Lastly, there is a brief section on the common reasons for cattle to be found dead.

Clinical Examination, Including History Taking

The clinical examination is the vital start for making a diagnosis in cattle practice. The respiration rate in the normal adult animal is 12–30 breaths/min, with a quicker rate of 20–24 breaths/min in calves. The pulse rate, which should normally be 60–80 beats/min can be taken from the coccygeal artery at the same time as taking the rectal temperature, which should be between 38 and 39 °C. Also,

while in this area of the animal, an abnormal pulse in the urethra of male animals can be felt. The normal pulse rate in calves lies in the range of 70–120 beats/min and the normal rectal temperature is between 38.5 and 39.5 °C. Auscultation of the heart should reveal a steady rhythm with a pulse being seen in the lower third of the jugular being normal. Careful lung auscultation should reveal a lack of sounds in the normal animal. Subcutaneous oedema, which is abnormal, will be seen below the mandibles, on the brisket and in front of the udder. The mucous membranes can be checked in the vulva of females or in the conjunctiva of both sexes. The eyes should be checked for abnormalities and any ocular discharge. The mouth should be checked for excess saliva and for abnormal lesions on the mucosa of the lips and tongue. Auscultation of the rumen should reveal contractions every 20 or 30 s. A resonant ping on auscultation of the left flank is abnormal, as is a splashing on simultaneous ballottement and auscultation of the right flank. The consistency of the faeces can be checked on rectal examination.

The history taken should include the type of animal and its age. Knowledge of the number in the group, together with the total number on the farm, is also important. It is useful to find out how long this group of cattle have been on the farm and whether their management has changed recently.

Obviously, the number affected by the condition under examination and any deaths that have occurred should be recorded as well. Asking for any other observations is useful. Farmer's ideas should not be disregarded.

Diseases of the Gastroenteric System

The predominant signs

- Diarrhoea
- Anorexia
- Pyrexia
- Vomiting
- Dysentery
- Tenesmus
- Excess salivation
- Lack of rumination

Diagnosis

The age of the animal, with a full history (including any alteration to diet), should be linked with any abnormal clinical signs to aid diagnosis. An adequate faeces sample – 70 g is recommended – should be taken as rectal swabs are not normally sufficient even for bacteriology.

Causes of enteric disease

- Viruses
- Bacteria
- Protozoa
- Endoparasites
- Poisoning
- Change of nutrition
- Miscellaneous (and unknown) factors

Enteric diseases caused by viruses and their treatment

Bluetongue disease

The causative organism, *Bluetongue virus* (BTV), is an *Orbivirus* with 24 serotypes, which tend to be restricted to certain areas. Various species of *Culicoides* midges are required as vectors. Replication of the virus has to occur in the vector. Serotype 8 first came to northern Europe in 2006 and caused the birth of 'Dummy type' calves. BTV is primarily a disease of sheep and goats, but the first recorded case in the UK was in a cow. Normally the virus is asymptomatic in cattle except for causing abortions and stillbirths with central nervous system (CNS) defects. If there are signs of clinical disease in cattle they are caused by endothelial damage and disseminated intravascular coagulation (DIC), and are shown as haemorrhage, ischaemia, inflammation and oedema. The lesions are common in areas subject to mechanical trauma and abrasion, e.g. the feet, mouth and eyes. There is fever up to 42°C. The diagnosis is confirmed by PCR for viral RNA. It can detect all 24 serotypes. There is no specific treatment for BTV. Antibiotics and non-steroidal anti-inflammatories (NSAIDs) are helpful. Nursing is vital and should include offering water and mushy food, and providing deep bedding out of the sun and heat. There are vaccines available which are monovalent for each serotype. Cattle require two doses separated by 2 weeks.

Bovine malignant catarrh (BMC)

This disease is rare in the UK but seasonally common in East Africa. It is caused by a group of herpesviruses, which include *Alcelaphine herpesvirus 1*, *Ovine herpesvirus 2* and *Caprine herpesvirus 2*. The most important is *Alcelaphine herpesvirus 1* which is carried asymptomatically by the wildebeest (gnu) in East Africa. In the UK, the sheep is the asymptomatic carrier. Affected cattle will have a high fever and acute ocular discharge with corneal opacity and erosions causing a high mortality. Treatment is hopeless. Differentiation from bluetongue and mucosal disease may be difficult clinically. Diagnosis is either with an ELISA or a PCR. There is no vaccine available.

Bovine papular stomatitis

This is a mild disease of calves which exhibits raised papules in the mouth and is caused by a *Parapoxvirus*. There are no lesions seen on the coronary band. The disease is self-limiting and there is no treatment or vaccine available. It is only important in case it is confused with FMD. See also the section on 'Viral skin diseases' under 'Diseases of the Integument' below.

Bovine viral diarrhoea (BVD)

BVD type 1 disease, caused by *Bovine viral diarrhoea virus 1* (BVDV 1) is normally associated with reproductive problems in adult cattle. There is also a BVD type 2 disease which can cause acute illness in cows and is usually fatal. The cows feel ice cold to the touch and have a low rectal temperature. They have profuse watery diarrhoea and death follows in a few hours. There is no treatment but there is a vaccine.

Cows infected with BVD type 1 during very early pregnancy will reabsorb the embryo and return to service. Cows infected in early and middle pregnancy will produce calves which are persistently viraemic (i.e. persistently infected (PI) calves). These calves may develop mucosal disease, which is invariably fatal. The calves or yearlings will be ill, sometimes with a fever. They will have erosions around the mouth and will be totally anorexic. A heparinized blood (Green top Vacutainer) test will reveal virus positive animals, i.e. PI calves, even before they manifest clinical disease.

See also *'Bovine viral diarrhoea virus (BVDV)'* as a cause of abortion under 'Diseases of the Reproductive System' below.

Coronavirus

This virus causes scouring in young calves and is implicated in causing 'winter dysentery' in adult cows. 'Winter dysentery' is misnamed as dysentery and is rare, but explosive diarrhoea will be seen in virtually the whole herd. There is no treatment or vaccine but recovery is swift. Coronavirus is commonly associated with scouring in calves. It can be confirmed by an ELISA on the faeces. Treatment is symptomatic, as well as using oral antibiotics to help the secondary infections. There is a vaccine for calves which can be given to cows 6 weeks before parturition to boost passive immunity.

There is also a vaccine which can be given orally directly to calves within 6 h of birth.

Foot-and-mouth disease (FMD)

This highly contagious disease is caused by an *Aphthovirus*. There are seven immunologically distinct serotypes; A, O, C, Asia1, South African Type (SAT) 1, 2 and 3. The signs will vary markedly in severity with the strain of virus, the breed of animal and the type of husbandry. The earliest signs are vesicles – fluid-filled sacs within the epithelium on the tongue, buccal mucosa and coronary band. There is marked excess salivation, lameness and pyrexia. There are vaccines available for all serotypes.

Rotavirus

Rotavirus is the most common virus causing scouring in calves worldwide. The disease has a high morbidity and a very low mortality. Diagnosis is confirmed by a PAGE test on the faeces. Treatment is symptomatic, i.e. by rehydration, as well as using oral antibiotics to help the secondary infections. There is a vaccine which can be given to cows 6 weeks before parturition, and passive immunity can be boosted by a vaccine given orally within 6 h of birth.

Enteric diseases caused by bacteria and their treatment

Actinobacillosis

This disease occurs worldwide and is called 'wooden tongue'. The causal organism is *Actinobacillus lignieresii*. Treatment with streptomycin daily for 5 days is often successful. See below under 'Diseases of the Integument', 'Bacterial skin diseases' for more information.

Actinomycosis

The disease occurs worldwide and is called 'lumpy jaw'. The causal organism is *Actinomyces bovis*. Treatment with streptomycin daily should be continued for a minimum of 2 weeks. See the under 'Diseases of the Integument', 'Bacterial skin diseases' for more information.

Calf diphtheria

This is an infection of the oral cavity caused by *Fusobacterium necrophorum*. The main sign is excess salivation with only a transient illness. It may develop into hard golfball-sized abscesses in the head region. Treatment will require these to be lanced, and antibiotics – normally a mixture of penicillin and streptomycin – to be injected im for 3 days.

Campylobacter jejuni *and* Campylobacter coli

These organisms can cause mild self-limiting enteritis in calves. No treatment is required and diagnosis can be confirmed on culture.

Clostridial disease

There are several separate clostridial species which affect cattle, causing different disease entities:

- Bacillary haemoglobinuria has been reported in the UK but is rare, although it is common in central Ireland. The disease is sometimes called bacterial redwater and is caused by *Clostridium (Cl.) novyi* type D. It occurs in areas of high rainfall, particularly when summers are wet. The signs shown include abdominal pain, jaundice and dysentery, and, as the name suggests, haemoglobinuria. Aggressive treatment is required with penicillin and fluid therapy.
- Blackleg is found worldwide. It is caused by *Cl. chauvoei*. The first sign is lameness. On examination, the animal will show a very swollen painful area over a wound. Treatment with high doses of penicillin and NSAIDs is rarely successful. There is a vaccine available. See also the section on 'Clostridial cellulitis' under 'Diseases of the Integument', 'Bacterial skin diseases'.
- Black's disease or infectious necrotic hepatitis is caused by *Cl. novyi* type B. The trigger factor is acute fluke infection, i.e. the migration of immature flukes through the liver, which is unusual in cattle. Acute fluke occurs in the autumn. Control can easily be carried out by vaccinating all animals against *Cl. novyi* type B. Fluke control is vital not only to prevent Black's disease but also to prevent the damage caused by the flukes in the liver.
- Botulism is caused by the organism *Cl. botulinum* which multiplies in the soil and in silage but not in the cow. The organism produces toxin outside the body. Therefore the severity of the disease will be related to the amount of toxin ingested. Diagnosis is not difficult if the pathognomic sign of a flaccid anus is seen. There is no specific treatment. Animals will recover if they can be kept alive with oral fluids.
- Enterotoxaemia is found in growing cattle which have overeaten. It is caused by *Cl. perfringens* type D. There is normally violent scouring. Treatment is with fluids and NSAIDs. Antibiotics are ineffective.
- Malignant oedema is caused by several clostridial organisms, namely *Cl. septicum*, *Cl. chauvoei*, *Cl. perfringens* and *Cl. novyi*. Animals can be found dead or *in extremis*. They show swellings, which are often gaseous. The disease may follow wounds, particularly to the vulva at parturition, and cause massive swelling of the hindquarters. Aggressive treatment with penicillin and NSAIDs may be successful if started promptly.
- Necrotic enteritis is a disease of calves caused by *Cl. perfringens* type C. It is a disease of suckler calves up to 4 months of age. The main signs are diarrhoea, dysentery, tenesmus, abdominal pain and pyrexia. These lead to dehydration and death. Treatment with intravenous fluids, NSAIDs and antibiotics is rarely successful.
- Sordellii abomasitis is caused by *Cl. sordellii*. It attacks the abomasum and releases lethal toxins causing so-called sudden death, but of course the animals do have a brief period of sickness. There is a vaccine available.
- Tetanus is caused by *Cl. tetani*. It is rare. Stiffness and rigor will be seen before the jaws become clamped together. Initial treatment should be large doses of

tetanus antitoxin (TAT) and also large doses of penicillin. Some practitioners think that injections of acetylpromazine reduce the symptoms but this has not been the author's experience. Animals may recover if they are given adequate nursing.

Escherichia coli (E. coli) *O157*

This is not a pathogen in cattle. However, it is carried by them and therefore carriers are a danger to man. The commensal bacterium of concern is VTEC 0157:H7. It causes no clinical signs in cattle.

Escherichia coli

Certain strains are pathogenic to calves particularly if they are the bacteria with the K99 antigen. These will cause septicaemia. The condition may be peracute so that death may occur before the calf is seen to scour. Most of the strains are resistant to ampicillin. Amoxicillin with clavulanic acid is likely to be the antibiotic of choice, together with rehydration and NSAIDs.

Johne's disease

Johne's disease, or paratuberculosis, is caused by *Mycobacterium paratuberculosis* (*M. avium* subsp. *paratuberculosis*). This chronic debilitating disease occurs throughout the world and causes chronic untreatable diarrhoea. It is spread to calves soon after birth but is only seen as a clinical disease in adults, normally after their second calf. The organisms may be seen in the faeces with Zeihl–Neelson (ZN) stain, but the gold standard for diagnosis is culture. Johne's disease is seen most commonly in the UK in Jersey cows. There is also a serological test, for which blood samples may be taken from the tail vein (see Fig. 3.1). There is a vaccine available.

Salmonellosis

The main causative organisms are *Salmonella typhimurium* and *S. dublin*; the former is highly zoonotic. The main condition is in calves but these organisms will cause acute diarrhoea and death in freshly calved cows. The faeces

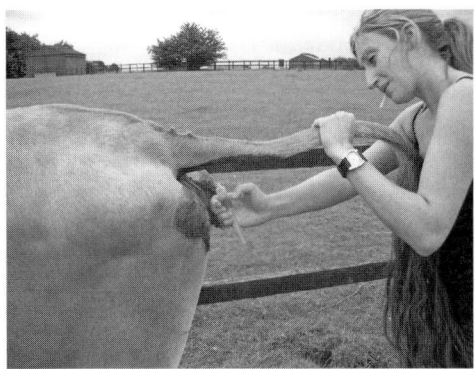

Fig. 3.1. Blood can be taken from the cow's tail vein in a test for Johne's disease.

have a distinct and unpleasant smell. Diagnosis is by culture of the faeces in enrichment media. Calves should be treated with rehydration and an appropriate antibiotic per os, e.g. amoxicillin and clavulanic acid, until culture and sensitivity results have been obtained. Cows should receive fluids per os using an Agger's pump, and parenteral antibiotics and NSAIDs. See also 'Salmonellosis' under 'Abortion and its causes' in the section 'Diseases of the Reproductive System' below.

Enteric diseases caused by protozoa and their treatment

Candida albicans

This yeast can cause diarrhoea in calves after prolonged antibiotic treatment. Peracute deaths from septicaemia have been reported. Treatment is stopping the antibiotic treatment, giving probiotics and fluid replacement.

Coccidiosis

The organisms involved in this disease are multiple but the most important are *Eimeria eznernii*, *E. bovis* and *E. alabamensis*. Tenesmus and diarrhoea, often containing fresh blood, are seen at about a month of age. Diagnosis is by counting oocysts in the faeces using a McMaster slide. Treatment should be rehydration and a coccidiostat, e.g. toltrazuril or diclazuril, orally. Decoquinate or monensin can be used in feed prophylactically (the latter is not licensed in the UK).

Cryptosporidium parvum

This organism is not restricted to calves and can cause diarrhoea in other species, including man. It causes diarrhoea in 2–3 week old calves. Diagnosis is from faecal smears stained with Giemsa. Treatment should be rehydration and oral halofuginone lactate.

Enteric diseases caused by parasites

Fasciolisis

In the UK, this condition is caused by *Fasciola hepatica* (the liver fluke). *F. gigantica* is found in Africa and Asia. The intermediate host in the UK is *Lymnaea truncatula* (the water snail). The normal form of the disease in cattle is chronic, with most of the flukes shed within 6 months, leaving the bile ducts irreparably thickened and even calcified. The principal signs are weight loss and diarrhoea, with raised liver enzymes. Diagnosis can be confirmed on a blood test with an ELISA. Eggs may be seen in the faeces and these are diagnostic but often, even in bad cases, eggs are not found. Treatment is with oral triclabendazole which kills adults and immature stages, clorsulon both by injection and as a pour on, and albendazole which only kills the adults.

Parasitic gastroenteritis (PGE)

The main parasitic nematodes causing PGE that are found in the UK are *Ostertagia ostertagia*, *Cooperia onocophora*, *Nematodirus helvetianus*, *Trichostrongylus axei* and *Haemonchus placei*, there are many other such species found throughout the world. These nematodes do not have an intermediate host and each tends to have different clinical manifestations.

O. ostertagia manifests as two separate clinical conditions, type 1 and type 2:

- Type 1 is the more standard form of PGE, with susceptible animals ingesting larvae later on in the grazing season. These become adults in the abomasum in the late summer, causing diarrhoea and ill thrift. High faecal egg counts (FECs) will be recorded. Anthelmintic treatment, unless there are resistant strains, will normally alleviate the problem.
- Type 2 follows type 1 in that larvae are ingested, but these do not become adults; rather they encyst in the mucosa of the abomasum in large numbers. The encysted larvae lie dormant until a trigger factor in the winter makes them all emerge together, when the animal will not only have severe diarrhoea but will be very ill and may even die. FECs will not be raised but diagnosis can be confirmed by a blood sample to measure serum pepsinogen. Treatment not only consists of anthelmintics but also of dexamethazone and antibiotics to try to reduce inflammation in the abomasal mucosa.

C. onocophora causes a standard form of PGE like *O. ostertagia* type 1, but normally slightly earlier i.e. halfway through July in the UK. *N. helvetianus* is the most common species in cattle worldwide. The eggs, which are very resistant to degradation, will accumulate on pastures for many months and infect calves in the next season. Severe signs of diarrhoea may occur before large numbers of easily recognized eggs (they are twice the size of those of other nematode species) occur in the faeces. *T. axei* is the very common small stomach worm which causes standard parasitic gastroenteritis worldwide. *H. placei* does not occur in the UK, but causes severe disease in tropical and subtropical countries. The disease and the diarrhoea may be so acute that the FEC will not have had time to rise to the massive levels seen later in the disease. Prompt treatment with anthelmintics is vital to prevent death.

Enteric diseases of unknown cause

Abomasal ulcers

These are seen in calves and the signs are colic, diarrhoea and melena – which manifests as black faeces. Treatment is symptomatic with a guarded prognosis.

Jejunal haemorrhagic syndrome

This is a sudden onset sporadic disease manifest by acute abdominal pain. There is rapid progression to shock, recumbency and death. A possible cause is *Cl. perfringens* type A. Treatment is symptomatic and rarely successful.

Vagal indigestion

This condition of cows used to be called 'well stomach' because when the rumen is auscultated the clinician hears a noise like a stone being dropped into a well. The rumen is atonic, perhaps because the vagus is damaged by an abscess in the mediastinum. Treatment is with oral rumen stimulants which offer doubtful efficacy and therefore the prognosis is poor.

Miscellaneous enteric conditions

Cleft palate

This congenital condition, which is usually bilateral, may be inherited. The clinician will be alerted to the condition by milk coming down the nose when the calf sucks. Diagnosis can be confirmed visually and euthanasia should be carried out.

Congenital erythropoietic porphyria

This is commonly called 'pink tooth' and occurs worldwide. It is an inherited disease related to a simple autosomal recessive gene. The teeth fluoresce in ultraviolet light. Vesicles and necrosis occur in unpigmented areas of the nose and mouth. There is no treatment and animals should be culled.

Pathogenic causes of diarrhoea in cattle

These can be classified by pathogen, age of affected animal or another incidence pointer, as shown below in Table 3.1.

Diseases of the liver

- Abscesses are a common finding in the liver of healthy cattle at slaughter (see Chapter 4).
- Black's disease (see above).
- Fasciolisis (see above).
- Fatty liver syndrome. This is a disease of dairy cows which are too fat at parturition, and their livers cannot cope with the demands of lactation. Treatment is with dexamethasone and glucose by injection iv and orally, in severe cases.
- Plant toxicity. Toxic plants include: blue-green algae (which contain *Cyanobacteria* spp.), bog asphodel (*Narthecium ossifragum*, found on marshy ground and dangerous in hay (Angell and Ross, 2011), fungi containing mycotoxins (mainly aflatoxins), *Panicum* spp. (grown as a fodder crop in tropical and subtropical areas and dangerous only when fed to excess), ragwort (*Senecio jacobea*, particularly dangerous to cattle in hay) and St John's wort (*Hypericum perforatum*, consumed after ditch clearing).
- Rift Valley fever (RVF) (mainly a disease of sheep and goats found in Africa, but causes abortion in cattle, see below).
- Tumours of the liver are rare (they are mainly adenomas or adenocarcinomas).

Diseases of the pancreas

Fat necrosis

The aetiology of this disease is obscure and in the author's experience it only occurs in the two Channel Island breeds of cattle. Large lumps of hard fat will be felt in the abdomen on rectal examination. The cows do not appear to be ill.

Diseases of the Neurological System

These can usefully be divided into three categories: conditions of calves; conditions of adult cattle; and ocular conditions.

Table 3.1. Infectious causes of diarrhoea in cattle.

Pathogen	Age group	Incidence pointer
Bovine viral diarrhoea	Adults	Abortion and linked to mucosal disease (see below)
Campylobacter jejuni and *C. coli*	Calves	Neonatal
Candida albicans	Calves	After prolonged antibiotic treatment
Coronavirus	Calves and adults	In adults, mainly in dairy cows in winter. Calves aged 3–21 days
Coccidiosis	Calves	4–6 weeks of age
Cryptosporidiosis	Calves	2–3 weeks of age
Escherichia coli	Calves	Neonatal, strains with K99 antigen are more pathogenic, may be peracute
Enterotoxaemia	Growing cattle	*Clostridium perfringens* type D, violent scouring
Fascioliasis	Yearlings and adults	Must have been grazing wet ground in the previous autumn
Johne's disease	Adult cows over 3 years of age	Infected soon after birth
Mucosal disease	Yearlings	Always persistently infected (PI)
Necrotic enteritis	Suckler calves up to 4 months	*Clostridium perfringens* type C
Parasitic gastroenteritis	Yearlings or 2 year olds which have been turned out for the first time	At grass in late summer or autumn
Rotavirus	Calves	Neonatal high morbidity, low mortality
Type 2 *Ostertagia ostertagia*	Yearlings or 2 year olds which must have been out grazing in the previous late summer or autumn	January to March
Salmonellosis	Cows and calves	*Salmonella typhimurium* in calves, *S. dublin* in cows and calves

Neurological conditions of calves

Bacterial meningitis

The most common isolates are *E. coli* and *Streptococcus* spp. The signs are ataxia, hyperaesthesia, neck pain, star gazing, wandering and vocalization. These will lead to recumbency, opisthotonous, convulsions and death. Treatment should be florfenicol 20 mg/kg iv twice daily and intensive nursing.

Brain abscess

This is likely to be caused by haematogenous spread of *Arcanobacterium pyogenes*. Diagnosis may be difficult as the calf will show neurological signs but may not have a raised rectal temperature. The choice of antibiotic is difficult. Trimethropin/sulfadiazine is suggested for a minimum of 10 days, together with NSAIDs.

Cerebrocortical necrosis (CCN)

In the author's experience this is the most common neurological disease of calves in the UK. Calves will appear blind and will wander around aimlessly. Treatment with thiamine, often in combination with other B vitamins, is very effective. The aim should be to give 350 mg thiamine hydrochloride (vitamin B_1) daily for 5 days. Ideally, the first dose should be given iv. The disease can be confirmed on post-mortem by observing the fluorescence of the brain under ultraviolet light.

Femoral nerve damage

This occurs in large calves which have a difficult parturition and are subjected to large amounts of traction in the final stages of delivery. Atrophy of the quadriceps soon becomes apparent with the calf having difficulty in walking. The prognosis is guarded and related to the severity of the clinical signs. Treatment is with NSAIDs and nursing.

Lead poisoning

Fifty years ago this was a common condition as there were still gates and doors painted with lead paint. The condition is rare today. Calves would lick the flaking paint and show acute neurological signs without a pyrexia. Treatment is an iv injection of calcium edetate (EDTA) to act as a chelating solution for the lead ions. This is very effective but should be given for 3 days to remove the lead that may still be in the gastroenteric tract.

Middle ear infection

Calves with this condition will have a head tilt, a staggering gait and a raised rectal temperature. If the infection has come from the outer ear, which is the normal manifestation, calves will show pain when the ear is squeezed and the clinician will perceive a crackling on palpation. Several organisms may be involved so a broad-spectrum antibiotic should be give parenterally together with aural antibiotics licensed for dogs. The prognosis is good. However, if the infection has come from a haematogenous spread with no outer ear infection, the prognosis is poor even with prolonged parenteral antibiotics.

Radial paralysis

This condition is common, and is usually a result of a calf being trapped in a gate or creep. It can also occur after a kick from a cow. The calf will be fracture lame, but when the leg is placed on the ground it will be able to bear weight on the affected leg without difficulty or pain. The calf should be given NSAIDs to reduce the inflammation but will normally learn to flick the leg forward as it walks and show a total recovery in 6 weeks.

Neurological conditions of adult cattle

Aujeszky's disease

Often called pseudorabies, this disease has a worldwide distribution but has been eliminated from the UK and many countries in western Europe. It is caused by a herpesvirus whose primary host is the pig. The main signs are intense pruritis, depression and lethargy. Diagnosis is from virus isolation and paired serum samples. There is no treatment. The disease is notifiable in the UK.

Bovine spongiform encephalopathy (BSE)

This condition was first diagnosed in the UK in 1986. It has been found in Europe, the Middle East, Japan, the USA and Canada. Cows become infected by eating infectious proteins in cattle feed contaminated from animal sources. Horizontal transmission is of minor importance. The incubation period can be many years. Animals are very unlikely to be infected under 2 years of age. The disease has an insidious onset with just a slight change of character. Full-blown signs of aggression and paraplegia are often brought on by parturition. Diagnosis other than that from clinical signs relies on histology of the CNS. The disease is similar to Creutzfeldt–Jakob disease (CJD) in man and is notifiable in the UK.

Listeria monocytogenes

L. monocytogenes causes a very serious zoonotic disease, with animals showing neurological signs, pyrexia and abortion. Animals can pick up the organism from other animals but the normal spread is from contaminated silage. The most prominent neurological sign is circling and a raised rectal temperature. Diagnosis can only be confirmed by culture from a cerebrospinal fluid (CSF) tap. Treatment should consist of high levels of oxytetracyclines and NSAIDs. See also 'Bovine iritis (silage eye)' under 'Ocular conditions' below, and 'Abortion and its causes' under 'Diseases of the Reproductive System'.

Nervous acetonaemia

This is a metabolic disease of dairy cows (see below).

Obturator nerve damage

This occurs during parturition of a relatively fetal oversized calf and may be linked to sciatic nerve damage (see below). The obturator nerve controls the motor function of the muscles that adduct the hind legs, so that the animal does the splits and lies down in sternal recumbency like a frog. Immediate treatment is vital to prevent further nerve damage; it should consist of NSAIDs and securing the hind legs with 'Somerset shackles'. These should be adjusted to prevent the legs from abduction by more than 40 cm for a large cow.

Rabies

This is caused by a rhabdovirus, and where the virus occurs is the most important cause of encephalitis in cattle, thanks to its zoonotic implications. Cattle are infected by a bite of an infected carnivore and invariably die. They exhibit both the dumb and the furious signs. Cattle are a particular danger to man as they excrete the virus in their saliva, which is produced excessively and gives the appearance of an oesophageal foreign body. There is no treatment but there is a vaccine available although it is not licensed in the UK. The disease is notifiable in the UK.

Sciatic nerve damage

Damage causing paralysis occurs in the pelvic canal during parturition. Both the sciatic and the obturator nerve may be damaged, causing ischiatic paralysis. The signs will include abduction of the hind legs together with the hock being overextended and the fetlock partially flexed. Treatment involving NSAIDs and a high level of nursing needs to be instituted immediately. The cow needs to be moved either outside if the weather is clement or on to a deep muck bed. The prognosis will be related to the severity of the clinical signs. A rising serum creatine kinase (CK) level indicates a very poor prognosis.

Ocular conditions

Besnoitosis

Apart from cysts in the sclera conjunctiva, this disease can be asymptomatic. Cattle can show an initial acute phase with generalized skin oedema, swollen lymph nodes and a reluctance to move. This may lead to a chronic phase of alopecia, skin thickening with wrinkles and cracks, and hyperpigmentation. Besnoitosis

has been reported in Africa, Asia and South America, and very sporadically in south-west Europe. The cat is the normal intermediate host, and infects cattle by contaminating feedstuffs. Biting insects may also spread the condition. Diagnosis is from the cysts in the sclera, which are pathognomic. Treatment is with oxytetracyclines and supportive nursing. See 'Protozoal skin diseases' under 'Diseases of the Integument' below, for further information.

Bovine iritis (silage eye)

This condition is seen in cattle fed silage contaminated with the bacterium *L. monocytogenes*, particularly when the silage is fed in 'ring feeders'. Normally both eyes are affected. Diagnosis can be confirmed by observing the iritis with an ophthalmoscope. Treatment is with a sub-conjunctival injection of atropine sulfate and dexamethasone.

Congenital cataracts

These occur as a result of an autosomal recessive gene seen in Friesians, Holsteins, Jerseys and Herefords.

Foreign bodies

These are normally oat flights (see Plate 1). Careful removal needs to be carried out under sedation and local anaesthesia.

Horner's syndrome

This is a syndrome-associated interruption of ocular sympathetic nerve pathways. The signs are miosis, enophthalmos and loss of sweat on the ipsilateral side of the muzzle. The normal cause is trauma to the neck or abscesses in the chest or behind the eye. If the root cause is an abscess that should be drained and the animal given antibiotics. If the cause is trauma, NSAIDs would be appropriate treatment.

Infectious bovine keratoconjunctivitis (New Forest eye)

This is the most common ocular disease in cattle in the UK. There are several theories on the cause. One eye is normally affected, with approximately 10% of affected cattle having some signs in the other eye. Initially there is excess lacrymation followed by corneal damage. The condition is spread by flies. Many animals will self-cure. There are various accepted treatments:

- long-acting antibiotic eye ointments
- sub-conjunctival injections of antibiotics
- parenteral injections of long-acting antibiotics

Squamous cell carcinoma of the third eyelid

This is the most common tumour affecting the bovine eye worldwide. It occurs in non-pigmented third eyelids, e.g. in Herefords, and is more prevalent in the tropics. If the condition is noticed early enough the third eyelid can be cut off with sharp scissors under sedation and local anaesthetic blocks. Provided the tumour can be removed totally leaving a margin on the third eyelid the prognosis is good. Otherwise, enucleation is required.

Thelazia *spp.*

These nematodes live in the lacrimal ducts and are spread by flies. They have a world-wide distribution mainly in the tropics and subtropics, and cause conjunctivitis and keratitis. Treatment is with ivermectins parenterally.

Vitamin A deficiency

This is rare except in totally barley-fed bulls and bullocks. There is a retinal degeneration which is irreversible.

Metabolic Diseases

These can also be viewed as a category of neurological conditions.

The predominant signs

- Anorexia
- Lack of rumination
- Ataxia
- Recumbency

Acetonaemia

This is also called ketosis as by definition there are raised levels of ketones in the blood and milk, which can be demonstrated in the latter by Rothera's powder turning purple. Acetonaemia is primarily a condition of dairy cows either too fat at calving and with an underlying insulin resistance or of cows given too low an energy diet. It may be secondary to some other condition, e.g. a left hand displacement of the abomasum (LDA). The normal signs are lethargy and poor appetite with a sweet-smelling breath which can only be smelt by some people. In unusual cases, nervous signs will be shown. Treatment is with dexamethazone together with treatment of the underlying cause.

Acidosis

This may be acute in cases of grain overload, or chronic with a diet low in fibre. The pH of the rumen will be low and this will depress food intake. This chronic form tends to occur in high-producing dairy cows or beef-fattening cattle fed entirely on grain. Diagnosis can be confirmed by measuring the pH of a sample of the rumen contents. Treatment is by adding bicarbonate to the food in the short term and by adding more fibre in the long term. In acute cases, animals should be given high volumes of electrolytes spiked with bicarbonate using an Agger's pump, with supportive injections of vitamin B. In peracute cases, e.g. when an animal has broken into a grain store, a rumenotomy should be performed to remove the rumen contents and replace them with electrolytes.

Hypocalcaemia

This is a disease of adult cows called 'milk fever'. Classically it occurs around parturition when there is a sudden drop in blood calcium levels. The case may be a true 'milk fever' around parturition, or in Jersey cows it may be brought on by oestrus. Feeding excess root crops, particularly the tops, will cause hypocalcaemia in growing and adult animals.

Also, poisonous plants containing oxalates, e.g. rhubarb, will cause hypocalcaemia. Diagnosis can be confirmed by measuring blood calcium levels. One 400 ml bottle of 40% calcium into the vein should be sufficient for treatment except in a very large cow. There is no evidence to confirm that the solution is better given at blood heat and slowly, but taking these precautions is prudent. If the cow is staggering but not recumbent, it is advisable not to try to give large volumes of fluid iv, and obviously it should not be put in a crush. Trying to inject a staggering cow is difficult and dangerous. The worst scenario is that some fluid will be injected perivascularly. This will make the cow move her head violently, and will either result in injury or the needle will come out of the vein. It is preferable to give the dose sub cut as this will achieve the same blood levels of calcium within half an hour. It is important that after treatment the cow is moved either on to deep muck or out on to the pasture and then propped up on to her brisket in sternal recumbency.

Hypomagnesaemia

This condition may cause the highest mortality of all conditions in beef suckler cows. It is rare in dairy cows. Magnesium levels in most suckler cows are on a knife-edge. Any upset to the absorption of sufficient magnesium by the small intestine will bring on hypomagnesaemia. The laxative effect of lush grass is the normal cause. Other causes of stress, e.g. oestrus or weaning of a calf, are sufficient to trigger the condition. The almost pathognomic sign shown by cows with hypomagnesaemia is recumbency and convulsions. Diagnosis can be confirmed by measuring blood magnesium levels or at post-mortem by measuring magnesium levels in the aqueous humour of the eye.

At the very onset, the clinician should warn the owner that the cow could die *at any moment* and that any treatment will be hazardous. It should also be stressed that although the level of magnesium in the blood will be raised by the treatment, irreparable brain damage may already have occurred.

Historically, in a cow having convulsions, clinicians used to inject 10 ml of a small animal euthanasia triple-strength barbiturate solution iv to calm her so that treatment was not so hazardous for the cow or the handlers. However, with the current legislation on veterinary medicines, this practice is not advisable. The first treatment is to inject a 400 ml bottle of 25% magnesium sulfate (this normally has a black top) sub cut. This should be well rubbed in and then a 400 ml bottle of 20% calcium borogluconate with 5% magnesium hypophosphite and 20% glucose monohydrate (this normally has a blue top) should be injected slowly iv. Nursing is important in hypomagnesaemia cases. Trying to maintain the cow in sternal recumbency is difficult but worthwhile.

Hypophosphataemia

This is an overdiagnosed condition of adult cows. The classical signs are recumbency, pain in the lumbar region and, on some occasions, there is haemoglobinuria. Diagnosis can be confirmed by measuring blood phosphorus levels. Treatment is 25 ml of 20% w/v of sodium toldimphos injected iv daily for 2 days.

Common trace element deficiencies

Cobalt deficiency

Cobalt is an ingredient of vitamin B_{12} which is synthesized in the rumen. Lack of cobalt is rare but will result in a vitamin B_{12} deficiency which in turn causes ill thrift and anaemia. Diagnosis can be confirmed on a heparinized blood sample. Cobalt is readily given in the diet or as a drench. Vitamin B_{12} is readily given by injection.

Copper deficiency

True copper deficiency is very rare but secondary copper deficiency due to high levels of molybdenum or sulfur in the diet is common. The signs seen are multiple. Initially, black animals will take on a ginger colouring and the hair will rough, then erosions on the mouth and diarrhoea will occur, and eventually animals will die. Diagnosis can be confirmed on a heparinized blood sample. As copper is stored in the liver, low copper blood samples will only be seen in cases of severe deficiency. Liver samples give a more accurate picture. Treatment is with boluses containing copper oxide needles, which are licensed in the UK, or with copper injections, which are licensed in other parts of the world.

Iodine deficiency

This condition, called goitre, is extremely rare but is still seen in calves in goitrogenic areas worldwide. The pathognomic sign is a swollen, non-neoplastic thyroid. Low-grade deficiency may result in sub-fertility or the birth of weak calves. Prevention by adding iodized salts to the diet is preferable to treatment.

Selenium deficiency

Selenium deficiency will readily occur in selenium-deficient areas. The deficiency can be linked to vitamin E deficiency. Equally, calves can be affected by vitamin E deficiency when selenium levels are normal. The deficiency is manifest as 'white muscle disease', which may give signs of muscular weakness or, if the heart is affected, sudden death. Treatment in the short term is with injections of selenium and vitamin E. In the long term, there are long-acting selenium injectable preparations.

Diseases of the Respiratory System

The predominant signs

- Dyspnoea
- Pyrexia
- Coughing

Diagnosis

- Age
- History
- Clinical signs

- Nasopharyngeal swabs
- Serology
- Faeces sample (70 g minimum is required for lungworm larvae)

Causes of respiratory disease

- Viruses
- Bacteria
- Fungi
- Parasites
- Miscellaneous factors

Respiratory diseases caused by viruses and bacteria, and their treatment

Bovine respiratory disease (BRD)

BRD is a syndrome affecting calves and growing cattle. Good animal husbandry is vital for its prevention and treatment. Vaccination and treatment with antibiotics and NSAIDs should always be secondary to changes in animal husbandry, particularly modifications to ventilation, prevention of draughts and lower stocking rates. Causative agents include the viruses and bacteria in the following list:

- *Bovine herpesvirus 1* (BHV 1) will cause respiratory disease, particularly in older growing cattle, which is called infectious bovine rhinotracheitis (IBR). It will also cause the reproductive disease infectious pustular vulvovaginitis (IPV). The respiratory form of the disease manifests as serious pyrexia with an ocular and nasal discharge. Remarkably, the clinical course of the disease is much improved by injections of a combination of penicillin and streptomycin. The disease is readily detected by serology, which can be used in herd eradication schemes. There are good vaccines which are available either as live vaccination for intra-nasal or im use or as attenuated dead vaccination for sub cut injection. Care should be taken to use a marker vaccine if later eradication schemes are envisaged. See also '*Bovine herpesvirus 1* (BHV 1)' as a cause of abortion under 'Diseases of the Reproductive System' below.

- *Bovine respiratory coronavirus* (BRCV) has only recently been recognized as a serious potential respiratory pathogen. It now needs to be considered when investigating a BRD outbreak.
- *Bovine respiratory syncytial virus* (BRSV – or just plain RSV) is a very serious pathogen, particularly for young growing cattle – either suckler calves or concentrate-fed animals. It causes serious pyrexia, coughing, and nasal and lacrimal discharge. Dyspnoea and mouth breathing is a feature of advanced cases. Passive immunity helps but does not prevent the disease. There are good vaccines available.
- *Bovine parainfluenza virus 3* (PI3) is a paramyxovirus which causes relatively mild disease signs but is a prime initiator for secondary bacterial infections. There are good vaccines available.
- Infectious bovine rhinotracheitis (IBR) is caused by BHV 1 (see above).
- *Mannheimia haemolytica* (formerly *Pasteurella haemolytica*) is probably the most important bacterial pathogen in the BRD complex. It can cause disease in its own right without a viral initiator. It is the main pathogen causing 'shipping fever'. It is actually sensitive to penicillin in high doses even through it is a Gram-negative rod. However, there are a large number of other suitable antibiotics which are perhaps more effective and have a considerably longer action. NSAIDs are very useful. There are vaccines available.
- *Pasteurella multocida* is a bacterium that is also often found in the 'shipping fever' complex. It is also seen as a secondary to BRSV and PI3 infections in younger calves. It can cause pneumonia in its own right. Like *M. haemolytica* it is sensitive to high levels of penicillin, but more modern antibiotics and NSAIDs would be more appropriate for treatment.
- *Arcanobacterium pyogenes* is found at the end stage of a BRD case, i.e. it is a tertiary pathogen. Although it is sensitive to antibiotics *in vitro* the bacteria are infective in

pus-filled abscesses. Euthanasia is the only option.

- *Histophilus somni* is a serious bacterial pathogen in its own right but is often linked with *M. haemolytica*. The bacteria can cause BRD on their own or be secondary to a virus. *H. somni* often occurs later on in the disease process and is difficult to treat with antibiotics. Changing the type of antibiotic used and NSAIDs are helpful treatments.
- *Mycoplasma* spp. include *M. disbar* and *M. bovis*. These are emerging pathogens in BRD. They synergize with other pathogens and cause fatal disease. Oxytetracycline is the antibiotic of choice. They will also infect the joints, causing acute lameness in young cattle which are already systemically ill. NSAIDs are very worthwhile treatment. The species are not included in any vaccines.
- *Ureaplasma* spp. may have a secondary role in BRD but it is not clear how important they are in respiratory disease. They are more important in reproductive disorders.

Bovine tuberculosis

This very important zoonotic disease is found throughout the world and is notifiable in the European Union (EU), USA and elsewhere. It primarily affects the respiratory tract and associated lymph nodes. Historically, it was very important when it affected the udder and caused contamination of the milk. The main causative organism is *Mycobacterium bovis*, but other *Mycobacterium* spp. are also found. The disease can be spread by other wild mammals, e.g. badgers in the UK and opossums in New Zealand. It is a chronic wasting disease, only causing a cough and respiratory signs in the later stages. Peripheral lymph nodes may be enlarged. The disease is transmitted by the respiratory and ingestion routes. Herd screening is not easy as the standard comparative avian and bovine tuberculin intradermal test, as used in the UK, reveals false positives. The gamma interferon blood test is used as a follow-up. There is no treatment and affected animals should be slaughtered as soon as possible.

Contagious bovine pleuropneumonia (CBPP)

This very serious cattle disease is caused by *Mycoplasma mycoides mycoides* and is notifiable in the EU and the USA. It is found in Africa, India and China. It causes severe respiratory signs of coughing and an elbow abducted stance. There is a carrier state which can be confirmed by routine serology testing. On the whole, treatment with oxytetracyclines should be carried out after careful evaluation as this may increase the number of carrier animals.

The shipping fever complex

This is a specific serious respiratory condition that is separate from BRD. It is caused by *M. haemolytica* and *Pasteurella multocida* as noted above, and follows a stress, usually transport. Treatment is with oxytetracyclines and NSAIDs, and this is normally successful so more modern and expensive antibiotics are not required. There is a vaccine available.

Respiratory diseases caused by fungi and their treatment

Aspergillosis

This is extremely rare but will occur in very badly ventilated cattle sheds when mouldy straw is used. Actual hyphae will be seen in the lungs of this invariably fatal condition. A more common condition is a hypersensitivity reaction to the fungal spores which will give signs of acute respiratory distress similar to 'fog fever' in adult cattle. Fresh air and dexamethazone are the required treatment.

Respiratory diseases caused by parasites and their treatment

Lungworm (parasitic bronchitis)

This occurs 3 weeks after ingesting *Dictyocaulus viviparus* larvae. The excellent oral vaccination against this condition, which uses irradiated larvae, is sadly being neglected with the use of pour-on ivermectin-type anthelmintics. The animals at risk are 2 year old breeding heifers and, of course, adult cows. Lungworm causes devastating effects in naive adults, with very marked violent coughing. (Plate 2). Mortality may be as high as 10%. Treatment with anthelmintics, antibiotics and NSAIDs is often not very effective, with many survivors being left with irreversible lung damage.

Miscellaneous respiratory diseases, their causes and treatment

Anaphylaxis

This has a sudden onset of severe dyspnoea and muscle tremors. The rectal temperature will be raised to 42°C. The occurrence is normally linked either to a recent injection or is found in a dairy cow heavy in milk with a massively stocked udder. If the latter is the cause milking out will prompt a swift recovery. In other cases, animals should be injected with dexamethazone iv, or if pregnant with NSAIDs iv.

Fog fever

There are many theories on the aetiology of this condition of interstitial pneumonia. The theory with the most credence is that of a toxicosis resulting from the ingestion of large quantities of L-tryptophan in lush autumn grass. The disease occurs only in adults and the main sign is respiratory distress, with the rectal temperature remaining normal. It is a disease of beef suckler cows, and the affected animals tend to be separate from the rest, and are quieter than normal. Animals may be found dead or die following exercise. Care should be used in rounding up animals for treatment, which is far from evidenced based. Apart from more normal therapies, e.g. antibiotics, NSAIDs, steroids, etc., atropine and methylene blue have been advocated. In reality, the advice must be to stick to antibiotics and NSAIDs. The prognosis is guarded.

Inhalation pneumonia

This can occur when a cow is drenched carelessly with a liquid medicine, e.g. liquid paraffin or vegetable oil. It can also occur with a misplaced Agger's pump. General anaesthetics (GAs) in adult animals are particularly hazardous. Inhalation pneumonia can occur in untreated 'milk fever' cases which have become bloated in lateral recumbency. The signs will vary from violent coughing to death depending on the volume of liquid inhaled. Treatment would consist of antibiotics and NSAIDs.

Diseases of the Circulatory System

Circulatory diseases with various causes and their treatment

Anthrax

This serious zoonotic disease is caused by a Gram-positive spore-forming bacterial rod called *Bacillus anthracis* and is notifiable in most parts of the world, including the UK. Ingestion is the most common method of infection, and there is very rapid extracellular multiplication of the bacteria, with toxin production and sudden death (although the author has seen a case that recovered which had been promptly treated after diagnosis by a colleague). Diagnosis is confirmed on staining a blood smear with McFadyen's stain and seeing the rectangular rod-shaped bacteria with the blue-staining capsules.

Bleeding disorders

These are relatively rare and therefore represent a considerable diagnostic challenge for the clinician (Bell, 2011). In disorders of primary haemostasis, only a small amount of blood loss occurs from an injury site before a fibrin clot is formed by secondary haemostasis. Petechiae will be seen in the mucosa. In disorders of secondary haemostasis, large-volume bleeds will be seen in the body cavities. Primary disorders will cause thrombocytopenia, which is seen in acute bracken fern toxicity, acute infection with BVD virus, trichothecene mycocytosis, bovine neonatal pancytopenia (typically in calves under 1 month of age showing pyrexia and unexplained haemorrhage from the nose), ingestion of bone-marrow suppressive substances, e.g. furazolidone (now prohibited in the EU), and inherited bovine thrombopathia in Simmental cattle. Secondary disorders are seen in inherited deficiency of coagulation factor XI, Warfarin poisoning and mouldy sweet clover poisoning. Treatment is with blood transfusions (see Chapter 4).

Bovine leucosis

This is sometimes called bovine lymphosarcoma. There are two separate diseases recognized: bovine enzootic leucosis and bovine sporadic leucosis. Bovine enzootic leucosis is linked with a retrovirus and is spread by direct contact and dirty needles. It is a notifiable disease in the UK and is confirmed by agar gel immunodiffusion (AGID). The disease has been eradicated in most EU countries but is found in North America. Bovine enzootic leucosis is normally seen in older cattle, where it causes widespread tumours. There is no treatment. Bovine sporadic leucosis is seen in young growing calves, which exhibit swollen lymph nodes, salivary glands and thymuses. The disease causes rapid emaciation and death, and is confirmed at post-mortem.

Bovine petechial fever

This disease in endemic in Kenya and is caused by the blood parasite *Ehrlichia ondiri*. It is transmitted by an unknown arthropod vector from the bushbuck, *Tragelaphus scriptus*. The signs are petechial and ecchymotic haemorrhages on all the mucus membranes. There is some immunity as the disease only seems to infect animals brought into endemic areas. The treatment is with oxytetracyclines.

Cor pulmonale

This sporadic condition is right-side heart failure, normally following chronic pneumonia. The treatment is centred on the original cause of the condition together with frusemide as a diuretic.

Dilated cardiomyopathy

This is an inherited condition found in Holstein cattle. The signs are slow-developing peripheral oedema and pleural effusion, typically in 2–3 year old cattle. Diagnosis can be confirmed on ultrasonography. There is no realistic treatment and animals should be slaughtered.

Endocarditis

This is normally vegetative and caused by *Arcanobacterium pyogenes*. Diagnosis will be confirmed by auscultation and observing the peripheral signs which will vary according to which valve or valves are affected. The most common sign is engorged jugular veins. Treatment is a very prolonged course of antibiotics which seldom cure the disease. If the cow improves it is important that she receives full antibiotic cover at her next calving.

Heartwater

This is caused by a rickettsia, *Ehrlichia ruminantium*, which is spread by *Amblyomma* spp. ticks. It occurs in tropical Africa, the Caribbean, South and Central America and tropical parts of the USA. The disease is normally acute with a high fever and an increased vascular permeability, which causes hydropericardium and hydrothorax. These signs lead on to fatal neurological signs. Diagnosis is confirmed by the presence of the organism in Diff-Quik stained brain smears. Treatment is with high doses of oxytetracycline. Control is through effective tick control and vaccination.

Lightning strike

This assumes an over-importance in farmers' minds in the UK as it normally is the only condition which their cattle are insured against. Sudden death in groups of cattle without signs of a struggle after a storm is reasonable evidence of lightning strike, particularly if they are all in contact with a wire fence. Burn marks may be seen on the medial aspects of the legs and haemorrhagic streaks will be seen on careful skinning.

Lyme disease

This condition is caused by the spirochaete *Borrelia burgdorferi* and is a worldwide zoonosis. It is not primarily a disease of cattle but will cause joint infection, which may be an immune-mediated response. Cattle will have swollen joints on their lower limbs and will be stiff on movement. Diagnosis is by PCR. Treatment with oxytetracycline for 3 weeks together with NSAIDs has been suggested.

Mycoplasma wenyonii

This condition is not fully understood and it is thought to be spread by arthropods or needles from mass vaccination procedures (Strugnell and McAuliffe, 2012). The main clinical signs in the UK are hind limb oedema, pyrexia and painful, swollen udders in dairy cows, with reduced fertility in stock bulls. Clinical signs gradually resolve and a full recovery may take 10 days or longer. Diagnosis is from fresh blood smears taken in a clean environment and stained with Giemsa. Treatment with 3 days of tylosin at 5 mg/kg im is said to be more effective than oxytetracycline at 10 mg/kg im.

Circulatory diseases caused by protozoa and their treatment

Anaplasmosis

The main organism causing this disease is *Anaplasma marginale*. It is tick borne and occurs in the tropics and subtropics. The main signs are pyrexia and anaemia. Diagnosis can be confirmed by thin blood smears stained with Giemsa. Treatment is with oxytetracyclines or imidocarb dipropionate. Prevention is by tick control.

Babesiosis

This disease does occur in the UK but is much more important in other areas of the world, mainly in the tropics and subtropics. It is spread by ticks of various species. The main causative organisms are *Babesia bigemina* and *B. bovis*.

The disease is characterized by acute fever, anaemia and recumbency. Haemoglobinaemia and haemoglobinuria are only seen in the later stages of the disease. Diagnosis can be confirmed by thin blood smears stained with Giemsa. Treatment is with diminazene aceturate or imidocarb dipropionate. The latter is licensed in the UK as the product Imizol injection (imidocarb 85 mg/ml). Prevention outside the UK is carried out by tick control.

Theileriosis

This tropical or subtropical tick-borne disease follows 10 days after exposure to infected ticks so weekly dipping or spraying with acaricide will normally prevent the disease. The most important type is East Coast fever (ECF) which is found in East and Central Africa. ECF is caused by *Theileria parva parva* and is spread by *Rhipicephalus appendiculatus*. ECF has a high morbidity and a high mortality. There is a less virulent strain of the parasite, *T. p. bovis*. *T. p. lawrencei* causes a similar disease but can only be spread from buffalos to cattle but not from ox to ox. The main presenting signs for all types of theileriosis are high fever and swollen peripheral lymph nodes. Diagnosis can be confirmed by seeing Koch's blue bodies in lymph node smears. Treatment with buparvaquone is very effective if given in the early stages of the disease. An immunization using an infection-and-treatment regime is used in some areas of East Africa.

Trypanosomiasis

The majority of trypanosomiasis cases occur in areas where the tsetse fly is found as this is the vector for all *Trypanosoma* spp. that affect cattle. *T. vivax* causes peracute disease, pyrexia and rapid death. *T. brucei brucei* causes an acute disease which, if untreated, will result in death. *T. congolense* causes a more chronic disease with anaemia and weight loss. Diagnosis is confirmed by thick and thin blood smears stained with Giemsa. Treatment is with diminazene aceturate, homidium bromide and chloride, and isometamidium chloride. The latter also has some prophylactic value but does not treat *T. b. brucei*.

Diseases of the Urinary System

Post-parturient haemoglobinuria

The aetiology of this rare sporadic condition which is found worldwide is not known. Affected animals often have hypophosphataemia and hypocupraemia. It tends to occur in older high-producing dairy cows within 4 weeks of calving. Animals will have haemoglobinuria and anaemia. Treatment is supportive with fluids, injections of phosphorus and copper boluses orally.

Pyelonephritis

This is normally an ascending infection caused by *E. coli* or *Corynebacterium renale* in recently calved cows, and found worldwide. The main signs are pyrexia, pain on urinating or palpation of the left kidney, if affected, on rectal examination. Diagnosis can be confirmed by ultrasonography or culture of the urine taken by catheterization of the bladder. Treatment is with high doses of antibiotics, penicillin for *C. renale* or enrofloxacin for *E. coli*. A minimum of 3 weeks of treatment is suggested.

Renal amyloidosis

This rare sporadic disease is characterized by deposits of amyloid throughout the organs of the body, but particularly in the kidney. There is proteinuria and chronic wasting with diarrhoea shown if the liver or bowel is affected. Diagnosis is not easy, but urine creatinine and urea nitrogen are elevated. Kidney biopsy is definitive. There is no treatment.

Diseases of the Reproductive System

Abortion and its causes

Akabane

This condition is caused by an *Orthobunyavirus* (*Akabane virus*) and is spread by several species of mosquito and biting midge. It occurs in the tropics and subtropics, namely in northern Australia, Japan, Korea and South Africa, and the author has seen it in the Middle East. It causes congenital abnormalities in full-term calves as well as abortion, but other than these signs adults are normally asymptomatic. There is a vaccine available.

Arcanobacterium pyogenes

This bacterium is rarely isolated and is found in late-term abortions. There is no vaccine available.

Bacillus licheniformis

This is a rare cause of abortion and is associated with the feeding of poor-quality forage. The cow is not ill but the bacterium is isolated from the fetus or the placenta. There is no vaccine available.

Bovine herpesvirus 1 *(BHV 1)*

This virus will cause abortion after 150 days post service. There is venereal spread of a strain of virus which appears to be different from the virus that causes respiratory signs. Animals which have aborted are then immune. There is a vaccine, which is not licensed in the UK, which should be given to heifers before service when at risk from the disease.

Bovine viral diarrhoea virus *(BVDV)*

BVDV may cause infertility problems related to early embryonic death, but abortion is rare. The virus will cause diarrhoea in adult cows and mucosal disease in calves infected *in utero* (these calves are PI). Infected cows will test serologically positive but virus negative, unlike the PI calves. There are very effective vaccines available.

Brucellosis

This is caused by the bacterium *Brucella abortus*. The disease has largely been eradicated in the EU and totally eradicated in the UK, where it is notifiable. It is highly contagious via the products of abortion and is a zoonosis. It will cause late abortion storms in naive cattle. There are two vaccines available, one of which does not interfere with the serology used for eradication programmes. Diagnosis is by bacteriological examination of the fetus, the placenta and milk, or by the detection of antibodies in blood or milk.

Campylobacter fetus *subsp.* veneralis

This is an obligate bacterial parasite of the reproductive tract and cannot survive outside the host for any appreciable time. Normally it causes early embryonic death. This can be reduced by blanket injections to the cows of streptomycin. Bulls can be cleaned by preputial washing with an oily preparation of streptomycin for 3 days.

Chlamydophila abortus

This bacterium is a common cause of abortion in sheep, but is extremely rare in cattle. However, it is important as it is a zoonosis.

Coxiella burnetii

This bacterium causes Q fever which does occur sporadically in cattle causing late abortions and stillbirths. It is found worldwide (except in New Zealand). Diagnosis is best by histopathology and staining with a modified ZN stain. The organism is spread in milk, placenta, urine and faeces, and is zoonotic. At the time of writing there is no cattle vaccine but there is a vaccine for goats.

Leptospira icterohaemorrhagiae

This organism is very rare but is associated with a serious systemic illness in cattle, which will show clinical jaundice. In some instances, the pyrexia from the systemic disease will cause an abortion. In other instances, the organism will be isolated from the abortion products.

Leptospira *serovar Hardjo* (L. borgpetersenii *serovar Hardjo* and L. interrogans *serovar Hardjo*)

These bacteria will cause abortion but more commonly cause infertility. They are associated with transitory illness in cows which show a 'milk drop' syndrome. The condition is readily diagnosed on serology. It can be spread from infected urine and infected ditches, and also from infected sheep which are symptomless carriers. It is a zoonosis. There are good vaccines available.

Leptospira *serovar Pomona*

This organism is not a primary cattle pathogen and is found in many mammalian species. It has been isolated in rare instances from aborted cattle fetuses.

Listeria monocytogenes

This bacterium causes primarily a neurological pyrexic, zoonotic disease. Abortions are normally sporadic but can affect up to 20% of the herd at any stage of gestation. Death of the fetus occurs 2 days before the abortion so the fetus is normally decomposed. The disease is normally associated with the feeding of silage. Treatment with antibiotics is helpful. There is no vaccine available.

Mycotic abortion

Aspergillus fumigatus is the main causal organism of mycotic abortion. Infection comes from eating mouldy bedding or feeding stuffs. The organism spreads in the bloodstream to the placenta, and causes late abortions. Diagnosis is by demonstration of the fungus in the placenta, which has 'ringworm'-like lesions.

Neospora caninum

This protozoan was first seen in dogs and spreads from them by the faecal–oral transfer to cattle. It has only recently been associated with bovine abortion. The organism is common in the UK but it may not be as common as serology might suggest. The definitive diagnosis is from immunohistochemistry of fetal brain tissue. This will differentiate *N. caninum* from *Toxoplasma gondii*. The main method of spread is vertical transmission from infected dams to congenitally infected calves. There is no vaccine available.

Parachlamydia acanthamoeba

This bacterium was first found in Switzerland causing suppurative and necrotizing placentitis. It is now found in southern Scotland. It can be diagnosed on PCR. It may have zoonotic implications.

Rift Valley fever

This viral disease caused by a bunyavirus is found in Africa and the Middle East. The main method of spread is by *Aedes* mosquitoes. The abortion rate can be 100%, with 10% of adult cattle dying, and showing icterus and pyrexia. Diagnosis can be confirmed with serum and heparanized blood that show high titres and by virus isolation. There is no treatment but there is a vaccine available.

Salmonellosis

This is a rare cause of abortion and might just be the raised temperature from a systemic infection, but in some instances *S. dublin* or *S. typhimurium* are isolated from the fetus or the placenta. The spread is via the contaminated environment. There is a vaccine against *S. dublin* available.

Schmallenburg virus *(SBV)*

The *Orthobunyavirus* that causes this disease of cattle is named after the town of Schmallenburg in North West Germany where it was first discovered in August 2011. By the time of writing, it had spread to most of Western Europe. SBV is spread by *Culicoides obsoletus* and *C. dewulfi* and is reportable but not notifiable in the UK. Clinical signs seen in cattle include fever, reduced milk yields, inappetence, weight loss and diarrhoea. These signs are transitory, but the most important result is the formation of congenital abnormalities if the virus affects the cow when 8–16 weeks pregnant. The abnormalities seen are limb contracture, brain abnormalities and a twisted neck (see Plate 3). These may result in the need for an embryotomy or a Caesarean section. Cows after parturition do not appear to be shedding virus.

Ureaplasma diversum

This mycoplasma is found in healthy animals and so its role in causing abortion is unclear. It is certainly transmitted venereally, but it is likely that it requires another agent to cause an abortion.

Wesselsbron disease

This viral disease, found in Africa, is caused by an arthropod-borne (mainly *Aedes* spp. mosquitoes) *Flavivirus* (*Wesselsbron virus*) which causes abortion and a fatal disease in neonatal calves. It is zoonotic and difficult to differentiate from RVF.

Endometritis

This condition is seen commonly post calving, particularly if there has been fetal membrane retention. The normal causal organisms are *Arcanobacterium pyogenes*, *Streptococcus* spp. and *E. coli*. In the acute form, the cow will be ill, show pyrexia, have swollen hocks and a bloody smelly vulval discharge. Treatment would be penicillin parenterally and NSAIDs. In the chronic form, the cow will appear normal except for a purulent smelly vulval discharge. Treatment should be aimed at bringing the cow into oestrus with a prostaglandin injection. Uterine washouts were recommended historically but show poor evidence of efficacy.

Mastitis

Mastitis can be attributed to contagious or environmental pathogens or, in the case of summer mastitis, to the fly *Hydrotaea irritans*.

Contagious pathogens

- These are *Staphylococcus aureus*, *Streptococcus dysgalactiae*, *S. agalactiae*, *Corynebacterium bovis*, coagulase-negative *Staphylococcus* spp. (these often colonize the teat canal and are opportunist pathogens), *Mycoplasma bovis*, *M. californicum* and *Mycoplasma* spp.
- They cause inflammation and pain in the udder, as well pyrexia and painful and swollen hocks.
- A milk sample should be taken for culture and sensitivity before treatment is started and then this treatment can be modified when the results are known.
- Although short milk withhold periods are important in dairy cows, effective antibiotic treatment is more important in the long term, not only for the affected cow but also for the rest of the group – bearing in mind that these pathogens are contagious.
- It is important to use the same antibiotic administered into the mammary gland as is used parenterally.
- *Mycoplasma* spp. present in the udder are not controlled by antibiotics.
- NSAIDs are useful in treatment.
- Dexamethazone should be used with care, making sure that the cow is not pregnant and the organism is being controlled by the antibiotic.
- There is a vaccine available against *S. aureus*.

Environmental pathogens

- These are *E. coli*, *Klebsiella pneumoniae*, *Streptococcus uberis*, *Pseudomonas aeruginosa*, *Bacillus cereus*, *Pasteurella* spp., *Candida* spp. and *Aspergillus* spp.
- *E. coli* and *K. pneumoniae* are both very serious pathogens which normally infect newly calved cows. They both produce toxins which cause a peracute disease called 'toxic mastitis'.
- Toxic mastitis is a specific disease syndrome often causing acute toxicity before mastitis is seen in the udder, and culture of the milk may often be unrewarding.
- Only 30% of affected animals are likely to survive toxic mastitis.
- Treatment of mastitis caused by environmental pathogens should involve NSAIDs and fluid therapy. Antibiotics suitable for use against Gram-negative bacteria are normally given parenterally and into the udder but many authorities consider that this is hardly worthwhile

as the organisms have produced the lethal toxins and been destroyed.

- There are many ideas put forward for fluid therapy. The author favours giving large volumes of electrolytes with an Agger's pump.
- Prevention measures include dry cow therapy, teat sealants and vaccination against *E. coli*.

Summer mastitis

- This occurs in dry cows and in-calf heifers but rarely in maiden heifers.
- The author has on rare occasions seen it in the mammary tissue of bulls.
- The disease, which is bacterial, is spread by the fly *Hydrotaea irritans*, which has a predilection for trees.
- There is a sequence of events; initially the udder is colonized by *S. dysgalactiae*, there is a slight swelling and the animal will be only slightly ill with a pyrexia. If treatment with antibiotics, normally penicillin, is initiated immediately, the disease will not progress further and the infected quarter will be saved.
- If the animal is not treated, other bacteria, namely *Arcanobacterium pyogenes*, *Peptococcus indolicus*, *Bacteroides melaninogenicus* and *Fusobacterium necrophorum* will colonize and the animal will become ill and the quarter will be lost, even with antibiotic treatment.
- At this stage, the udder discharge will be creamy and malodorous, alerting the clinician to the poor prognosis for the udder.
- Animals will be stiff behind and often their hocks will swell so treatment with NSAIDs as well as antibiotics would be appropriate.
- Prevention is with dry cow therapy, teat sealants and fly control.

Mummified fetus

The aetiology of this condition is obscure; in fact, there may be two conditions with different causes. The most common manifestation is the cow which has been diagnosed as in calf but never develops normal udder enlargement, i.e. does not 'bag up' for calving at the expected date. Rectal examination of the uterus will reveal an enlargement but no cotyledons or fremitus. Only if clinicians are certain of service dates, and are 100% certain that there has been no subsequent unrecorded service, should prostaglandin injections followed by dexamethazone be given. These mummified chocolate non-malodorous fetuses of about the size of a hare are difficult to abort. After the abortion, the cow should be served at the first oestrus as this has been shown to be the most fertile. The second much more unusual manifestation – after a prolonged pregnancy – is felt on rectal examination as a bag of bones either in the uterus or actually in the vagina. This small calf is mummified but also purulent and malodorous. The calves can be pulled out of the vagina or are easily aborted with a prostaglandin injection. It is possible that the second scenario is just a sequel of the first scenario which has been invaded by pus-forming bacteria.

Pyometritis

This condition causes confusion as literally it means 'pus in the uterus', and might be muddled with endometritis which occurs post-parturition (see above). The main cause of pyometritis is *Trichomonas fetus* which is spread by the bull and results in death of the fetus. The fetus often remains dead in the uterus bathed in pus. Diagnosis is by rectal palpation or rectal ultrasonography. There is no serological test. Treatment is with prostaglandin injections. Prevention is by using artificial insemination (AI).

Udder oedema

This occurs in high-producing dairy cows and, particularly, in heifers immediately before calving. Inducing calving with a prostaglandin injection may be warranted to prevent damage to the udder.

Udder rot

The cause of this condition is not clearly understood, but it is associated with cows with enlarged mammary glands. Inflammation and infection occur between the udder and the hind leg. This irritates the cow which then starts to lick the area regardless of any creams or sprays applied. This licking becomes an obsession and can even result in the licking off of a teat if it becomes involved. Parenteral antibiotics and dexamethazone may be helpful, but the latter should be used with care as these animals are often pregnant.

Diseases of the Locomotory System

Viral diseases

Bovine ephemeral fever (BEF)

This is caused by a rhabdovirus and transmitted by *Culicoides* spp. and *Anopheles* spp. It occurs in Africa (where it is called 'three day sickness'), Asia and Australia. Animals will be pyrexic and recumbent with a serous nasal, lacrimal and salivary discharge. There may be dyspnoea. Mortality is low and animals normally recover with good nursing. There is no treatment. Infection can be confirmed by paired serum samples.

Deficiency diseases

Rickets

This is a chronic condition of younger growing calves suffering from vitamin D deficiency, unlike osteomalacia which is a chronic condition of older cattle suffering from phosphorus deficiency. The diaphyses of bones

are shorter and broader than normal and the cortices are increased in width. Animals will be lame and will respond to injections of vitamin D in the early stages of the disease.

Diseases of the Integument

Viral skin diseases

Bovine papular stomatitis

This is caused by a *Parapoxvirus*, *Bovine papular stomatitis virus* (also called Parapoxvirus bovis-1). It mainly occurs in young cattle as papules around the muzzle. It is self-limiting. The disease is a zoonosis that causes 'milker's nodule'.

Herpes mammillitis

This is caused by *Bovine herpesvirus* 2. It only occurs on the udder and is seen as crusty lesions which predispose to mastitis. The lesions are painful, but self-limiting.

Lumpy skin disease

This is caused by a *Capripoxvirus* (*Lumpy skin disease virus*). It is spread by flies. It is seen in European dairy cattle in Africa (Fig. 3.2). There is a generalized disease causing a fever. The whole body is covered in raised plaques which look like hairy tufts. Mortality is low and the disease is self-limiting.

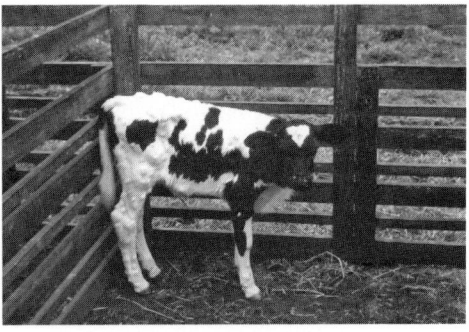

Fig. 3.2. A calf with lumpy skin disease.

Pseudocowpox

This is caused by a *Parapoxvirus, Pseudocowpox virus* (also called Parapoxvirus bovis-2). It is the most common teat infection in cattle. Like bovine papular stomatitis, the disease is a zoonosis. The 'milker's nodule' formed is indistinguishable from that caused by Parapoxvirus bovis-1. The infection is self-limiting.

Vesicular stomatitis

This is caused by a *Vesiculovirus*. It is seen in North, Central and South America. Vesicular erosions will be seen in the mouth, on the feet and on the udder. Clinical signs are very similar to those of FMD. Diagnosis is by virus isolation. The infection is self-limiting.

Bacterial skin diseases

Actinobacillosis

This is caused by *Actinobacillus lignieresii* and is classically called 'wooden tongue', but lesions may be found all over the head and neck. Animals will salivate excessively; and the tongue will be swollen and painful. Large nodules have been reported on the legs and abdomen in Norfolk, UK. Diagnosis can be made on Gram-stained impression smears which will show the Gram-negative short rod-shaped bacteria, or by culture. Treatment is with prolonged doses of streptomycin given im daily and is normally successful.

Actinomycosis

This condition is caused by *Actinomyces bovis* and is classically called 'lumpy jaw' as it is an infection which affects the mandible but is also seen in the maxillary bone. The pathognomic sign is a hard painful bone swelling which is actually osteomyelitis, and often has pus-draining tracts connecting to the skin. Treatment is with prolonged doses of streptomycin given im daily and is rarely fully successful.

Clostridial cellulitis

This condition is caused by a mixture of organisms which include *Cl. septicum*, *Cl. chauvoei* and *Cl. sordellii*. The condition also has several manifestations and names, including malignant oedema and blackleg. These are peracute and very painful conditions causing crepitus and sloughing. Treatment with penicillin and NSAIDs needs to be immediate and aggressive to save the affected animal.

Dermatophilosis

This is a very serious skin condition in the tropics which is caused by *Dermatophilus congolensis* and called streptothricosis. The whole of the dorsal surface of the animal will be covered with crusts over pus-filled ulcers. The condition is contagious but the author suspects that a predisposing condition is required as well as the organism. Streptothricosis is a zoonosis. Treatment is with antibiotics parenterally and with oily creams topically. The condition called rain scald in the UK is a similar but less severe disease and mainly restricted to equines. It is not zoonotic.

Staphylococcal skin disease

This disease, which is caused by *Staphylococcus aureus*, causes folliculitis and furunculosis anywhere on the body. A trigger is required to initiate the rare condition which responses well to antibiotics provided that a sensitivity test has been carried out.

Protozoal skin diseases

Besnoitosis

This is caused by *Besnoitia besnoiti*. It occurs in Africa but has been reported in the Middle East, Southern Europe and South America. It is spread by flies and cat faeces, and is a serious disease seen as acute lethargy and pyrexia. There are large painful oedematous plaques. Cysts will be seen on the conjunctiva which will yield the protozoa; these can be seen under the microscope. Although the disease rarely kills animals, they are normally destroyed on account of the emaciation. There is no realistic treatment.

Fungal skin diseases

Dermatophytosis

The main pathogen causing dermatophytosis (or 'ringworm') in cattle is *Trichophyton verrucosum*. This is the most common skin disease of cattle worldwide, and it is also a very contagious zoonotic disease. The organism can remain in woodwork for many years. The disease is self-limiting on the animal and will disappear in 16 weeks without treatment, except in animals suffering from another debilitating condition, e.g. chronic pneumonia. There are skin preparations, such as enilconazole, available for treating show animals. The oral antibiotic griseofulvin is highly effective but has been banned in the EU for use in food-producing animals. There is a vaccine available which can be used from 2 weeks of age in the face of an outbreak and this has a therapeutic effect.

Parasitic skin diseases

Biting flies

There are a large number of species that attack cattle worldwide. These include: *Haematobia irritans* (the horn-fly), *Stomoxys calcitrans* (the stable fly), *Tabanus* spp. (the horsefly), *Simulium* spp. (the black fly) and *Glossina* spp. (the tsetse fly). Control is with topical deltamethrin.

Chorioptic mange

This is caused by *Chorioptes bovis*, which is a mite found worldwide. It causes thickened scaly areas around the tail and on the legs. The mites can easily be seen on brushing the scaly areas into a Petri dish and examining them under low power with a microscope. Treatment is with pour-on ivermectin preparations.

Demodectic mange

This type of mange, which is caused by *Demodex bovis*, is rare and pruritic, and is seen worldwide. It is seen as pus-filled follicles on the body, which will contain mites that can be

seen in smears under the microscope. Treatment is with 2% trichlorfon dips every other day for three treatments.

Dermanyssus gallinae

This mite, which is found on poultry worldwide is pruritic on cattle. Control is with topical deltamethrin.

Myiasis

This is called 'fly strike' in the UK and is only seen in cattle with a wound, as secondary 'fly strike' (see Plate 4). In tropical areas, it can be caused by primary-striking screw worms. Treatment must include destroying the maggots with cypermethrin and treating the wound.

Pediculosis

Lice are the most common and important ectoparasites in cattle. They cause marked pruritis and subsequent hair loss from rubbing. There are divided into sucking lice – *Linognathus vituli*, *Haematopinus eurysternus* and *Solenopotes capillatus*, and biting lice – *Damalinia bovis*, in the UK. They can be seen with the naked eye but are more easily seen with a magnifying glass. There are many other species worldwide. The distinction into sucking and biting lice is important as certain products kill only sucking lice. Topical eprinomectin will kill both types.

Psoroptic mange

This is caused by the mite *Psoroptes ovis* and results in acute pruritis. It is rare in the UK, but is common in feedlot cattle in the USA. Topical eprinomectin is a useful treatment as it can be used in lactating cows with no milk withhold.

Sarcoptic mange

This is caused by the mite *Sarcoptes scabiei* var. *bovis* and is exceedingly contagious. It is highly pruritic and causes large thickened skin folds. Any skin scraping made needs to be deep to find the mites. The condition can be treated with topical eprinomectin; in refractory cases this needs to be diluted one to one with DMSO (dimethyl sulfoxide) and painted on to the lesions at weekly intervals.

Tick infestation

Ticks are vectors of important diseases as well as causing anaemia in their own right. The most important tick affecting cattle in the UK is *Ixodes ricinus*, but there are over 600 species of tick worldwide, mainly in the tropics. Ticks on cattle are controlled by dipping or spraying with acaricides. This has to be carried out weekly in East Africa to prevent ECF.

Warble fly infestation

Warble fly (*Hypoderma bovis*) infestation has been eradicated in the UK, but still occurs elsewhere. The fly lays eggs on the legs of cattle in the late summer. The egg hatches into a larva which bores through the skin and makes its way through the body until it reaches the back where it forms a nodule. The larva bursts through the skin as a large maggot in the late spring and falls to the ground, where it pupates. Control is carried out by killing the larvae in the cattle in the winter and early spring using ivermectins.

Nutritional skin diseases

Vitamin C-responsive skin disease

Traditionally this condition is seen in 2–3 month old dairy calves which lose hair all around their tails and hind legs following a bout of calf scours. Weekly injections of multivitamins are said to improve the condition. The author has doubts on the evidence for this treatment. There is another condition of unknown origin, anagen defluxion (which also involves hair loss), which may have a similar aetiology.

Zinc-responsive skin disease

This is seen in growing cattle as alopecia and scaling of large areas of skin, with no parasites, fungi or bacteria found. Diagnosis is difficult as zinc levels often appear to be normal

(blood samples must be taken in containers not having rubber stoppers). Improvement is seen when a diet with adequate zinc levels is fed.

Miscellaneous skin diseases

Frostbite

This will occur at the tips of the ears and on the end of the tail in extreme conditions, particularly in calves. Animals should be brought inside and any affected areas should be treated with oily creams.

Mast cell tumour

These are rare but will occur as fast-growing individual nodules in young adult cattle. They are invariably malignant and normally will have spread to the draining lymph nodes before being shown to the practitioner. There is no treatment and humane slaughter should be carried out.

Photosensitization

This is not uncommon, particularly in black and white cattle, where it affects only the white areas of the skin, causing inflamed areas which soon become large chronically crusted areas. The traditional explanation is ingestion of a plant toxic to the liver, e.g. St John's wort. This will undoubtedly cause the condition but toxic plants are found rarely and often the condition is only seen sporadically with many other unaffected animals. Treatment is with injections of vitamin B to help the liver (liver enzymes are only infrequently raised), oily creams applied topically, fly control and keeping the animal out of the sun.

Subcutaneous emphysema

This is an accumulation of gases under the skin and between tissue planes. These can be of air and benign following a laparotomy, but the condition can be very serious following a wound or needle injection which has been contaminated with *Clostridia* spp. In the latter case, the animal will be very ill and the prognosis is very poor. Aggressive treatment with penicillin and NSAIDs will at best result in a large skin slough.

Urticaria

This is called 'blain' or 'hives' and is an acute skin reaction to histamine release as an allergic response. Traditionally, it was thought to be a dietary allergy, but this is unlikely and the condition is much more likely to be a reaction to an insect bite. It will regress spontaneously or more rapidly following dexamethazone injection iv (although clinicians must check pregnancy status before treatment).

Common Causes for Cattle to be Found Dead

Iatrogenic causes of sudden death

The term 'sudden death', as normally used, is a misnomer. In reality, sudden death usually means that death has occurred since the animal was last seen. The owner will very rarely see an animal die. It is even rarer for the clinician to see death. Sadly, when such deaths do occur it is usually at the time of veterinary treatment. The likely causes of these iatrogenic deaths in cattle are shown in Table 3.2.

Reasons for animals to be found dead

As indicated above, true sudden deaths are very rare. Possible causes of such sudden deaths in cattle are shown in Table 3.3.

Table 3.2. A list of possible iatrogenic causes of sudden death.

Anaphylaxis from administration of medicines
General anaesthesia
Massive haemorrhage (this could occur at parturition where there is no human involvement)
Intra-arterial injection
Intravenous (iv) injection (particularly with calcium/magnesium solutions)
Sedation (particularly after iv xylazine injections)

Table 3.3. A list of the possible causes of sudden death.

Anthrax
Chemical poisons
Clostridial disease
Drowning (this may occur during a stampede into water by thirsty cattle)
Electrocution (can occur in the milking parlour or robot milker)
Hypomagnesaemia
Lightning strike
Poisonous plant intake
Ruptured uterine artery

4

Cattle Surgery

Introduction

The chapter starts with a discussion on the basic procedures used for analgesia, sedation and anaesthesia in cattle practice. This is followed by an account of surgical conditions and procedures which is organized by system, with sections on the gastroenteric system, the neurological system, the urinary system, the reproductive system, the locomotory system and the integument. Lastly, there is a brief section on euthanasia.

Analgesia

There are no licensed opiates for use in cattle in the UK. Xylazine gives profound analgesia but is also a potent sedative (see below). Therefore the cattle clinician has to rely on nonsteroidal anti-inflammatory drugs (NSAIDs), of which there are several licensed for cattle (see Chapter 2, Cattle Medicines: Anti-inflammatory preparations).

Sedation

The universally available sedative in all ages of cattle is xylazine. The dose is 0.05–0.2 mg/kg im or 0.03–0.1 mg/kg iv. The latter has a much

quicker onset of action and is more reliable. Younger animals need lower dosages: 0.5 ml of a 2% solution im will give heavy sedation for a young calf; 6 ml of a 2% solution iv will provide heavy sedation for a cow; 2 ml of a 2% solution will give mild sedation for a cow for minor procedures, e.g. foot trimming in a crush. Recumbent animals, particularly heavy bulls after administration of xylazine, need to be placed in sternal recumbency and receive regular checking.

Anaesthesia

General anaesthesia in adults

In adult cattle, administering a general anaesthetic (GA) is a very hazardous procedure, and is especially so in large bulls. However, many procedures can be carried out on the standing restrained animal or the heavily sedated recumbent animal using regional anaesthesia, so a GA should be avoided if possible. If a GA has to be performed, the animal should be starved for 12 h and denied water for 6 h. It should be premedicated with atropine at 30 mcg/kg and xylazine at 0.1 mg/kg iv. A stun dose of ketamine at 1.1 mg/kg should be given on recumbency. The animal should have the largest endotracheal tube available passed into the oesophagus and the cuff should be inflated. An appropriately sized endotracheal tube should be passed into the trachea and the cuff should be inflated. Anaesthesia should be maintained on halothane or isoflurane. It should be recorded here that neither atropine nor ketamine are licensed for cattle in the UK. Recovery from anaesthesia should be supervised. Both endotracheal tubes should be kept in position until a swallowing reflex is attained, and then the tube in the trachea should be removed first. The animal should be propped up in sternal recumbency.

General anaesthesia in calves

Milk and solid food should be withheld for 12 h before GA in a calf, which should be premedicated with xylazine at 0.05 mg/kg followed 5 min later by ketamine at 1.1 mg/kg. The calf will remain fully anaesthetized for 10 min. If longer anaesthesia is required the animal should be intubated and maintained on halothane or isoflurane. The endotracheal tube should only be removed on recovery when the calf shows a swallowing reflex.

Regional anaesthesia

Cornual block

- This block will anaesthetize the horn and the surrounding skin.
- 5 ml local anaesthetic will be required for calves and 15 ml for adults.
- Divide the distance between the eye and the horn into three and inject below the temporal ridge a third of the distance nearer to the eye.

Epidural block

- This should really be termed a caudal epidural block in cows as it only anaesthetizes the tail, vulva and the caudal part of the vagina.
- It will not prevent a calving cow from straining.
- Inject up to 10 ml local anaesthetic through the sacrococcygeal space with a 3 cm 18G needle pointing ventrally and cranially in the direction of the udder.
- 2 ml of a 2% solution of xylazine can be added to prolong the action when reducing prolapses.

Inverted L block

- This can be used for Caesarean sections, rumenotomies and laparotomies.
- Up to 200 ml local anaesthetic can be used in total for the skin and musculature.

Lower limb block

- This can be used to anaesthetize the fetlock and below on either front or hind limb.
- The animal needs to be sedated and firmly secured in lateral recumbency, preferably in a rotary foot trimming crush.
- A tourniquet is placed above the carpus or tarsus (a roll of bandage should be placed either side of the Achilles tendon).
- A prominent vein should be located in the metacarpal/metatarsal region.
- The area should be clipped and surgically prepared.
- A small bleb of 1 ml of local anaesthetic should be placed under the skin over the vein with a 23G needle.
- After 5 min, a 21G needle is inserted into the vein and 30 ml (for a cow, but a smaller volume can be used in calves) local anaesthetic is very slowly injected iv.
- In 5 min the whole area below the tourniquet will be anaesthetized. The anaesthesia will continue for 45 min and cease as soon as the tourniquet is released.

Paravertebral block

- This is very useful to block the flank in dairy cows, but placing the needles is not easy in fat beef cows.
- The aim is to block the dorsal and ventral branches of the spinal nerves as they emerge from thoracic vertebra 13 (T13) and lumbar vertebrae 1, 2 and 3 (L1–L3).

- Clean the area along the back from the last rib caudally for 20 cm.
- The hair is best left so a small clip mark can be used to mark the point of entry of the 10 cm spinal needle with internal stilette.
- Initially locate the transverse process of L2.
- In a normal cow, the process from the first lumbar vertebra cannot be felt.
- The initial mark is 5 cm from the midline on a line between the end of the transverse process and the caudal point on the vertical process of L2.
- Clip a 1 cm diameter circle and infiltrate 3 ml of local anaesthetic with a short 21G needle under the skin.
- Make a second mark in a similar position using the end of the transverse process and the caudal point on the vertical process of L3.
- Infiltrate 3 ml local anaesthetic under the skin.
- Make a third mark the same distance cranial to the first mark as the second mark is caudal to the first mark.
- Infiltrate 3 ml local anaesthetic under the skin.
- The fourth mark is made the same distance cranial to the third mark.
- Infiltrate 3 ml local anaesthetic under the skin.
- Grasp a spinal needle with both hands.
- One hand holds the butt of the needle and the other hand holds the shaft of the needle with a sterile swab.
- Pass the needle vertically through the skin in the middle of the most caudal mark and the needle should strike bone in 5 cm in a dairy cow with a condition score of 3.
- Infiltrate 5 ml local anaesthetic after removing the stilette.
- If bone is not struck, the needle should be withdrawn 3 cm and redirected 1 cm cranially.
- This should be repeated until bone is felt.
- Once bone is felt and 5 ml local anaesthetic has been infiltrated, the point should be walked caudally until the edge of the bone is felt.

- 10 ml local anaesthetic should be infiltrated at this point.
- The point of the needle should then be pushed ventrally and the sensation of piercing a membrane will be felt.
- 10 ml local anaesthetic should be infiltrated at this point.
- Exactly the same procedure is carried out through the two marks cranial to the most caudal mark.
- The injection is different through the most cranial mark as the block is for the spinal nerve emerging from T13.
- This is cranial to the transverse process of L1 and so the needle needs to be walked cranially when bone is located.
- This procedure will require approximately 112 ml local anaesthetic. At least 15 min should be allowed for the block to take effect.

Retrobulbar block

- This is required for (eye) enucleation.
- Local anaesthetic in the form of tropicamides is first instilled into the conjunctiva.
- Using a 7.5 cm spinal needle 10 ml local anaesthetic is infiltrated behind the eye in four places – medially, laterally, ventrally and dorsally.

Teat blocks

- These are required for any teat surgery.
- Sedation should be given first as the clinician is at risk.
- 10 ml local anaesthetic solution should be instilled into the teat cistern through the teat canal with a syringe without a needle.
- This will anaesthetize the mucosa.
- Then a ring block should be placed under the skin of the udder around the top of the teat.
- A small gauge needle should be used and, after the initial injection, the needle should only be placed in anaesthetized tissue.
- Up to 20 ml local anaesthetic can be used.

Surgical Conditions of the Gastroenteric System

Abscess in the mediastinum

This may cause bloat in growing cattle that have had pneumonia. The gas is easily relieved with a stomach tube, but the bloat will return and may be life threatening. The treatment is to create a small valvular rumen fistula. This is placed in the centre of the para-lumbar triangle on the left flank, in the same position as the trocar and cannula described below. The area is clipped and surgically prepared, and 5 ml local anaesthetic is instilled under the skin and into the muscle layers. A 3 cm incision is made through the skin and underlying tissue. The two muscle layers are incised and torn in the direction of their fibres for 2 cm. The rumen is grasped and withdrawn through the incision after piercing the peritoneum. The rumen is then anchored to the skin with eight single sutures of monofilament nylon. These should be removed in 10 days, leaving a small fistula which will allow the escape of gas but not of rumen contents. These contents seem repellent to flies and myiasis does not seem to be a problem after the initial healing.

Actinobacillosis of the oesophagus

This should be treated with daily doses of streptomycin for a minimum of 5 days. A trocar and cannula may be required.

Bloat as a result of choke

Normally, diagnosis of choke will not be a problem if the animal has access to potatoes or another root feeding stuff on account of the drooling of saliva and signs of bloat (Fig. 4.1). Confirmation should be obtained that there has been no effort to remove the obstruction with a pipe and therefore there is no danger of perforation of the oesophagus, which will result in a fatal mediastinitis. If the farmer has not tried to remove the obstruction, there are three options:

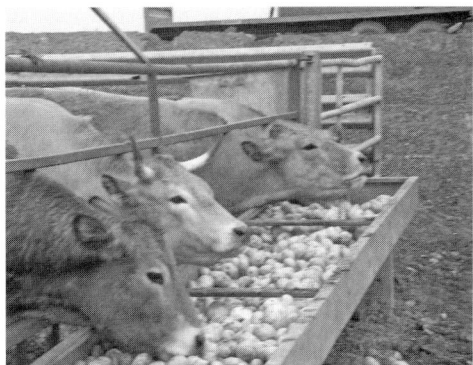

Fig. 4.1. Cattle should not be fed whole potatoes unless they are on the ground.

1. Insert a trocar and cannula in the left-hand para-lumbar fossa. If in doubt, always place it lower than the middle of the equilateral triangle to make allowances for the bloat. Unless the animal is flat out and on the point of death, trim a 2 inch diameter circle of hair and inject 5 ml local anaesthetic under the skin and into the muscle. After 5 min cut a 1 inch incision with a scalpel blade through the skin. Then stab the muscle layers with the trocar and cannula (Red Devil Type) and twist in a clockwise direction until the flange of the cannula is flush with the skin. It is important not to remove the trocar prematurely and release the gas or the rumen wall will fall off the end of the cannula. After removing the trocar give it to the farmer so that he/she can use it to clean out the cannula should it become blocked. The obstruction will soften and be swallowed within 48 h. Care should be taken not to remove the cannula until there is 100% certainty that there is no obstruction remaining. If there is concern that the animal is becoming dehydrated, then oral electrolytes can be given via the cannula. Antibiotic cover and NSAIDs should be given appropriately.
2. Pass a probang and try to dislodge the obstruction. There is an inherent danger of oesophageal perforation during this process, as mentioned above. However, on applying careful firm pressure with a probe, success – if a potato is causing the choke – is 80% achievable. If the obstruction cannot be moved then a trocar and cannula must be inserted.

3. If the obstruction can be felt in the neck, in adults it is possible to remove it per os. The animal should be given xylazine 4 mg/500 kg im and restrained in a crush. A running noose is applied to the neck caudal to the obstruction and kept tight by an assistant. The head is restrained by a bulldog clip, not a halter. A Drinkwater gag is placed in between the cheek teeth and held in position by the tongue with one hand. The other hand is then pushed into the mouth and down into the oesophagus, and the obstruction grasped by the nails and withdrawn to the outside. It is vital that the obstruction is not released into the pharynx or it will be reswallowed.

If the farmer has tried to move the obstruction it is important that the dangers of this are explained. If there has been blood seen on the pipe used by the farmer then the animal could be slaughtered for human consumption by an 'on farm kill and bleeding' before immediate transfer to an abattoir. If any medicines have been administered then humane destruction should be carried out. If no blood has been seen a trocar and cannula are placed in position as described above.

Bloat without choke

In cases of rumen tympany – or bloat without choke – when there is not a foreign body obstructing the oesophagus, massive salivation is not seen and a stomach tube or a probang can be passed into the rumen to relieve the tympany and confirm that the animal is not choked.

The different types of bloat without choke are as follows.

Chronic bracken poisoning

The actual cause of the bloat in this case is a tumour in the oesophagus.

Fore-stomach obstruction

This is often caused by the ingestion of plastic bags and baler twine and is related to feeding of big bale silage. Animals will lose their appetite but not have pyrexia. The rumen will sound sluggish and there will be moderate tympany. Difficulty may be experienced in passing a stomach tube. Diagnosis may be difficult but will be confirmed on rumenotomy (see below). Dosing with liquid paraffin may be tried but is rarely successful.

Frothy bloat

This is normally caused by overeating of clover or by ingestion of potatoes and pea straw or pea silage at the same time. A trocar and cannula should be placed in position. A vegetable oil or proprietary solution should be given down the cannula.

Tetanus

The bloat will be mild and not life threatening per se, although the disease is serious (see Chapter 3).

Traumatic reticulitis

This may cause mild bloat and mild pyrexia. The rumen movement will be sluggish and be accompanied by a grunt. Traditionally, a pain response can be elicited by placement of a beam under the sternum just caudal to the elbows and lifting it. This may not be necessary to establish a diagnosis. Before treatment by rumenotomy, as described below, is attempted, careful auscultation of the heart should be carried out. If there is evidence of a fluid splashing sound, this will indicate a pericarditis. Surgery should not be carried out in that case as it will not be successful. Humane destruction is recommended. Some clinicians advocate the giving of specially prepared magnets by mouth. These may be helpful, but not if the pericardium has already become infected.

Intestinal torsion

Intestinal torsion or volvulus is rare in calves and adult cattle. Diagnosis may be aided by ultrasonography. Rectal examination will reveal gas-filled small intestinal loops in adults. Animals will be shocked, and have a subnormal rectal temperature. There will be rumen stasis and total inappetence. Surgery in young calves could be attempted under GA, and in adults standing and with a paravertebral block. Welfare must be considered and euthanasia may be the best option.

Intussusception

Intussusception of the small intestine is seen in calves. They will be acutely ill and have a subnormal temperature. In some cases, they will survive with medical treatment consisting of antibiotics and NSAIDs. In theory, a diagnosis could be made with ultrasonography early enough for successful surgery to be an option. This is outside the author's experience.

Left-sided displacement of the abomasum (LDA)

This is a condition of dairy cows 3–6 weeks post-partum that is related to inappropriate feeding. The cows will have a poor appetite and lower than expected milk yield. The rectal temperature will be normal. The pathognomic sign is a ping sound heard with a stethoscope on the left side over the caudal ribs when the skin is flicked with the finger. Clinicians may have to search over quite a large area. The sound is made by the gas-filled abomasum. In certain cases, if the abomasum is not filled with gas, no ping will be heard. Diagnosis can then be confirmed by listening behind the ribs on the left-hand side with a stethoscope while ballotting the lower flank with the knee. If there is displacement of the abomasum a tinkling sound will be heard. It is likely that there will be secondary ketosis to this condition. This secondary ketosis is treated with 40 mg dexamethasone iv or im, while the cow can be treated surgically to get her appetite back.

Other possible methods of treatment are described below.

A single-flank surgical method

A small lower right flank incision is made in the normal manner. The surgeon reaches across under the anterior rumen and grasps the abomasum, which is then drawn over to the right flank and anchored there within the inner suture line. This is difficult for a clinician with short arms, or if the abomasum is full of gas. The incision is then closed in the normal manner.

A double-flank surgical method

A small flank incision is made on both sides in the normal manner. The clinician on the left side of the animal passes the abomasum after deflation under the anterior rumen to a second clinician on the right side, who anchors the pylorus to the body wall within the suture line. The two incisions are closed in the normal manner.

Medical treatment

Various medicines can be tried, e.g. for an adult cow, 300 mg metoclopramide iv or 2 g choral hydrate/500 ml warm water as a drench.

Rolling

The cow is cast into lateral recumbency lying on her left hand side using Roeff's method (Fig. 4.2). As she is rolled into full dorsal recumbency her abdomen is vigorously pummelled. The ping from the abomasum will then be heard to the left of the midline. Pummelling is continued as she is rolled on to her right side. The abomasum will be heard to the right of the midline. The cow is then

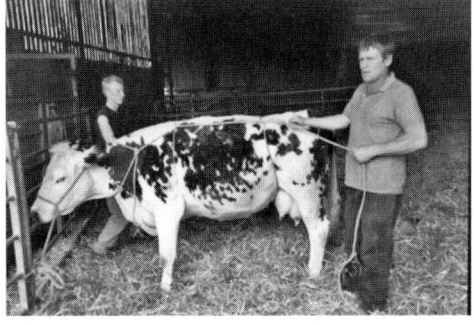

Fig. 4.2. Roeff's method of casting a cow into lateral recumbency.

allowed to stand, and 20 l electrolytes are then pumped into her rumen with an Agger's pump. She then should be encouraged to eat good-quality fibre food, ideally grass.

Stitching the abomasum to the ventral body wall

A small lower right flank incision is made in the normal manner. After locating the greater curvature of the abomasum a 2 m length of thick monofilament nylon is threaded 30 cm along junction of the omentum and the wall of the greater curvature of the abomasum with a 10 cm straight-cutting suture needle, leaving a 1 m length at the caudal end. With the end of the suture needle guarded, the surgeon enters the abdomen and follows the abdominal wall down to the most ventral point just caudal to the xiphisternum. The needle is then quickly pushed through the peritoneum, linea alba and body wall, grasped by an assistant under the belly of the cow and pulled through. A fresh sterile straight suture needle is attached to the 1 m length of suture material on the cau-dal end of the abomasum. This is then is taken into the abdomen and pushed through the body wall 15 cm caudal to the other end and grasped by an assistant. With the surgeon aligning the greater curvature of the abo-masum to the body wall the assistant pulls up on the two lengths of monofilament nylon and ties them together so the abomasum is firmly anchored to the abdominal wall. The surgeon then closes the body wall in the nor-mal manner. The nylon suture, like the skin sutures, is removed in 10–14 days.

Toggling

The initial procedure is same manner as roll-ing. When the cow is in dorsal recumbency and the abomasum can be heard, the toggles are inserted. After surgical preparation, the first toggle is placed into the abomasum using a special trocar and cannula near to the xiphisternum. Care is taken not let too much gas escape up the cannula before it is removed. The second toggle is inserted a hand breath caudal to the first. The two tog-gle ties are tied loosely together. The ties are removed in 14 days.

Left-sided volvulus of the abomasum

This is often accompanied by moderate-to-severe ischaemia of the abomasal wall (Grosche *et al.*, 2012). The affected animals will show more severe signs than those affected by displacement. Peritoneal fluid analysis will be helpful in differentiating the two conditions. Those affected with volvulus require immediate surgery.

Liver abscess

Abscesses are commonly seen on the livers of cattle at the slaughterhouse, while the animals appear well and healthy. However, some liver abscesses may be large and cause a septicaemia, when the animal will be ill and pyrexic. Such cattle should be treated with antibiotics for a minimum of 10 days. In most cases, the abscesses will be walled off and settle down, but in a few cases they will continue to enlarge and the animal will continue to show bouts of pyrexia. Liver enzymes are likely to be raised and it may be possible to visualize the abscesses by ultrasonography. Mindful of meat-withhold periods, clinicians should give the animal antibiotics and then if it is well send it for slaughter after the withhold period is over. If this plan fails, then a laparotomy should be performed. The abscess should be drained to the outside with a sterile tube attached to a needle. Often these cases will then respond well if given long-term antibi-otics. Liver abscesses can also bring about haemoptysis. The pathogenesis involves the abscess causing infiltration of the vena cava to form a septic thrombus. This enters the pulmonary arterial system and causes embolic pneumonia. Abscessation in the lung may then erode the arteries in the lung and cause haemoptysis. Prognosis in these cases is extremely poor, with some cases causing instant death from a massive haem-orrhage. If the animal is not shocked or pyrexic, it may be sent for immediate slaughter, hopefully for human consump-tion. Otherwise humane destruction should be advised.

Rectal prolapse

This condition is extremely rare in cows. It is seen in calves with tenesmus from a coccidiosis infection. This latter condition must be treated as well as returning the prolapsed rectum. The calf should be given an epidural with 2 ml local anaesthetic and 0.5 mg xylazine. After cleaning, a purse-string suture of braided nylon should be laid around the anal ring. The prolapse should be reduced and the suture tied tightly around a single finger. Appropriate antibiotics and NSAIDs should be given. The suture should be removed in 10 days.

Right-sided displacement of the abomasum (RDA)

Unlike animals with an LDA, these cows are very ill. They will have subnormal rectal temperatures. Rumen movement will be absent. If the abomasum is dilated and dorsal, a resonant ping will be heard on the right hand side on tapping with a finger and listening with a stethoscope in a similar manner that used in LDA. Medical treatment of adult cows with 300 mg metoclopramide iv may be effective. However, these cases normally have a grave prognosis, particularly if there is a fluid splash heard on ballottement on the right side. Surgery may be attempted, if the cow is not too ill; otherwise, euthanasia is indicated. The cow is given antibiotics and NSAIDs. The right-hand side of the cow is surgically prepared after paravertebral anaesthesia. The abdomen is opened about halfway down the flank. A laparotomy is performed, as differential diagnosis from caecal volvulus (see 'Torsion of the caecum' below) is not easy. On locating the large fluid/gas-filled abomasum it is drawn to the abdominal wall. Two large stay sutures of uterine tape are placed 10 cm apart on the greater curvature. The abomasum is drawn to the abdominal wall and, if possible, through it. If this is not possible it is packed round with large sterile swabs. The abomasum is opened and drained, and then closed using a continuous layer of inverting sutures of polyglactin. The stay sutures are removed when the surgeon is satisfied that the abomasum is adequately closed. The abomasum is pushed down to the ventral midline and the abdomen is closed in the normal manner. The cow is given 300 mg metoclopramide iv.

Rumenotomy

There are various frames or rubber sleeves available for this operation, which is indicated in cases of traumatic reticulitis and forestomach obstruction (see above). The procedure described here is Goetz's method, which can be performed just with basic surgical equipment. The cow is given antibiotics and NSAIDs. The left-hand side of the animal is surgically prepared after paravertebral anaesthesia. The abdomen is opened vertically for approximately 15 cm in the middle of the para-lumbar triangle. The surgeon can carry out a digital search of the outside of the rumen to check for any penetrating sharp foreign bodies. The rumen is stitched to the peritoneum approximately 3 cm inside the abdomen with a continuous suture of polyglactin. When the surgeon is satisfied that there is an adequate seal between the peritoneum of the rumen and the peritoneum of the body wall, the rumen can be opened with a large enough incision to allow the surgeon's forearm into the rumen. The rumen and the reticulum can then be searched for sharp and bulky foreign bodies, which can then be removed. The rumen can then be closed with a continuous layer of inverting sutures of polyglactin. The musculature and the skin can be closed in the normal manner.

Torsion of the caecum

This is a rare condition and normally it is only recognized by the time the cow is too shocked to survive surgery. The animal will show severe colic and a splash on auscultation on the right flank. Diagnosis may be aided by ultrasonography. The cow is given antibiotics and NSAIDs. The right-hand side of the animal is surgically prepared after paravertebral anaesthesia. The abdomen is opened about halfway down the flank. A laparotomy is performed to confirm the diagnosis. If the caecum appears to be viable then the torsion can be corrected. Normally, there is ischaemic damage and so either the organ is removed, involving extensive surgery which is outside the author's experience, or euthanasia is performed. There is a condition of intussusception of the tip of the caecum which is possible to cure with careful resection of the damaged part of the organ as the caecum can be brought through the abdominal wall for careful surgery. The non-viable tip of the caecum is removed outside the cow to reduce contamination. The organ is closed by two layers of continuous inverting sutures of polyglactin and is carefully replaced in the abdomen which is flushed with solutions of antibiotics. The musculature and the skin can be closed in the normal manner.

Umbilical hernia

Umbilical hernias are common. They have a high heritability and so repair should not be carried out in bulls unless they are castrated at the time. Normally, animals with a hernia will be left without surgery. They should be castrated and fattened. It is reasonable to repair an umbilical hernia in a heifer which is being kept for breeding on the understanding that her progeny will not be kept for breeding. Repair of umbilical hernias should be delayed until the calf is at least 2 months old because often, with increasing age, there is little reason to repair them as the abdominal opening becomes relatively small. If no more than three fingers can be inserted into the abdominal opening the hernia can be closed with an elastrator ring. The calf should be placed in dorsal recumbency. Raising the hernia sack to ensure there are no bowel contents in it, a rubber ring is placed as near to the abdominal wall as possible. Antibiotic cover, NSAIDs and fly control should be maintained for a minimum of 10 days. If the abdominal opening is larger than three fingers wide, a full surgical operation will need to be carried

out under GA. The calf should be prepared as described above under GA, and the area should be clipped and surgically prepared. An elliptical skin incision is made around the hernia sack. With blunt dissection, the skin is removed. With great care, and also using blunt dissection, the hernia sac is undermined from the abdominal wall without entering the abdomen, so that there is a rim of 1 cm around the orifice. Sterile nylon mesh is then sutured to the abdominal ring over the orifice with continuous stitches of monofilament nylon. After closing the wound with a continuous layer of subcuticular sutures of absorbable material, the skin is closed with single horizontal mattress sutures of monofilament nylon. The wound is covered with antibiotic spray. The calf should be confined for a minimum of 10 days and receive antibiotics and NSAID cover.

Surgical Conditions of the Neurological System

Removal of the eye

In all cases where there is no chance of the eye condition in any disease or traumatic problem recovering, enucleation should be considered on welfare grounds. It can be carried out under heavy sedation, normally using 10 mg/500 kg xylazine, which will cause recumbency. Some surgeons prefer lighter sedation at 4 mg/500 kg with the animal restrained in a crush. A retrobulbar block should be performed. The eyelids should then be sutured together and the whole area clipped and surgically prepared. A careful incision is then made through the skin parallel to the upper eyelid margin but not entering the conjunctival sac. Using blunt dissection the eye muscles are sectioned around that half of the eye. The same procedure is then carried out to the lower half of the eye. Eventually a pair of curved scissors can be used to section the optic nerve and the eye can be removed. The remaining socket can then be obliterated with sub-cuticular suturing with absorbable material and the remaining eyelids can be sutured with non-absorbable material. The animal should receive antibiotics and NSAIDs for a minimum of five days.

Squamous-cell carcinoma of the third eyelid

These only occur in non-pigmented third eyelids and are more common in the tropics. If the tumour has only invaded the third eyelid they can be removed simply with a pair of curved blunt-ended scissors after a local block, making certain that there is a margin between the cancer and the healthy tissue. If the tumour has invaded the conjunctiva as well as the third eyelid, the eye should be removed.

Surgical Conditions of the Urinary System

Infected urachus

Persistent patent urachus is usually a congenital condition as the urachus fails to close at birth. If it occurs a few days after birth it is likely to be as a result of a septic omphalophlebitis. Differentiation is important as treatment is likely to be different. If the urachus remains patent at birth, it can be ligated immediately. The animal should receive antibiotics for 10 days and a careful check by the clinician should be carried out after that period.

In the event of the urachus not closing with this treatment or if it has become patent some days after birth as a result of infection, more aggressive surgery needs to be carried out. The calf should be anaesthetized and placed in dorsal recumbency. The site is surgically prepared. The abdomen is opened so that the urachus can be traced back to the bladder. It should be sectioned and the bladder closed with a double layer of continuous Lembert sutures of an absorbable material. The umbilical vessels should be ligated proximally to any infected and diseased tissue. This tissue should then be totally removed. The abdomen should be closed with interrupted

sutures of monofilament nylon. These all should be laid individually before any are tightened in a 'vest over pants' configuration. Only when the practitioner is satisfied that there are enough sutures to close the abdomen, and that no small intestine is trapped, should the sutures be tightened. It is very important that no extra sutures are added after this because of the danger of perforation of the small intestine. A subcuticular layer of continuous sutures of an absorbable material should be laid before the skin is closed with interrupted horizontal mattress sutures of monofilament nylon. It is necessary that the animal receives aggressive antibiotic treatment until 10 days after the surgery when, if the sutures are clean and dry, they can be removed. If there is any doubt, they should be left in place and further antibiotic treatment should be given.

Obstructive urolithiasis

The welfare of the bullock must be at the forefront of the clinician's mind. Animals should not be put through painful surgical procedures just for monetary gain. The use of muscle relaxants is extremely rarely successful and catheterization of the urethra is impossible. Surgery or euthanasia must be performed as soon as possible on welfare grounds. Bladder rupture will occur within 48 h, and urethral rupture with urine escaping into the tissues may occur sooner than that. Immediate slaughter for human consumption is rarely an option as unless the diagnosis has been made very quickly the carcass will be condemned because it will be uraemic.

Prolapsed prepuce

This is a condition which occurs in *Bos indicus* breeds of cattle which have a pendulous dewlap and pendulous prepuce. The prepuce gets damaged and then prolapses. The bull should be given antibiotics and NSAIDs. He is then sedated with a high dose of xylazine (0.1 mg/kg iv) so that he becomes recumbent. The prepuce and surrounding area is surgically cleaned. Local anaesthetic is infiltrated in a ring block around the skin on the end of the prepuce. (Some authorities prefer to do this whole procedure with the bull standing, and using an internal pudendal block, but the author has found this block far from satisfactory and the surgery extremely difficult and dangerous underneath such a large heavy animal.) The penis is grasped and secured by a loop of soft bandage. After careful examination, the surgeon should decide on the amount of damaged prepuce to be removed. This should be as small as possible as there is a real danger that the penis will not be covered if too much prepuce is resected. Four stay sutures should be placed in the prepuce caudal to the part to be removed. These are required so that when the damaged prepuce has been removed, the surgeon can orientate where the two ends of the prepuce should be sutured. The damaged part of the prepuce should be resected and the remaining prepuce sutured back in position with a layer of small interrupted sutures of polyglactan, using the stay sutures as markers. The bull should be given sexual rest for 2 weeks.

Rupture of the penis

This can occur in three ways:

- Direct trauma from a mature bull jumping a gate or solid fence. A large swelling will be seen in the area cranial to the scrotum. There is a danger of adhesions forming and preventing the bull from having an erection. There are two schools of thought on treatment which are diametrically opposed, but no evidence base for either view.
  - That the bull should have sexual rest for 2 months and be allowed to work again when all the swelling has dispersed.
  - That the bull should be encouraged to have an erection twice weekly to prevent fibrous adhesions from forming.
- Rupture of the penis from pressure and damage from a urinary calculus in a dry-fed fattening steer. There will be massive

swelling in front of the scrotal area but not involving the scrotum. These cases have a hopeless prognosis and should be humanely destroyed as soon as possible.
- Rupture of the penis from necrosis of the tissues caused by infection with a *Clostridia* sp. outside the penis following surgical castration. Diagnosis is difficult as there will be swelling from the prepuce caudally around the scrotum and up to the anus. The animal will be very ill. Some animals will recover if they are treated with antibiotics and NSAIDs. It is important to establish drainage from the scrotal incisions. Once penile rupture has occurred, then the prognosis is hopeless. This can be confirmed by urine coming from the scrotal incisions. The condition can be avoided by not performing open castrations in areas where horses have been.

Urethrostomy

The bullock should be restrained in a crush. An epidural should be given. Appropriate antibiotics and NSAIDs should also be given. The area below the rectum is surgically prepared, and the penis located just below the anus. A linear incision is made over the penis and it is drawn through the incision by blunt dissection. The penis is then incised and the urethra is located within it. The urethra is then sutured to the skin with multiple small sutures of monofilament nylon leaving an orifice of at least the size of a finger. Urine will flow out and the bladder should be flushed with warm sterile water to remove any further stones. The wound should be cleaned daily and the stitches removed in 10 days.

Urethrotomy

Historically, clinicians used to perform a urethrotomy rather than a urethrostomy as the animal was sent for slaughter as soon as the withhold period had been reached for any medicines given and the smell of urine could no longer be discerned. The author is concerned about such a procedure from a welfare and an ethical point of view.

Urinary calculi

Urethral obstruction from urinary calculi may occur in steers fed on a concentrate diet. This obstruction will quickly turn to bladder or urethral rupture, renal failure and death. Early diagnosis is very important. The signs are:

- lethargy
- anorexia
- abdominal straining
- the urethra will be felt pulsing just ventral to the rectum
- the hairs around the prepuce will be dry
- diagnosis can be confirmed by ultrasonography

Surgical Conditions of the Reproductive System

Surgical conditions of females

Problems at or associated with parturition

- Relative fetal oversize, including damage to the pelvic canal
- Foetal malpresentation, including twins
- Uterine torsion
- Metabolic disease affecting the cow, causing recumbency
- Hydrops amnion or hydrops allantois
- Fetal abnormalities, e.g. schistosoma reflexus or bulldog calf syndrome, or viral deformities, e.g. Schmallenburg disease

Note that all these problems will be worse if the animal has been calving for a considerable time and the calf is rotten. With abortions, clinicians should be aware that there is not the urgency that there is with a full-term fetus. Animals should receive antibiotics and NSAIDs but be given up to 48 h to dilate.

Once the clinician has diagnosed the problem, a plan needs to be formulated. A trial of labour may be carried out, and if a vaginal delivery is totally impossible then a decision has to be made:

- Caesarean section
- embryotomy
- euthanasia

The very worst scenario is for an embryotomy to be unsuccessful and a Caesarean undertaken as a last resort, as this may be also unsuccessful and result in the death of the cow or euthanasia. Welfare *must* always be at the top of the agenda in such a situation. Caesarean sections have a poor success rate if:

- the calf is rotten
- the cow is exhausted
- the clinician is exhausted
- there is inadequate trained assistance
- the facilities are poor

CAESAREAN SECTION   A Caesarean box will be required (see Chapter 1). The cow should be restrained so that if she goes down she can remain in that position. A rope should be attached to her right metatarsal bone and brought out under her belly so that this can be pulled if she does go down to make sure her left flank is uppermost. Most surgeons prefer the cow to be standing. A large area in her left flank should be clipped and surgically prepared. With an assistant holding her tail up like a flag, a regional block (an inverted L block) should be injected. The tail should then be secured so that it cannot contaminate the wound.

The cow should be given 10 ml clenbuterol solution, 30 mcg/ml iv. Antibiotics and NSAIDs should also be given. The author favours a mixture of penicillin and streptomycin, which gives good uterine penetration and can be continued daily by the farmer. Some practitioners give an epidural anaesthetic but the author has not found that to be beneficial. Before surgery, it is important that any calving ropes have been removed.

A 35 cm incision should be made through the skin and the abdominal muscles in the left para-lumbar fossa, taking care not to penetrate the rumen. Ideally, the calf in the uterus should be manipulated using a calf's limb (this is normally a hind limb with a calf in an anterior presentation) to bring the uterus to the incision (see Plate 5). An incision should be made along the greater curvature of the gravid horn of the uterus from the calf's foot to the point of the hock. The foot should be pulled from the uterus and secured with a sterile calving rope. This procedure should be repeated with the second leg.

The calf should initially be pulled upwards, and then after it is half out it should be rotated so that the ventral surface of the calf is facing downwards. Assistants or a pulley block attached to the roof can be used to exteriorize large calves. Should it not be possible to bring the uterus to the incision, then the uterine incision along the greater curvature can be made in the abdomen with an embryotomy knife. As soon as the calf or calves are out of the uterus, it should be closed with a continuous row of inverting Lembert sutures using an absorbable suture material and a non-cutting needle (assistants should be left to revive the calf or calves). If the fetal membranes can easily be removed, they should be removed before suturing, otherwise they should be left to be passed later *per vagina*.

The uterus should be checked carefully to ensure that it is completely closed before it is returned to its correct position in the abdomen. A vial of 5 mega units Crystapen dissolved in 20 ml water for injection should be syringed into the abdomen. This need not be done if the cow has received antibiotic cover before the operation commenced. The first layer of abdominal musculature, together with the peritoneum, should be closed with a continuous layer of mattress sutures with absorbable suture material using a cutting needle. Half a vial of 5 mega units Crystapen dissolved in 20 ml water for injection should be syringed down the suture line. The second layer of abdominal musculature should be closed with a continuous layer of mattress sutures with absorbable suture material using a cutting needle. Half a vial of 5 mega units Crystapen dissolved in 20 ml water for injection should be syringed down the suture line. As before, these two Crystapen treatments need not be carried out if antibiotic cover has already been given. The skin should be closed with a layer of interrupted mattress sutures of polypropylene number 1 on a swaged (the suture material is attached to the suture material) reverse-cutting needle. The incision site should be sprayed with oxytetracycline spray (Fig. 4.3). The cow should be given 10 IU oxytocin im to involute the uterus.

HUNG CALF Often, a calf which has stuck at the hips can be delivered by slight rotation with renewed traction. Prolonged severe traction (equivalent to three men) will result in damage to either the sciatic or the obturator nerve and should be avoided. Caesarean section is obviously not an option. Thus, fetotomy is the only answer. The author has never been unable to deliver a live hung calf. If the calf is not dead, euthanasia of the calf should be carried out. Fetotomy is not a real problem provided certain procedures are followed:

1. The loop of wire should be placed round the trunk as far *caudally* as possible. This is helped by some traction on the calf and by pushing the embryotome into the cow's pelvis, which will make the next cut easier.
2. The trunk should be cut through with steady long sawing strokes. The cranial part of the calf up to the lower lumbar area can then be removed.
3. Having replaced the caudal end of the calf into the cow's uterus, a heavy introducer, or a closed bull ring attached to a thin calving rope, should be placed over the dorsal aspect of the

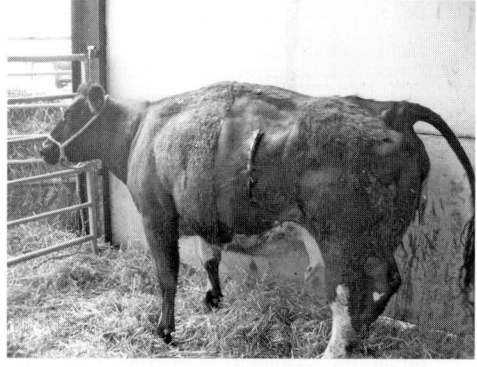

Fig. 4.3. Caesarean section in a cow: the final incision is sprayed with oxytetracycline spray.

calf and dropped between the calf's legs. Then reach in ventrally and grasp the bull ring.

4. The embryotomy wire should be tied *securely* to the calving rope and pulled into the cow and out again.

5. Before starting the second cut it is necessary to *make sure* that the wire is exactly in the middle of the calf's pelvis. The danger is that if it is to the side, the second cut will only cut off one hind leg and the calf's pelvis will be as wide as ever.

6. The two parts of the hindquarters are now easily removed separately.

HYDROPS UTERI Two forms of this condition are recognized: hydrops amnion, when excessive fluid is present within the amniotic sac; and hydrops allantois, when the allantoic sac is involved. At term in the normal cow, approximately 20 l of fetal fluids are present in the uterus, with three-quarters of this in the allantois. In hydrops uteri, over ten times that volume may be present. If the cow is in good condition, she can be left to come to calve normally. However, if she is in poor condition, parturition should be induced with a prostaglandin injection. Uterine drainage has been advocated prior to parturition to lessen the shock of such a large amount of fluid being lost at one time, although the danger of causing a uterine infection by this means is great and, on balance, it is better to let the cow calve naturally.

PROLAPSED CERVIX This condition is extremely rarely seen post-partum. It is normally a pre-parturient non-urgent condition (see Plate 6). The cow should be restrained in a crush. An epidural should be given but sedation is rarely necessary. A Buhner suture, untied, should be put in place before replacement. It can be tightened immediately after replacement. A bow should be used rather than a knot, so that if parturition is suspected the suture can be left in place while an examination is carried out. If the cow is not parturient the bow can be retied as a knot without replacement of the suture. Normally, antibiotics and NSAIDs are not required. This condition will *always* recur, so further pregnancies are not recommended.

PROLAPSED UTERUS While cattle practitioners have an understanding of when euthanasia might be appropriate in cases of uterine prolapse, it can be difficult to give a reliable assessment of the prognosis on the first examination (Gregory, 2011). It is even more difficult for less experienced members of the profession (see Plate 7).

The following criteria indicate a poor prognosis for cows with uterine prolapse:

- Cow was prolapsed more than 6 h before successful uterus replacement.
- Cow had signs of parturient nerve damage.
- Uterus was difficult to replace. The ease of replacing a uterus is related to the time taken to replace it. A survey of cattle practitioners (Ball and Gregory, 2007) found that the average time taken to replace a uterus was 22 min. However, in cows that later died, the average time taken to replace the uterus was over 30 min.
- Cow still down 30 minutes after uterine replacement.

Prognosis is hopeless if three of these criteria occur together at the same time, in which case the cow should be euthanized. If the cow is still recumbent after 24 h the chances of recovery are very poor, and the cow should also be euthanized in this case. Practitioners should have a serious discussion with the cow owner, so that a joint decision can be made to avoid unnecessary suffering.

There are two causes of prolapsed uterus:

1. The primary cause in high-producing dairy cows is hypocalcaemia.
2. The primary cause in beef cows is relative fetal oversize, which causes trauma at parturition.

If there is any danger of the cow dying of hypocalcaemia, then treat this condition first. Cows may die from internal haemorrhage after rupture of one of the very large uterine arteries. It is advisable to sedate any fractious cows with xylazine, and an epidural anaesthetic is vital. If the cow is standing, two helpers should hold up the uterus in a clean parturition gown. If the cow is recumbent, two helpers should arrange the back legs to stick out straight behind the cow. When this has been accomplished, one of the helpers should sit astride the cow facing backwards holding the tail up like a flag. The uterus should be cleaned but any attached membranes should be left *in situ*. The uterus is worked back into the cow using a variety of techniques, while making sure that it is not twisted. The smooth dorsal endometrium, which has no cotyledons, is a good guide. Some practitioners try to put the smaller inverted horn of the uterus in first; others push in the body of the uterus from the sides. Patience and perseverance is vital. It is very important to ensure that the uterus is totally back in the correct position.

Rarely is the human arm quite long enough to carry out this procedure. There is a special instrument available, which is like a rubber boxing glove on a long rod. However, a bottle is normally adequate. A large dose of oxytocin, 10 IU/100 kg iv, should be given immediately after replacement. In theory, there is no need to stitch the vulva, but it is a good insurance policy. A single 'Buhner suture' of uterine tape is ideal. A long Seaton needle is inserted into the skin at the ventral end of the vulva. It is pushed carefully in a dorsal direction subcutaneously and slightly laterally to emerge ventral to the anus. The tape is treaded and withdrawn. This repeated for the other side of the vulva. The two ends are tied tightly so only two fingers can be inserted into the vulva. The owner is advised to remove the suture in 48 h. NSAIDs should be given iv and repeated as required. Antibiotics should be given and repeated for a further 5 days. It is claimed that prolapsed uterus greatly reduces subsequent fertility and that in the unlikely event of a subsequent pregnancy the condition will reoccur. This has not been the experience of the author.

POST-PARTUM ARTERIAL HAEMORRHAGE   This type of haemorrhage is usually from the uterine artery and massive blood loss can be seen lying behind the cow. The pulsating vessel can be felt *per vagina*, and is normally only a forearm length from the vulva. Trying to ligate this vessel is difficult. An easier procedure is to grasp the vessel with a pair of artery forceps or a disposable umbilical clamp. Either of these can be left in the cow. A revisit should be made to the cow in 48 h to retrieve them. Sadly, haemorrhage can occur into the abdomen, and the cow will appear to die before the cowperson's eyes. Antibiotic treatment of post-partum haemorrhage is very important, and cover must be continued for a minimum of 10 days to prevent the danger of secondary haemorrhage which, in the author's experience, is always fatal.

Cows with massive haemorrhage are obviously in shock. The use of normal or hypertonic saline is not worthwhile; whole blood is required. This is not an easy situation. While there is no danger of mismatching blood, unless repeated transfusions are carried out, the donor needs to be selected for temperament and lack of pregnancy. If there are decent crush facilities, available sedation of the donor is not required, as local infiltration over the mid-jugular region will be sufficient. The site should be prepared aseptically. A cut is made through the skin with the vein *not raised*. A small trocar and cannula are pushed through into the raised jugular – the trocar used for the toggling procedure for anchoring the abomasum is ideal. The 5 l of blood that are required will take 5 min to drain out. It should be collected in a container holding 0.5 l sterile water with 20 g sodium citrate; heparin should not be used as any excess will delay clotting time for the recipient and make the situation worse. There are 5 l plastic containers available that have a top to allow a large bloodline to be inserted. The blood should be infused into the recipient over a 20 min period with a 14G catheter.

UTERINE TORSION   In the cow, this occurs at parturition (unlike in the mare), except in exceedingly rare circumstances, when the torsion is in the neck of the uterus, as in the mare, when the cow will show signs of colic and not be parturient. The history will be that of a calving cow 'not getting on with it'. Diagnosis is straightforward on vaginal examination, as the condition is wrongly named: it is in fact a torsion of the vagina. In some cases, it is possible to rotate the calf *per vagina* with the cow standing, although this is very difficult. An easier approach is to roll the cow, with the help of three people. If she is standing, she should be cast using Roeff's method and then rolled *in the direction of the twist*. Usually, when the torsion is resolved, the cervix will only be partly dilated. Many textbooks advise waiting to allow cervical dilation to occur, but in my experience (Duncanson, 1984) and that of others (Pearson, 1971) this *does not occur*. Instead, the cervix becomes indurated. Therefore, I advise dilating the cervix with slow traction without any delay. Caesarean section should, in the author's opinion, be the very last resort in cases of uterine torsion.

Removal of supernumerary teats

The heifer calf should be turned upwards so that her rear end is resting on the ground. Careful examination is made of the teats so that the correct supernumerary teats are located. A small pair of Burdizzos are clamped at the base of the supernumerary teat and then removed. A cut is made with a pair of blunt-ended scissors in the groove left by the Burdizzos. The wound is sprayed with oxytetracycline spray.

Teat amputation

The animal should be sedated using a dose of xylazine, e.g. 4 mg/500 kg im, so that the animal is calm but not recumbent. The teat is anaesthetized with a teat ring block. After 15 min, the area is prepared surgically. The teat is removed with a bold incision with a scalpel. There will be at least two arteries bleeding which will need to be tied off. If the reason for the amputation is sepsis, then the teat canal should be left open to allow drainage. It there is no sepsis or mastitis, the skin should be closed with simple interrupted non-absorbable sutures. The cow should be given antibiotics for 5 days.

Teat lacerations

If the wound does not penetrate the teat cistern, these lacerations should be closed with a row of simple interrupted non-absorbable sutures after suitable anaesthesia and surgical cleaning. The teat should then be covered with special teat adhesive tape bandage which will allow milking with a machine without pain to the cow. If the wound penetrates the teat cistern or if the cow is being suckled the chance of healing is very low. Clinicians are advised to try to prevent mastitis with intramammary and parenteral antibiotics, together with the use of a teat cannula to allow milk drainage. Repair of the teat can then be undertaken at a later date when the cow is dry. This will involve a layer of continuous sutures of absorbable material to close the teat wall and mucosa, and an outer layer of simple interrupted non-absorbable sutures for the skin. Surgical sterility and antibiotics are very important.

Teat obstructions

If there is total obstruction high up between the milk cistern and the teat cistern, then these cases should be left alone as any attempt to clear them will cause chronic mastitis. If the obstruction involves the teat orifice, but there is milk in the teat cistern, surgery can be attempted. The teat should be anaesthetized after the cow has been sedated with 4 mg/500 kg xylazine so that she is calm but still standing. Depending on the size of the obstruction (often called a pea), and any attachment, different methods can be tried to remove it:

1. If the pea is small and not attached an attempt can be made to remove it by drawing two 20 ml syringes, held tightly together, down either side of the teat, to create pressure of milk to burst the pea through the teat orifice.
2. If this fails, or the pea is large, the teat orifice should be enlarged by the use of a McLean's teat knife first.
3. If the pea is pedunculated, it will need to be removed with a spiral teat instrument. This should be wound up into the teat cistern through the teat orifice so that it ensnares the pea. It is then sharply withdrawn through the teat canal.

With all these methods, antibiotics are essential.

Transmissible viral fibropapillomatosis

This condition is commonly referred to as warts and will be seen in the vulva of females, and the penis and prepuce of bulls. They are spread venereally. The age of the affected animal is very important. In both bulls and heifers under 3 years of age, regression and total cure is the norm. In old animals, the prognosis is guarded. Surgical debulking and laser treatment may be successful.

Uterine abnormalities

APLASIA The common manifestation is a single horn aplasia as seen in 'white heifer disease'. This occurs when a roan shorthorn bull is crossed with a roan shorthorn female. The resulting offspring will be in the ratio of two roan to one red to one white. The white females will have aplasia and will be infertile. Diagnosis can be made per rectum and affected animals should be fattened.

DOUBLE CERVIX This condition is rare and is usually first noticed when a heifer receives AI as this will prove difficult to accomplish. Pregnancy will normally occur after natural service. Parturition often occurs without interference, but it may be necessary to section a band of tissue. Subsequent parturitions should be normal.

FREEMARTIN This occurs 95% in female calves when twinned with a bull calf. It can occur if the twin bull calf dies early in the pregnancy and is concealed in the fetal membranes of the female calf when it is born normally. The ovaries and uterus do not develop properly and the animal is infertile.

VAGINITIS This may cause initial problems with diagnosis as the post-parturient cow will present with a pustular vulval discharge, similar to chronic endometritis. Careful examination of the vagina will reveal infected lacerations from damage caused by parturition. *No further trauma* should be caused to the vagina. A rectal examination will reveal whether there is an endometritis and a retained corpus luteum, which should be treated appropriately. The vaginitis should be treated with penicillin in beef cows but with cephalosporin in dairy cows. The cow should be re-examined with care before service.

Surgical conditions of males

Castration

In the UK, if a calf is more than 2 months of age it is illegal to castrate it without local anaesthesia. Depending on the size of the calf and the facilities available, the decision as to whether to use sedation, antibiotics and pain relief in the form of NSAIDs should be taken. Local anaesthetic should be placed in the cord at the neck of the scrotum and under the skin in the scrotum.

BLOODLESS CASTRATION
- The Burdizzo should be applied to a single cord in the neck of the scrotum and left in position for 30 s.
- The cord should then be crushed a second time as a safety precaution.
- The cord of the second testicle should be crushed in a similar manner.
- The crushing lines of the second testicle should not be continuous with those of the first.
- It is prudent to examine calves after 2 months to confirm that both the testicles have regressed.

OPEN SURGICAL REMOVAL
- After cleaning the scrotum, an incision is made in the scrotum laterally continuing down to the tip and just into the testicle.
- The testicle is then removed through the tunics using a twisting motion so that the cord is pulled out of the animal.
- This is repeated on the other side and the wounds are sprayed with an oxytetracycline aerosol.
- It should be noted that an emasculator should not be used as haemostasis is not a problem even in large calves. The use of an emasculator increases the risk of post-operative sepsis.
- It should also be noted that there have been extremely rare reports of the elastic cord of an emasculator retracting into the abdomen and causing strangulation of the small intestine, although this is so extremely rare that the danger should not be considered.

- The owner should be instructed that there is an added danger in using an open removal method in calves which are housed where horses have been, as there is a high probability that they will develop a life-threatening clostridial infection post-operatively.

RIG CASTRATION In the author's experience, there are no true rigs – animals with abdominal testicles – seen in cattle practice. The animals presented have had an attempt made at castration which has either failed or only been partially successful. Careful examination should be made of the scrotal area. A report should be made to the owner of what is present, whether the animal is fertile and how the problem can be solved.

If an elastrator ring has been wrongly placed, i.e. distally to one or both testicles, they will be felt as normal-sized testicles but they will be close to the abdominal wall and the scrotum will be absent. These animals are unlikely to be fertile (in fact in Australia the scrotum is purposely obliterated with an elastrator ring to form a bull with a 'short scrotum'), although they will be sexually active. If a Burdizzo has been ineffectually applied to one or both testicles, they may or may not be normal size but they are likely to be fertile.

The owner has to make a decision on what he/she requires the clinician to do, bearing in mind the expense and possible surgical complications – which are mainly as a result of the lack of good drainage from the incisions. If the owner opts for castration, this has to be carried out by an open surgical method. The calf should be given antibiotics, NSAIDs and sedation. Local anaesthetic should be placed under the skin at the lowest point, where the scrotum should have been. The testicle should then be squeezed into the area where the scrotum should have been. An incision is made over and into the testicle, just through the tunics. The testicle is pulled, twisted and removed. If necessary, the second testicle is treated in the same manner. The wounds are sprayed with an oxytetracycline aerosol. The owner is warned that the animal could be fertile for 2 weeks, but this is unlikely.

Corkscrew penis

The likely aetiology corkscrew penis is trauma as this is a condition of bulls that have been used for service. Diagnosis can be made by observation of service. There is no surgical method of correction, but semen can be collected by artificial insemination (AI).

Inguinal hernia

Inguinal hernias are rare in calves, and are caused by a recessive genetic disorder. Therefore, they should only be repaired after castration. The left side is more commonly affected. If there is strangulation, then the animal will show colic-type pain, but this is very rare. Normally, the calf appears healthy, and can be reared for normal slaughter for human consumption.

If requested, the hernia can be repaired after a closed castration. The calf should be given antibiotics and NSAIDs. After sedation with 0.05 mg/kg xylazine, the animal should be given a GA with 2 mg/kg ketamine. With the calf in dorsal recumbency, the area is surgically cleansed in the normal manner. A skin bleb of 5 ml local anaesthetic is placed over each testicle and an instillation of 2 ml local anaesthetic is put into each spermatic cord. A careful scrotal incision is made over the testicle, taking care not to incise the tunics. The testicle is drawn through the skin incision, milking any abdominal contents back into the abdomen. When the surgeon is 100% certain that this has been accomplished, two large pairs of artery forceps are placed over the cord. The proximal pair is then removed and a transfixing ligature is tied in the groove left by the artery forceps. If this surgery is being performed on a large calf, then a pair of emasculators should replace the distal pair of artery forceps. When the testicle has been removed, the skin should be sutured with horizontal mattress sutures. Similar surgery should be carried out on the other side.

Persistent penile frenulum

This is a congenital condition which is likely to be inherited, so treated bulls should not be used as pedigree stud animals. Surgery is straightforward and requires sectioning of the frenulum (the band of tissue pulling back the tip of the penis).

Surgical Conditions of the Locomotory System

Bovine progressive degenerative myeloencephalopathy (BPDME)

This often called the 'weaver syndrome'. The first signs are ataxia of the hind legs. The condition is only seen in Brown Swiss weanlings. It leads to recumbency, and euthanasia is the only course of action.

Carpal bursitis

This occurs after repetitive low-grade trauma between the carpus and the front of the feeding trough. Traditionally the condition was treated by the fluid being drawn off aseptically and the joint injected with corticosteroids, before the animal's leg was tightly bandaged. In the author's experience, this never results in a cure and the fluid returns even if the original cause has been removed. As the condition is not painful, it is better to leave the lesion alone.

Contracted tendons

This congenital condition is likely to be inherited. It can be corrected by manually straightening the leg so that the calf is weight bearing as many times a day as possible. The weight of the calf will correct the condition and no splinting or surgery will be required. In the author's experience, if the leg cannot be straightened these are difficult cases to manage and have a poor prognosis. There is a body of veterinary opinion which recommends high doses of oxytetracycline by injection, but there is no evidence of the efficacy of this treatment. Splinting is not an option because if the legs cannot be straightened, even with an anaesthetic, the splint and bandage would have to be so tight that

pressure necrosis would occur. There is a surgical option that could be carried out which might include sectioning the superficial and the deep digital flexor tendons, but the author has only carried this out in foals and the procedure is beyond his experience in calves.

Digital dermatitis

This is caused by *Treponema brennaborense* sp. nov. and is highly contagious. It is mainly a disease of dairy cows and is particularly associated with standing in slurry. One or more feet may be affected and the pain causes serious lameness. Treatment is topical antibiotics and bandaging. Prevention is footbathing in a solution of 1 g/l Linco-Spectin (lincomycin + spectinomycin, which is licensed for pigs and poultry as an antimicrobial but can be used as a footbath solution under the cascade principle).

Flying scapulas

This is a bilateral rupture of the serratus ventralis muscles and is an extremely rare condition. It occurs in poor-doing 4–8 month old calves. The whole of the fore-end of the calf drops so that the backbone is no longer parallel to the ground. There is no actual treatment, but with adequate nutrition and treatment of the underlying problem that is causing them to be in a poor condition, they will continue to grow and put on weight.

'Foul in the foot'

The causal organisms are *Fusobacterium necrophorum* and *Bacteroides melaninogenicus*. Muddy conditions or dirty yards encourage the spread of this infection which is contagious, but often appears sporadically. The affected animal will be lame with a swollen foot. Treatment is with penicillin in beef cows and young stock, but with cephalosporins in lactating dairy cows to reduce milk wastage.

Fracture of sacral/coccygeal vertebrae

This occurs as a result of oestrus activity. The affected cow will show the characteristic stance of the 'elephant on a ball', with knuckling of the hind fetlocks. Treatment with NSAIDs has a very guarded prognosis.

Fracture of the pedal bone

This can occur in any pedal bone, but seems to be much more common in the front medial claw and is often bilateral, which makes the aetiology obscure. Animals adopt a pathognomic cross-legged stance. Diagnosis can be confirmed with radiography. Fixation is not required but healing is accelerated by applying a wood shoe to the unaffected claw. Rest should be encouraged, together with added calcium and phosphorus in the diet.

Hip dislocation

The prognosis for this condition gets worse the longer the hip remains dislocated. Replacement requires five strong people as well as the surgeon. For surgery, a clean dry draught-free area is required with a firmly fixed pole to which the cow can be anchored. Sedate the cow with 0.1 mg/kg xylazine iv. Inject antibiotics and NSAIDs. Clip and surgically prepare an area bounded by the spine and the stifle, and the hip bone and the pin bone. Induce anaesthesia with 2 mg/kg ketamine iv. Tie a rope to the bottom of the good leg and pull on this as the cow goes down so that she falls with the affected leg uppermost. The cow needs to fall with her back to the fixed pole. Anchor the animal to the pole with a rope placed between the uppermost leg and the udder like a sling.

Make a local line anaesthetic block 30 cm long from the major trochanter, distally along the cranial edge of the femur, and make an incision along this line. Cut through the fascia lata and the gluteobiceps muscle. With blunt dissection, get a hand around the cranial surface of the proximal femur and around the caudal edge of the proximal femur. Dissection is complete when the surgeon can feel the head of the femur cranially and the acetabulum caudally. The surgeon should remove any blood clot and debris from the acetabulum and check that it is not fractured. If there is a fracture, the cow should be destroyed as the femur will never remain in the acetabulum.

Apply traction to the distal limb, exerting steady increasing pressure in a distal direction, as well as rotating the leg internally by putting weight on the stifle, i.e. downward pressure with the surgeon's knee. With a hand in the incision wound, the surgeon can feel how close the head of the femur is to the acetabulum, and direct more traction accordingly. Once the leg has been pulled enough, it will fall into joint quite easily. The most difficult part is applying sufficient traction. Close the incision with sufficient layers to remove the dead space. Apply 'Somerset shackles' to the cow's metatarsals before she attempts to rise. Assist her to stand on recovery. She should not be allowed on concrete or to walk very far for 10 days.

Hock bursitis

This is caused by long-term damage from lying in unsuitable cubicles (see Plate 8). The animal should immediately be moved to a freshly strawed dry yard or outside. Provided the hock joint has not become infected, animals will recover with antibiotics and NSAIDs. If the joint has been infected, the prognosis is seriously guarded.

Interdigital hyperplasia

This is seen in all types of adult cattle, but seems to be particularly important in bulls. The animals are not lame per se, but only when there is infection in the hyperplasia. Practitioners are put under pressure to remove the hyperplasia from between the claws. Careful counselling is required as the surgery is not difficult, but heavy sedation in older bulls is hazardous and the condition often recurs. Ideally, the surgery should be carried out in a rotary foot crush. After the area has been anaesthetized by a regional block, leaving the tourniquet in place, it should be surgically prepared. The whole of the hyperplasia should be removed with a scalpel. Some clinicians burn out the hyperplasia with a dehorning iron, but in the author's experience regrowth occurs more rapidly after burning. No suturing is necessary, but a tight bandage supporting padding between the claws should be applied. The animal should receive antibiotics and NSAIDs. The foot should preferably be redressed at regular intervals, approximately every 3 days, in a suitable crush. If this is not available, redressing should be carried out at longer intervals as repeated heavy sedation is not without risk. The bandage can be removed after 2 weeks with the animal put on a clean pasture or in a clean straw yard.

Joint ill

This is a condition of young calves, particularly if they have not received adequate colostrum. One or more joints will become swollen and infected. There are several possible organisms that may cause the disease. Traditionally, these were thought to gain entry at birth through the navel and so dressing the navels of newborn calves with iodine or oxytetracycline spray is recommended. It is now known though that organisms can gain entry from a dirty udder through the tonsil. Treatment is with high doses of antibiotics, normally a daily penicillin/streptomycin combination by injection and NSAIDs. Treatment should be maintained for a minimum of 10 days. If improvement is not noticed after 3 days the antibiotic should be changed.

Laminitis

This condition should really be called a coritis as it is a non-septic condition of the corium not of the laminae. It can occur as an acute condition resulting from grain overload, but the more usual manifestation is a chronic condition of both dairy and beef cattle fed on high-concentrate diets. Hooves react to hoof

testers and, in chronic cases, haemorrhagic areas will be seen on the soles. Treatment relies on changing the diet and treating the foot conditions resulting from the laminitis, e.g. white line disease, appropriately.

Osteochondritis dissecans (OCD)

This is a disease of rapidly growing young bulls that causes lameness. It can occur in a variety of joints, with perhaps the hock being the most common. Diagnosis will be from joint effusion backed up by ultrasonography. The author has no experience with treatment but would assume that arthroscopy under GA and joint medication would be worthwhile. The prognosis would be very guarded.

Osteomyelitis

This is a specific disease entity normally in the spine or the hock of young calves which is caused by Gram-negative rods, typically *Salmonella dublin*. Calves will be hunched or lame and with pyrexia, but not necessarily scouring. Diagnosis can be confirmed by radiography. Treatment is with daily enrofloxacin injections and NSAIDs. The prognosis is fair.

Progressive ataxia

This is seen in Charolais cattle in the UK, North America and Kenya. It has never been reported in France. It occurs in yearling cattle and it may take 6 months to progress to recumbency. Slaughter for human consumption should be carried out before the signs become severe.

Progressive myelopathy

This is an inherited condition mainly seen in Murray Grey cattle in Australia. It is caused by an autosomal recessive gene. Calves are ataxic at birth and become recumbent. Euthanasia is indicated.

Recumbent/downer cow

Recumbent cow

By definition, a recumbent cow is one that cannot get on to its feet. The causes in the UK are many:

- abdominal catastrophe
- acute acidosis
- acute babesiosis
- hypocalcaemia
- hypomagnesaemia
- hypophosphataemia
- traumatic injury, e.g. obturator paralysis (Fig. 4.4)
- toxic mastitis
- toxic metritis
- salmonellosis

Abdominal catastrophe includes uterine rupture, true uterine torsion, RDA, caecal torsion, small intestinal torsion and acute peritonitis; any of these conditions may show signs of colic so recumbency may be intermittent.

DOWNER COW This is a recumbent cow in which the cause is not known. She will appear to be bright and have a normal rectal temperature. Her pulse will be normal. She will be chewing the cud. She will be eating and drinking. Her rumen movement will be normal. By definition, her blood calcium, magnesium and phosphorus levels will be normal. It is likely that the cause is damage to peripheral nerves and muscles. Treatment will be NSAIDs and nursing. This should include making sure the cow is lying on deep muck or out at pasture. In the winter she must be protected from bad weather conditions. The cow must be rolled every 6 h.

The main problem for the clinician is the prognosis. This is vital, not only on account of welfare but also economics. Some years ago, the British Cattle Veterinary Association (BCVA) carried out a survey of downer cows. They recorded a wide range of parameters to see whether there was any statistical evidence for any of them to be used as prognostic indicators. Interestingly, the most useful was the judgement of an experienced cattle practitioner. The only other worthwhile indicator was creatine kinase (CK) levels. If CK levels continue to rise, the prognosis is very poor. Therefore, with downer cows it is worthwhile to take a serum sample on the first visit. To save expense this should be stored in the refrigerator. If the cow is still recumbent in 2 or more days a second sample should be taken. Both samples can then be analysed. If the CK level has risen, the clinician is fully justified in recommending humane euthanasia.

Removal of a digit

This procedure should be considered by clinicians if there is chronic septic arthritis in one intra-phalangeal joint. The operation is welfare friendly. It is best to carry out the surgery under light sedation and with a regional block. A tourniquet is required for both the regional block and the operation. The animal is given preoperative antibiotics and NSAIDs. The foot is trimmed to remove any overgrown horn. The whole leg below the middle of the metacarpus or metatarsus is clipped and surgically prepared.

A length of embryotomy wire is positioned between the cleats. With an assistant holding the affected cleat with a pair of hoof testers, the cleat is sawn off with the wire at

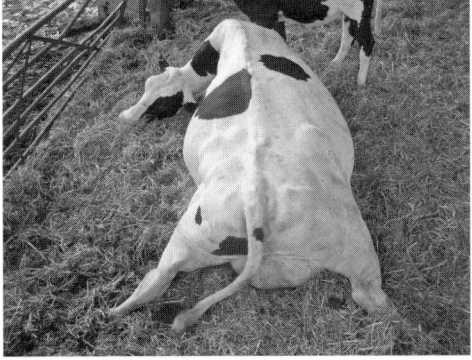

Fig. 4.4. Obturator paralysis in a cow.

a 45° upward angle. This cut will be made in the middle of the second phalange. The stump is then dressed with a suitable antibiotic cream and covered with a suitable dressing. The whole foot and leg to mid carpus/tarsus is bandaged with soffban and standard bandages. These are covered with gaffer tape, taking care that the tape does not actually touch the skin. The animal is kept under antibiotic and NSAID cover for a minimum of 10 days. The dressing should be changed twice in this period. If a good healthy bed of granulation tissue has been formed a lightly protective bandage can be applied.

Rupture of the gastrocnemius muscle

This condition is rare but occurs in overweight mature bulls. The animal will be weight bearing bilaterally on its hocks and its hind cannon bones. Immediate euthanasia is indicated.

Sacroiliac luxation

This is a condition of cows and is normally the result of damage at parturition or oestrus. The animal will not be recumbent but there will be knuckling of the hind limbs and the vertebral column will appear to be dropped in relation to the tuber coxae. Animals may show some improvement with time and NSAIDs. A rectal examination should be carried out before service to make sure there is no narrowing of the pelvic canal which would prevent normal parturition.

Sand cracks

Horizontal sand cracks

These are seen in cattle of all ages and occur after a stress in the life of the animal. This stress may be a period of very poor nutrition, e.g. a drought in range cattle, or a disease, e.g. foot-and-mouth disease (FMD) in Africa, or it may occur in a cow carrying twins but still suckling her previous year's calf. The crack

will go all the way round the claw and may occur in several claws. Lameness will occur when either the crack becomes infected or causes physical pain. Animals should receive antibiotics and NSAIDs when appropriate. The condition will only be resolved when all the horn distal to the crack has been removed, either by wear or trimming, and the healthy horn is weight bearing.

Vertical sand cracks

These will occur in two ways, either from the top when there is damage to the coronary band or from the bottom as a result of damage to the sole and wall. In both instances, there is likely to be lameness from infection and physical movement above the underlying sensitive tissue. If there has been damage to the coronary band, stability is vital, so that in the first instance the claw and the foot must be kept bandaged for at least 3 weeks. If there is no improvement, the sand crack should be widened from the proximal end and the claw and foot bandaged again. If there is still no improvement, two farrier's sand-crack clips should be hammered into the claw under sedation. The prognosis for healing must be guarded. If the sand crack is coming from the sole, the prognosis is much more favourable; the wall can be trimmed back in a V shape from the bottom of the crack and it will grow out.

Septic pedal arthritis

This is a very painful condition and needs prompt radical treatment either with removal of the digit (see above) or a 'street nail operation' (see below).

Shoulder bursitis

This is caused by trauma to the cranial point of the shoulder and will result in sudden-onset lameness. Normally there is pain on palpation of the affected area and also pain when the foreleg is extended caudally. NSAIDs are helpful and a full cure will occur in 6 weeks.

Sole ulcer

These occur on the caudal aspect of the sole and require cleaning and bandaging. Often the condition starts with penetration of the sole by a sharp flint. Continuous standing in slurry potentiates the condition. With antibiotic and NSAIDs as treatment the chances of healing are good, but in bad cases infection may spread to the joint, which is actually not far from the sight of the ulcer, and cause septic pedal arthritis (see above).

Spastic paresis

This is an inherited condition seen in 3–6 month old cattle. One hind leg will be held off the ground in an extended position. On movement the leg will be swung outwards and then forwards. It is not a painful condition and so NSAIDs are ineffective. Partial neurectomy of the tibial nerve is described for treatment, but the author has had a very poor success rate with this and considers euthanasia to be the welfare-friendly option.

Spastic syndrome

This is a progressive condition of old and overweight bulls. They will stop serving and stand with their hind legs stretched out behind them. There is no treatment and euthanasia is indicated.

Spinal muscular atrophy

This is an inherited disorder of Brown Swiss calves. The condition is not seen at birth but some few weeks later. Animals will have marked muscle loss in the hind legs and will become recumbent. Euthanasia is the only course of action. The condition might be linked to BPDME, which is also seen in Brown Swiss calves.

Stifle joint damage

This normally occurs suddenly in older animals and is related to ligament rupture, usually of the cruciate ligaments. Welfare must be considered as although these cases will improve with time and NSAIDs, the prognosis is very guarded.

Stone in the foot

The foot need to be raised in a crush to make a thorough examination (Fig. 4.5).

'Street nail operation'

This is an alternative treatment to claw removal for septic arthritis of the distal phalangeal joint. The foot is anaesthetized with a limb block and thoroughly cleaned. A wooden shoe is applied to the unaffected claw. A hole, approximately 1 cm in diameter, is made in the caudal aspect of the sole up through all the underlying tissues into the septic joint between (phalanges) P2 and P3. As much debris and infection as possible is flushed out and the hole is packed with gauze impregnated with antibiotics. The whole foot is bandaged with waterproof tape on the outside. The bandage is changed twice weekly until healing takes place. The animal is given antibiotics and NSAIDs for a minimum of 10 days.

Super foul

The aetiology of this condition is not clear. It is probably combined infection of the organisms causing 'foul in the foot', i.e. *F. necrophorum* and *B. melaninogenicus*, together with the spirochaete species that causes digital dermatitis (*T. brennaborense*). Treatment should be by bandaging the foot with gamgee soaked in a solution of lincomycin and spectromycin, and giving parenteral injections of lincomycin, tylosin or tilmicosin (tilmicosin may only be administered in the UK by a veterinarian). Clinicians should be mindful of the cascade principle and milk withhold periods.

White line infection

This is an ascending infection and can be linked with a vertical sand crack (see above).

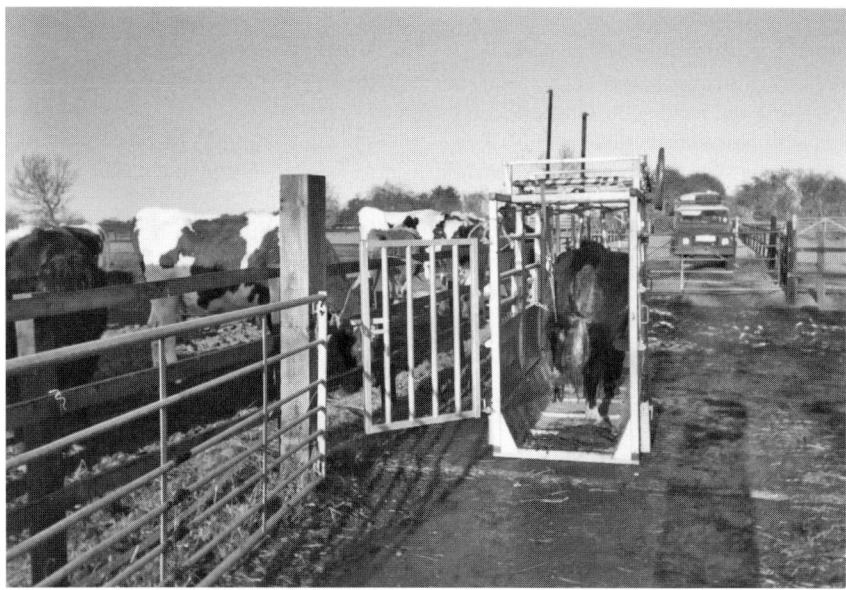

Fig. 4.5. Raising a cow's foot in the crush.

The black area of infection, which often contains very small stones, must be cut out with a hoof knife and the claw and foot bandaged. The animal should be given antibiotics and NSAIDs.

Surgical Conditions of the Integument

Bull ring insertion

This procedure is best carried out in young bulls which are small enough to go into a crush or, if a bull crush is available, then the procedure can safely be carried out on larger bulls. Otherwise, the bull should be secured with two halters, one on back to front, through a strong gate (Fig. 4.6), and given a low dose of xylazine (4 mg/500 kg im). This dosage will not be sufficient to make the animal recumbent. Local insertion of local anaesthetic in the nasal septum is not appropriate.

The size of bull ring must be suitable for the bull, e.g. 7.5 cm for a young bull. A bull ring that is too large is easily caught up on something and ripped out by the bull. A hole should be made in the nasal septum, ideally with a 'bull punch', or if this is not available, with a trocar and cannula. When using a trocar and cannula, the cannula should be left *in situ* to guide the open bull ring through the hole. After insertion, the bull ring should be completely snapped shut so that the small brass screw can be inserted without any danger of cross threading. When the screw is completely in place, the extra piece of brass can be snapped off. Antibiotics and NSAIDs are not required.

Dehorning of adults

This procedure should be avoided by carrying out disbudding on calves (see below), but if it is required clinicians must be mindful of the welfare problems. The animal must be secured in a crush and receive sedation and pain relief with 4 mg/500 kg im xylazine. This dosage will not be sufficient to make the animal recumbent. Cornual local anaesthetic blocks should be placed and allowed 15 min to fully anaesthetize the horn.

The horn can be removed with embryotomy wire, a saw or guillotine shears.

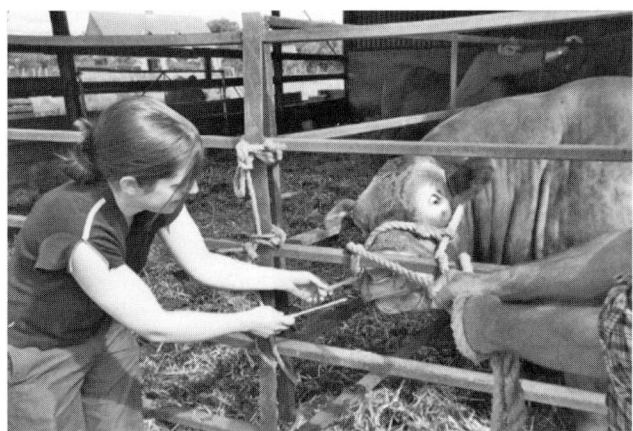

Fig. 4.6. Bull well secured with two halters through a gate before insertion of a bull ring.

Haemorrhage will be extensive and needs to be controlled, although the author has never encountered death or other problems from loss of blood except at 10 days after the operation when infection caused a total slough and death from exsanguination. Haemorrhaging can be controlled in several ways: (i) with hot irons, which has the added advantage of reducing pain as the nerve endings are destroyed; (ii) by a tourniquet of string around the crown of the head and tied between the horns, which is fairly effective but has the disadvantage that a certain amount of horn needs to be left to tie the tourniquet and this must be removed in 24 h; (iii) by ligaturing the corneal artery as it runs ventral to the horn, which can only realistically be carried out if the horn has been removed with a wide margin of skin by sawing; and (iv) by blocking the arteries as they emerge from the corneal bone with matchsticks.

Infection is a real problem, both around the base of the removed horn and in the sinus connecting the horn to the frontal sinus. Local application of oxytetracycline spray may prevent problems, but parenteral antibiotics should perhaps be given. If the sinus does become infected, parenteral antibiotics, NSAIDs and flushing will be required. *It must be stressed that although practitioners can carry out the surgery totally without pain, there will be considerable postoperative pain.* In mixed groups of animals,

those without horns should not be left with recently dehorned animals as fighting will cause further haemorrhage. Haemorrhage will occur in a few hours as the blood pressure – which has been lowered by the xylazine – returns to normal. The procedure should not be carried out in the summer months without very strict fly control as maggots are then a certainty.

Disbudding

Ideally, this should be carried in a special calf crush. If this is not available, a low dose of xylazine (0.5 mg/100 kg) will be helpful. A corneal block should be placed and given a minimum of 15 min to take effect. A red-hot disbudding iron should be placed on the horn-bud for 10 s. This should be repeated until the clinician is sure that all the corneal tissue has been destroyed. If calves have been left so that a large horn bud has grown, this should be removed before the application of the hot iron.

Tail amputation

This procedure should only be carried out if the tail has been damaged. The tail should be anaesthetized by a caudal epidural block and surgically prepared. A tourniquet should be placed at the tailhead with a roll of bandage in the ventral tail groove. A sight for amputation should be selected so that all the damaged tissue can be removed, leaving a minimum of 2 cm of healthy skin. The incision through the coccygeal vertebra should be made between two vertebrae and this should be at least 2 cm cranial to the skin incision so that skin closure is not interrupted by bony tissue. The tail should be well bandaged before the tourniquet is removed. The bandage should be covered with waterproof duct (duck) tape firmly anchored to the tail. Antibiotics should be given for 10 days and the dressing changed twice before suture removal at 10 days post-operation.

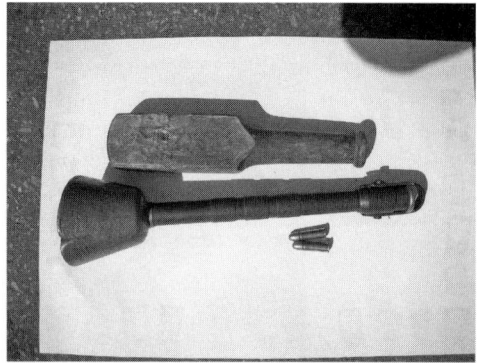

Fig. 4.7. A .310 bell gun for euthanasia.

Euthanasia

Use of a firearm with a free bullet

This is a very satisfactory method of euthanasia in adult cattle. However, in the UK, the operator must either be a veterinary surgeon with a current firearms licence for the weapon concerned or a licensed slaughterman with a similar firearms licence. The only exception to this is for the veterinary surgeon or the licensed slaughterman to use a shotgun (a smooth-bored gun, which is differentiated from a firearm proper) with permission of the owner of the shotgun.

There is no hard and fast rule on the size of the bullet or the bore of the shotgun. Operators should use their judgement. With adult cattle, a .310 or .320 calibre gun would be suitable (Fig. 4.7). With a younger animal, a .22 calibre would be safer and adequate. Equally a twelve-bore shotgun would be suitable for an adult.

It must be remembered when using a shotgun that the end of the barrel needs to be a minimum of 6 in. from the skull and can be up to 3 ft away. A 4.10 shotgun would be suitable for a calf. The location of the position is the same for a firearm or a shotgun. It is a point in the middle of a cross made between the ears and the eyes on the opposite side of the face. The position of any horns should be

disregarded. It should be stressed that the animal's head should be adequately restrained and no personnel should be behind the animal. With either of these methods, the animal should die instantaneously. There is no need to sever the carotids.

Use of a captive bolt pistol

This used to be the standard method of euthanasia in slaughterhouses. A captive bolt .22 pistol is fired into the brain by directing the shot into the middle of a cross made by two lines from the animal's ears to its eyes. The animal is immediately bled out by severing all the major vessels in the neck. This method can be used for adult animals. No firearms licence is required. If the animal is not for human consumption and is not bled out, it is very important that it is pithed to destroy the brain and spinal cord immediately after stunning. Farmers should be given a short training course if this method is going to be used on farm for the euthanasia of calves.

Chemical euthanasia

This is likely to be the method of choice for veterinarians without a gun and a licence. Good advice would be to use sedation first using im xylazine administered with a 3 cm needle (12 ml of a 2% solution for an adult animal).

The client should be warned that the animal might make a moaning noise. This is not from pain but from the effect of the drug. When the animal is in lateral recumbency, completion of euthanasia can be carried out by injecting 50 ml of a solution containing 400 mg/ml quinalbarbitone and 25 mg/ml cinchocaine hydrochloride or 180 ml of triple-strength barbiturate iv into the jugular vein. The reasoning for this approach is that it is not easy injecting large volumes iv into a standing animal. Chemical euthanasia can be used in calves. Once again, they should be sedated with a large dose of xylazine and then killed on recumbency with a solution containing 400 mg/ml quinalbarbitone and 25 mg/ml cinchocaine hydrochloride or triple-strength barbiturate iv into the jugular vein. The dosage used can be calculated on a *pro rata* basis.

5

Sheep and Goat Medicine

_____

Introduction

The author is well aware that sheep and goats are very different animals and that many authorities who he respects advise that they are not run together on account of the dangers of parasitism and clostridial disease. However, in vast areas of the world these animals are run together in huge herds/flocks, and in the UK they are kept in large numbers of small-holdings where, through lack of land, they have to cohabit. In the main, the diseases of the two types of animal will be discussed together, with any differences highlighted.

The chapter is organized by system, with sections on diseases of the gastroenteric tract, diseases of the neurological system, metabolic diseases (which can also be viewed as a category of neurological diseases), diseases of the respiratory system, diseases of the circulatory system, diseases of the urinary system, diseases of the reproductive system and diseases of the integument. The last section briefly covers common reasons for sheep and goats to be found dead.

Diseases of the Gastroenteric System

The predominant signs

- Diarrhoea
- Anorexia
- Rumen stasis
- Abdominal pain
- Salivation
- Pyrexia (rare)
- Vomiting (extremely rare)
- Dysentery (rare)
- Tenesmus (rare)

Diagnosis

When trying to reach a diagnosis of diseases of the gastroenteric tract it is important to know the age of the animal, and to have as full a history as possible, including any alteration to the diet. The clinical signs will need to be observed, and a faeces sample should be obtained (for most tests 70 g of faeces is required).

Causes of enteric disease

- Viruses
- Bacteria
- Protozoa
- Endoparasites
- Poisoning
- Problems relating to nutrition

©G.R. Duncanson 2013. _Farm Animal Medicine and Surgery: For Small Animal Veterinarians_ (G.R. Duncanson)

Enteric diseases caused by viruses and their treatment

Bluetongue disease

The causative organism, *Bluetongue virus* (BTV), is an *Orbivirus* with 24 known serotypes which tend to be restricted to certain areas. The vectors are various species of *Culicoides* midges. BTV first replicates in the local lymph nodes, causing a viraemia which normally lasts for 3–5 days, but can be up to 30 days in sheep and 60 days in goats. The virus causes endothelial damage and disseminated intravascular coagulation (DIC), which give rise to the clinical signs of haemorrhage, ischaemia, inflammation and oedema. The lesions are common in areas subject to mechanical trauma and abrasion, e.g. the feet, mouth and eyes. There is a fever up to 42°C. There are often respiratory signs and abortion in both sheep and goats. The diagnosis is confirmed by PCR for viral RNA.

When treating affected animals all handling should be gentle with as little movement as possible. There is no specific treatment. Antibiotics and nonsteroidal anti-inflammatory drugs (NSAIDs) are helpful. Nursing is vital, and should include offering water and mushy food, and providing deep bedding out of the sun and heat. Affected animals will never return to full production. There are vaccines available for the individual serotypes. The disease is notifiable in the UK.

Foot-and-mouth disease (FMD)

This extremely contagious disease is caused by an *Aphthovirus*. The signs will vary markedly in severity with the strain of virus, the breed of animal and the type of husbandry. The disease spectrum will range from inapparent infection which is detected only by subsequent flock sero-surveillance through to high morbidity outbreaks with very noticeable diseased sheep and goats.

The main signs are lameness and reluctance to move. Over 90% of sheep will have foot lesions and sudden severe lameness will be very evident. Whole groups will frequently lie down and be very unwilling to rise. Excess salivation is rarely seen in sheep but is seen commonly in goats. A thorough examination of the whole flock or herd will reveal the typical erosions and ulcers on the mouths and feet of a considerable number of animals. The earliest signs are vesicles – fluid-filled sacs within the epithelium. The fluid is clear, slightly yellow and slightly viscous. The vesicles are thin walled and therefore very transitory. There will be a radical drop in milk yield in milking sheep and goats. Lambs and kids suckling their mothers will be crying and hungry.

Recovery in sheep is quick, with the disease passing through the flock in a few days. Recovery is not quite so quick in goats. There are vaccines available in some countries, but in the UK the disease is notifiable and controlled by a slaughter policy.

Malignant catarrhal fever (MCF)

This is a disease of cattle caused by a group of herpesviruses. These include *Alcelaphine herpesvirus 1*, *Ovine herpesvirus 2* and *Caprine herpesvirus 2*. The most important is *Alcelaphine herpesvirus 1*. The normal host of this virus is the wildebeest (gnu) in which the disease is asymptomatic. However, in the UK, the sheep is normally an asymptomatic carrier like the wildebeest in Africa. Diagnosis is either with an ELISA or a PCR. There is no treatment or vaccine available. The disease is not recorded in goats.

Nairobi sheep disease (NSD)

This disease of sheep and goats is caused by a *Nairovirus*. It is spread by ticks, mainly the brown ear tick (*Rhipicephalus appendiculatus*), which occurs in areas of eastern Africa. The disease is not found in the UK. This is a very acute disease, with illness shown within 5 days of being bitten by an infected tick. There is acute depression and a high fever. A mucopurulent haemorrhagic nasal discharge and haemorrhagic diarrhoea will be seen together with petechiae and ecchymotic haemorrhages in the mucosa of the mouth. Pregnant animals will abort. Diagnosis can be made on clinical grounds and confirmed by blood samples with an ELISA test. There is no treatment. The disease is notifiable in the UK.

Peste des petits ruminants (PPR)

This disease, which is related to rinderpest, is caused by a *Morbillivirus*. It is a disease with a high morbidity and mortality in sheep and goats. It is seen in Africa, the Middle East, Central Asia and the Indian subcontinent. It is not found in the UK, where it is notifiable. There is high fever with erosions on the mucous membranes of the mouth and eyes. There is acute bloody diarrhoea and also signs of pneumonia. Whole herds will quickly become infected and the majority will die. There is no specific treatment. However, oxytetracycline injections seem to reduce the number of deaths. NSAIDs may be useful. There is a vaccine available.

Rotavirus

Rotavirus infection is found in most farm animals in many countries. There are seven serotypes recognized, although their pathogenicity in lambs and kids is not clear-cut. They will definitely cause diarrhoea but often there is another pathogen isolated at the same time. This may be a bacterium, e.g. *Escherichia coli*, or a protozoan, e.g. species of coccidia. Clinicians cannot treat the virus so attention should be given to the other pathogen involved.

Enteric diseases caused by bacteria and their treatment

Bacillary haemoglobinuria

This disease has been reported in sheep in the UK but it is rare. It is actually primarily a disease of cattle in central Ireland. The disease is caused by *Clostridium (Cl.) haemolyticum*. It is a disease of older sheep and goats, which may be found dead or severely ill. The disease occurs in areas of high rainfall, particularly when summers are wet. The signs shown in sheep and goats include abdominal pain, jaundice and dysentery, and, as the name suggests, haemoglobinuria. Aggressive treatment with penicillin and fluid therapy, particularly whole blood, may be successful in pet sheep and goats.

Blackleg

This is primarily a disease of cattle. The disease in sheep and goats is extremely rare in the UK. It is caused by *Cl. chauvoei*. It follows shearing wounds and dog bites. The first sign is lameness. On careful examination, the animal will show a very swollen painful area over a wound. Treatment with high doses of penicillin and NSAIDs is rarely successful. There is a good vaccine available.

Black's disease or infectious necrotic hepatitis

This is caused by *Cl. novyi* type B. It occurs relatively commonly in sheep suffering from acute fascioliasis, i.e. the migration of immature flukes through the liver. Acute fluke occurs in the autumn. It is also seen in goats. Control can easily be carried out by vaccinating all animals against *Cl. novyi* type B. Fluke control is vital not only to prevent Black's disease but also to prevent the damage caused by the flukes in the liver.

Botulism

This disease is caused by the organism *Cl. botulinum* which multiplies in the soil and in silage, but not in the sheep or the goat. The organism produces toxin outside the body, and the severity of the disease is related to the amount of toxin ingested. Sheep are more resistant to the toxin than goats. Diagnosis is not difficult if the pathognomic sign of a flaccid anus is seen. There is no specific treatment, but animals will recover if they can be kept alive with oral fluids. See below under 'Diseases of the Neurological System', 'Neurological diseases of adult sheep' for more information.

Braxy

This disease only occurs in sheep not in goats. It is caused by *Cl. septicum*. The trigger factor is thought to be eating frosted root crops, which cause an abomasitis. This allows the entry of *Cl. septicum*. The organism is included in several polyvalent vaccines.

Enterotoxaemia

This is the most common clostridial disease in sheep and goats in the UK. It is caused by *Cl. perfringens* type D. The disease is normally manifest by sudden death in sheep. Goats will be found as sick, apparently lifeless, cold and moribund animals. There is no treatment. Control by vaccination is vital.

Escherichia coli (E.coli) *O157*

This zoonotic pathogen is not a pathogen in sheep or goats. However it is carried by them, and carriers are a danger to man. Farmers, particularly those with farms open to the general public, should take precautions.

Escherichia coli

Certain strains of *E. coli* are pathogenic to neonates born in poor conditions, particularly if they have not received an adequate amount of colostrum. *E. coli* with the K99 antigen will cause septicaemia. The condition may be peracute so that death may occur before the neonate is seen to scour. Some 40% of these strains of *E. coli* are resistant to ampicillin. Amoxicillin with clavulanic acid is likely to be the antibiotic treatment of choice.

E. coli plays a role in the syndrome called 'watery mouth'. Watery mouth outbreaks can be controlled by giving antibiotics by mouth or by injection soon after birth as a prophylactic. A better method of control would be to improve the husbandry practices. Similar advice should be given to large goat herds if *E. coli* infection becomes a problem.

Johne's disease

Johne's disease, or paratuberculosis, is caused by *Mycobacterium paratuberculosis* (*M. avium* subsp. *paratuberculosis*) and occurs throughout the world. The main sign is not diarrhoea but ill thrift. In all animals, once clinical signs develop the disease is always fatal. Euthanasia is the only option. The normal method of transmission is from dam to offspring soon after birth through colostrum, milk and faeces. Trans-placental infection can also occur, particularly in animals showing advanced signs of ill thrift.

The ELISA blood test is fairly sensitive once the animal shows signs of the disease, although it is too insensitive to be used as a screening test in clinically normal animals. Faecal smears stained with Ziehl-Neelsen (ZN) have a high specificity but a sensitivity of only 30% as shedding of the organism is very intermittent in small ruminants. The strains found in small ruminants are very difficult to grow in culture as they are particularly slow growing: it can take over 3 months to grow them. The use of liquid cultures may speed up a positive diagnosis, but 3 months is required for a negative result which may not be that sensitive.

Control of Johne's disease in goats is possible using the Weybridge vaccine. Kids should be given half the cattle dose into the brisket at less than 4 weeks of age.

Lamb dysentery

This disease of young lambs is caused by *Cl. perfringens* type B. Often the animals die before they develop dysentery. The only method of control is to have lambs born from fully vaccinated ewes. The ewes need to have received a booster injection 4–6 weeks before lambing. Obviously, the lamb needs to have received adequate colostrum in the first 12 h of life to achieve passive immunity. The disease is not seen in goats.

Malignant oedema

This disease is found in goats as well as in sheep. It is caused by several clostridial organisms, namely *Cl. septicum*, *Cl. chauvoei*, *Cl. perfringens* and *Cl. novyi*. Animals can be found dead or *in extremis*. They will show swellings, which are often gaseous. The disease may follow wounds obtained by rams fighting. It is often then called 'big head disease' (see below under 'Diseases of the Integument', 'Bacterial skin diseases' 'Clostridial cellulitis'). In goats, the organism may gain entrance at parturition and cause massive swelling of the hindquarters. Aggressive treatment with penicillin and NSAIDs may be successful if started promptly.

Sordellii abomasitis

This disease is caused by *Cl. sordellii*. It attacks the abomasums in sheep and has different manifestations in the various age groups. In young lambs over 3 weeks of age, it will cause acute abomasitis. In older lambs, it will cause sudden death from abomasitis. In adults, it will cause sudden death or abomasitis which leads to death often from ulceration and peritonitis. This latter manifestation is seen in goats. There is now a vaccine available which is recommended for both sheep and goats. As the same vaccine is prepared for cattle it should be pointed out that there are two different dosages, which is 2 ml per dose for cattle and 1 ml per dose for sheep. Goats should receive the sheep dose.

Struck

This disease, caused by *Cl. perfringens* type C, is common in sheep in Kent but very rare elsewhere in the UK. As the name suggests, it causes sudden death. There is no standard trigger factor, although this is likely to be the very heavily fertilized grass under fruit trees. *Cl. perfringens* type C has also been recorded in goats.

Tetanus

Sheep and goats are very sensitive to the organism of this disease, *Cl. tetani*. Stiffness and rigor will be seen before the jaws become clamped together. Initial treatment should be large doses of tetanus antitoxin (TAT) and large doses of penicillin. Animals may recover if they are given adequate nursing. All animals receiving surgery, i.e. open castration or disbudding, should receive TAT if they are not fully vaccinated.

Enteric diseases caused by protozoa and their treatment

Coccidiosis

The species of coccidia that cause this disease are species specific. Their primary site of infection is the ileum, but they also cause damage to the colon and the caecum. The gut wall is damaged by oedema. There is haemorrhage and villus atrophy, which reduces fluid absorption and causes diarrhoea. All species of *Eimeria* that are pathogenic to sheep have oocysts which are relatively small, e.g. no larger than 30 µm across. This is in contrast to the pathogenic coccidial oocysts in goats, which are 40–50 µm across.

The nutritional status of the lamb or kid is critical to infection and, of course, there are stress factors, e.g. transport, muddy conditions, particularly around the water supply, and a sudden change of diet, usually a flush of grass. Lambs and kids become infected with oocysts early in life but as there is a long prepatent period, often in excess of 28 days, clinical signs appear much later, after the infection has built up. Clinicians also ought to judge high oocyst counts with caution as they may be boosted by non-pathogenic species. At the other end of the spectrum, acute or even fatal disease may occur before significant numbers of oocysts of pathogenic species appear in the faeces. Laboratory findings must be linked with clinical findings.

Control of coccidiosis must be a balance. Animals need sufficient infection to produce immunity but not too much to cause clinical disease. Low stocking densities and good hygiene – with dry bedding, are both required in lambs and kids that are indoors. Decoquinate can be fed to the lambs or kids in their creep continuously over the 28 days when they are most at risk. Animals can be treated with diclazuril or toltrazuril. Whatever treatment is given to kill the coccidia it must be a recommendation that oral rehydration therapy is carried out at the same time for the badly affected animals.

Cryptosporidiosis

This disease is caused by *Cryptosporidium parvum*. It has a direct life cycle, with infection occurring by the faecal–oral route. Most commonly, the infection in lambs and kids is not an infection by one type of organism but a mixed infection with other pathogens. The highest mortality rates in lambs are at 4–10 days old. Kids are infected a little later, with the highest mortality rates occurring at 5–21 days old. Age-related resistance, unrelated to prior exposure, is observed in lambs. This does not occur in kids. Fresh blood may be seen in the faeces, but tenesmus is not a feature. In severe cases, the animal will be depressed and dehydrated. The condition is easy to diagnose as large numbers of oocysts will be seen in the infected faeces. ZN is a useful stain as the oocysts are small and relatively non-refractile.

Control of the condition requires attention to detail in all aspects of hygiene to lessen cross-contamination and auto-infection. Halofuginone lactate can be used for prophylaxis and treatment, and is licensed for use in cattle in the UK. It is available as an oral solution containing halofuginone lactate 0.5 mg/ml. The dose is 2 ml/kg daily for 7 days. It should be stressed that cryptosporidiosis is a zoonotic disease.

Giardia

This is a zoonotic pathogenic protozoan, which is transmitted by the faecal–oral route. It can affect lambs and kids over 4 weeks of age and will cause diarrhoea. Treatment should be orally for 3 days either with fenbendazole 10 mg/kg or metronidizole 25 mg/kg.

Enteric diseases caused by parasites and their treatment

Intestinal cestodes

Adult tapeworms occur worldwide. In the UK, *Moniezia expansa* occurs in both sheep and goats. The secondary host is an oribatid mite found on pasture. The prepatent period is 40 days. In large numbers these tapeworms may cause ill thrift, and intussusceptions have been reported on post-mortem. They are well controlled with albendazole. The metacestode stages of *Taenia multiceps* – referred to as *Coenurus cerebralis* – cause 'gid' in sheep and goats (see below under 'Diseases of the Neurological System', 'Neurological diseases of growing lambs'). They are found in the muscles and subcutaneous tissues as well as in the brain. The metacestode stages of *T. hydatigena* – referred to as *Cysticercus tenuicollis* – occur in sheep and rarely in goats. Hydatid disease, or echinococcosis, which is caused by *Echinococcus granulosus*, occurs frequently in sheep in the UK, but only rarely in goats.

Intestinal nematodes

These are extremely important in sheep and goats. The overuse of anthelmintics has brought on universal resistance to the standard three types of anthelmintic. It is vital that the newest class of anthelmintics (aminoacetonitrile derivatives) – represented by monepantel, which has recently been released – is not rendered useless by overuse and the build-up of resistance. No animal must be underdosed, so if animals are in a group it is important that the dose is worked out for the largest animal and that this is the dose which is used for the whole group. Certain anthelmintics have a narrow safety range, e.g. levamisole in goats, so it is important that accurate weighing and dosing is carried out.

Ewes and does have a post-parturient rise in infection. Anthelmintics can be used routinely at this time, but to limit the rise in resistant worms it is advisable for 10% of the ewes or does to be left untreated. It is prudent for these 10% to be either ewes with only single lambs or goats which are not high yielders. Otherwise, anthelmintics should *only* be used when it is necessary to prevent clinical disease. In this way, the rate of selection for resistance will be reduced, and the drug efficacy will be preserved for as long as possible. To do this it is important that the number of worms in refugia is increased (worms which are not selected by anthelmintic treatment are said to be in refugia). The larger the population of worms that are in refugia compared with the population of worms that are exposed to treatment, the slower resistance will develop.

After treatment, there are always some worms that survive in the host. These worms are resistant to the anthelmintic used. If the offspring of these worms are in the majority, then this resistance will develop rapidly. To prevent resistance developing, a substantial number of worms needs to be left untreated each time anthelmintics are used so that these non-resistant worms essentially provide the subsequent generations of worms. It is now considered that where sheep and goats are continually exposed to worms it is a good idea to have a few worms inside the animal to not only help develop a form of immunity but also to prolong the effectiveness of the available anthelmintics. Goats require particularly careful management as they do not appear to develop as good immunity as sheep.

Every holding and every group of animals must be considered separately. There should be no blanket treatments. It is vital to prevent resistant worms being brought on to a holding. Therefore, the aim with any new animals is total deworming. This may involve a combination of the 'old' three wormers given at the correct dosage (these may be given at the same time but not mixed) or the 'new' wormer, monepantel. There is also a new combined wormer licensed in the UK which employs two active ingredients: derquantel and abamectin. After drenching, the animals should be housed or at least kept off the pasture for 48 h to allow any still viable eggs to be shed. The new animals can then be introduced on to the originally grazed pasture to pick up the 'non-resistant' worms and thus dilute any resistant worms.

Controlled grazing methods will help to avoid infection. Any method of allowing pastures to rest will be beneficial as soil organisms, e.g. earthworms, dung beetles and nematophagous fungi, will reduce pasture burdens. Mixed species, e.g. rabbits and horses, will also be helpful. Cattle grazing will help too but there are some species of helminths that cross between cattle and sheep, or cattle and goats, so practitioners should not give blanket advice but continue to monitor the situation. Preventing close cropping of grass is good as rarely do worms climb more than 3 cm up the stems. The ideal control of pastures is to plough and have a break crop such as lucerne or kale. Making hay also helps to control pasture contamination considerably, but like resting a pasture for a year it is not totally effective. Only resting a pasture for 3 years can be considered totally effective, but zero grazing is the ultimate method of control and may be considered in large milking herds of sheep or goats.

There are no licensed products for goat treatment. General advice would be to use twice the sheep dose of benzamidazoles and avermectins, which have a wide safety mar-

gin, in goats. As stated above, levamisole does not have a wide safety margin, so the dose can be increased to one and a half times the sheep dose but no higher than this. Faecal egg outputs should be monitored. It is important to sample individuals and not a bulked-up sample, or the egg count will be diluted. Testing before treatment will provide information about the worm status of the group and whether anthelmintic use is necessary. Testing after treatment will show the efficacy or otherwise of treatment. It takes 3 days for all the eggs in the gastrointestinal tract to pass out, so if treatment is 100% effective there will be virtually no eggs present at that time. However, there is a shock effect of the anthelmintic in that it will stop egg production but not actually kill the mature worms. It is therefore prudent to wait for 2 weeks after treatment before sampling. Worms acquired after treatment will not normally produce eggs for 3 weeks. The practitioner can therefore advise the owner on the likelihood of anthelmintic resistance to the drug being used and the advisability of a change of drug.

Probably the most serious nematode in sheep and goats is *Haemonchus contortus*, which is a bloodsucking parasite in the abomasum. Figure 5.1 shows a ewe infected by this nematode. It will cause severe life-threatening anaemia in both species at all ages. Diagnosis by faecal worm egg output is normally too late. Clinical diagnosis by assessing the pallor of the mucous membranes is vital so that prompt anthelmintic treatment can limit the number of deaths.

Nematodirus battus is a very serious nematode which causes scouring in lambs. A heavy infection will cause profuse watery yellow-green diarrhoea, leading to severe dehydration and death even before eggs are seen in the faeces. The eggs are roughly twice the size of those of other intestinal nematodes found in sheep and are easily recognized. Historically, in the UK, *N. battus* affect 4–8 week old lambs which had been grazing on pastures grazed by young lambs in the previous summer. The eggs required a frost before they could become infective. The pattern is now changing, with infections occurring in older lambs. Pastures which

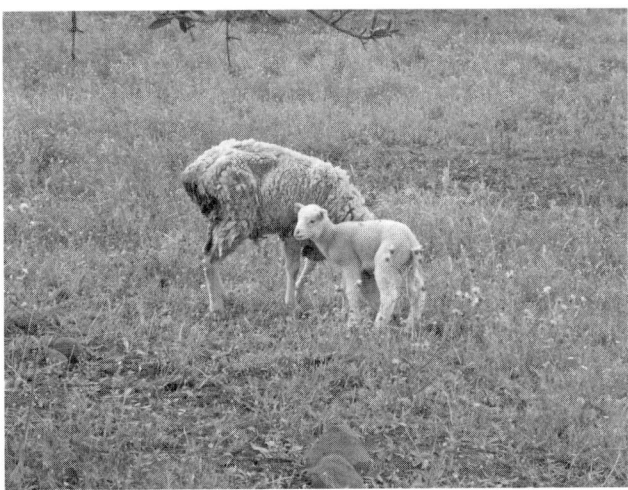

Fig. 5.1. Ewe with *Haemonchus contortus* infection.

have been grazed by young cattle or ewes are no longer safe. *N. battus* has now been found to be resistant to benzimidazole anthelmintics in the UK (Mitchell *et al.*, 2011). However, at the present time the benzimidazole anthelmintics are still recommended for treatment of *N. battus* as resistance is not yet widespread.

Trematodes

FASCIOLA HEPATICA This parasite, which causes fascioliasis, has shown a massive increase in prevalence in the UK. The distribution is dependent on the presence of the snail intermediate host, *Lymnaea truncatula*. This aquatic snail is now fairly ubiquitous. The levels of infection and incidence of disease are linked to the rainfall from May to October. The adult flukes in the bile ducts of cattle and sheep lay eggs in the faeces on to the pasture. In wetter summers, there is a massive shedding of cercariae on to the pasture during August to October. These encyst into metacercariae on the herbage and are ingested by the ruminant. The immature flukes migrate through the liver to the bile ducts. This is a dangerous stage, as there is massive damage to the liver, resulting in death. These deaths will occur from September to December. More chronic infections with adult fluke in the bile ducts occur in February and March. Sheep and

goats will be weak and anaemic. The classic sign is oedema in the mandibular space, often termed 'bottle jaw'.

In average rainfall years, all sheep should be dosed twice – in October and January – with a drug which is effective against immature stages of the fluke, e.g. triclabendazole. In some years, they will need to be dosed again in May. This can be with a combination roundworm and fluke drench in lambs which is used at this time only.

PARAMPHISTOMUM SPP. This is the rumen fluke and has been reported to cause clinical disease in adult sheep (Mason *et al.*, 2012). The sheep in this study were thin and had an acute scour, which in one case was haemorrhagic. Post-mortem showed large numbers of immature flukes in the duodenum with large numbers of mature flukes in the rumen, reticulum and omasum. The secondary host is an aquatic snail and the infection is thought to have originated in deer.

Gastric disorders

Acidosis

This occurs with grain overload. Signs will vary from mild abdominal discomfort and lethargy to acute collapse and death. In peracute cases, the animals will be found dead and show no sign of violent watery diarrhoea, which is the main sign in slightly less acute situations. All affected animals will show a lowered rectal temperature and an increased pulse. They will have toxic-looking mucous membranes. Antacid fluids should be given by mouth, ideally by stomach tube. Vitamin B injections, together with glucose, should be given iv.

Bloat

This occurs in sheep and goats as frothy bloat and the result of overeating legumes or clover. The animals will then become recumbent and die unless treated fairly rapidly. Treatment is best accomplished by stomach tubing to relieve the gas, if possible, and by passing vegetable oil down the tube to flatten the gas. If that is not possible, a trocar and cannula can be inserted into the left flank (see Chapter 6).

Gastritis

This causes severe pain which, in turn, causes vomiting. It will be seen in sheep and goats as a result of poisoning with certain plants, e.g. rhododendron (see Plate 9).

Rumen atony

This is seen in sheep and goats as a secondary sign caused by a primary lesion affecting the vagus nerve, e.g. inflammation of the mesenteric lymph nodes resulting from infection by *Mannheimia haemolytica* (formerly *Pasteurella haemolytica*). The animals will be off colour with pyrexia. Prognosis is guarded. Aggressive treatment with antibiotics and NSAIDs is required.

Rumen impaction

This is seen in sheep and goats which have consumed a toxic dose of acorns. Liquid paraffin may be helpful. Rumen impaction is also seen when large rumen papillomas cause problems with rumen emptying. There is no treatment for this condition. Rumen impaction is also seen if there are *Actinomyces bovis* granulomas at the caudal end of the oesophagus. The sheep or goat will be slightly off colour with some evidence of chronic bloat. The animal is not

normally pyrexic. Treatment is with daily doses of streptomycin which should be repeated for 10 days. Goats which have eaten something totally unsuitable, e.g. polythene string or cloth, will have rumen impaction. A rumenotomy may be required (see Chapter 6).

Diseases of the liver

Abscesses

These may form in the livers of sheep and goats either by haematological spread or by local invasion from the rumen. They may be caused by a variety of organisms. The most common organism in sheep is *Fusobacterium necrophorum*, and in goats it is *Corynebacterium pseudotuberculosis*. Clinically, the animals will be ill with pyrexia. Jaundice may be a feature. Diagnosis may be helped by raised liver enzymes, liver biopsy and trans-abdominal ultrasonography. Obviously, aggressive antibiotic treatment is required, but it is unlikely to be successful.

Black's disease

This is caused by *Cl. novyi*. It is mainly a sheep disease but is definitely seen in goats. Liver fluke infestation is required for this disease. See 'Black's disease or infectious necrotic hepatitis' under 'Enteric diseases caused by bacteria and their treatment' above for more information.

Fascioliasis

This is the most important liver disease in sheep and goats. See the section above on '*Fasciola hepatica*' under 'Trematodes', 'Enteric diseases caused by parasites and their treatment' for more information.

Plant toxicity

Certain plants can cause liver toxicity but this is rare.

Rift Valley fever (RVF)

This is caused by a bunyavirus (*Rift Valley fever virus*) which occurs in sheep and goats in Africa as well as in the Middle East.

The disease is spread by mosquitoes and maybe by other insects. It is also possible that there is direct spread from viraemic sheep and goats. The disease is most severe in very young lambs and kids and there is an extremely high mortality. Mortality is also fairly high in growing sheep and goatlings. The disease is normally mild in adults but always causes an abortion storm. All surviving animals develop a lifelong immunity.

Blood taken from a live animal and heart blood taken from a newly dead animal can be tested with an ELISA for confirmation of the diagnosis. Virus isolation will give a definitive diagnosis. There is no specific treatment. Administration of 30 ml of serum collected from convalescent animals given iv or ip may reduce mortality rates. This is a zoonotic disease and also causes abortion (see below under 'Diseases of the Reproductive System').

Tumours of the liver

These are rare in sheep and extremely rare in goats. They are nearly always formed from liver tissue, except for very rare melanomas which have normally started in the lungs and spread through the diaphragm. Primary liver tumours are rarely malignant and do not cause emaciation. Emaciation is only seen in malignant tumours which rapidly grow large and invade the lymph nodes.

Diseases of the pancreas

Pancreatitis

This may occur as a secondary complication to peritonitis or liver disease. The pancreas may also be infested with cysticerci from *Taenia* spp., whose primary host is a small carnivore.

Diseases of the Neurological System

Neurological diseases of neonatal lambs

Border disease

This disease is caused by a *Pestivirus*, which is also a cause of abortion. It can occur at any stage of pregnancy. The disease should be suspected if live lambs are born showing the pathognomic signs of a hairy coat and trembling. The shepherds call the lambs 'hairy shakers'. Other than abortion, the ewes show no other signs. If the lambs are not too badly affected they can survive and the neurological signs will gradually disappear. However, they will have significantly slower growth rates and carcass quality is affected.

Cerebellar hypoplasia or 'daft lamb disease'

The cause of the disease is unknown, but it is thought to have a genetic origin and be carried on a recessive gene. Degenerative changes in the Purkinje cells in various parts of the brain have been reported. Affected lambs show advanced neurological signs including opisthotonos, and have difficulty in maintaining their balance as their heads sway. Diagnosis should be made clinically. Histological examination at post-mortem may often be unrewarding. There is no treatment. If the lambs can suckle they may survive. Otherwise euthanasia is indicated.

Dandy–Walker malformation

The hypertensive hydrocephalus and domed skull of this malformation is readily recognized at birth. Euthanasia is indicated.

Hereditary chondrodysplasia

This has been termed the 'Spider Syndrome'. The lambs have twisted spines which cause considerable parturition problems. The condition, which is thought to be inherited, is common in 'Blackface' sheep and was first reported in that breed in Minnesota, USA. It is also found in 'Down' breeds in the UK.

Hypoglycaemia

This condition is, unfortunately, very common. It occurs as a result of failure to suck. This may occur as result of dystocia, particularly with oversized lambs. It may occur with multiple births when a lamb is neglected by its mother. If may also occur as a result of extreme weather conditions. Occurrence in all these instances can, in many cases, be avoided by good shepherding.

Treatment for the hypoglycaemic lamb is logical and straightforward. The shepherd must first decide whether the lamb is older than 12 h. If it is under 12 h old it should be given an adequate amount of good quality colostrum by stomach tube, or by a teat if it is still able to suck. The amount of colostrum depends on the weight of the lamb. A lamb weighing 3 kg or less requires 120 ml of colostrum. Most lambs require 180 ml of colostrum, and lambs over 5 kg require 240 ml. After the lamb has received this colostrum it should be warmed up to a core body temperature of 102°F. This can be accomplished in a variety of ways, either in a 'hot box' or with hot water bottles. Electric fan heaters should be avoided as they tend initially to reduce the core temperature further by latent heat loss. Colostrum can be warmed by conventional means or by using a microwave. The latter should be used on a very low setting, e.g. defrost, or it will denature the proteins.

If the lamb is over 12 h old it is much more likely to be hypoglycaemic. If its body temperature is below 99°F, it must receive glucose by ip injection *before* it is warmed up, or the last remaining reserves of glucose will be used up and the brain will be permanently damaged. A 20% glucose or dextrose solution should be used. This is easily prepared at the correct temperature by drawing up half the quantity required of a 40% solution (this is the normal strength of glucose solution supplied) at room temperature, into a 60 ml syringe. The other half of the solution is boiling water sucked up from a pan. The resulting warm solution can then be injected into the flaccid lamb ip using a 1 in. 19 gauge needle. The injection site is one finger's width from the midline and two fingers' width below the navel. The lamb is held up by its forelegs with one hand (remember that it is nearly dead or it would not require this treatment) with its body hanging down. The correct spot is marked on the fleece with a dot of blue antibiotic spray. The injection is then made at 45° from above towards the tail of the lamb. In this manner, the abdominal contents will not be damaged. It is sensible to give antibiotic cover by injection at this time as well.

The volume of the fluid depends on the size of the lamb. This should be roughly 10 ml/kg, i.e. 30 ml for a small lamb, 50 ml for a standard-sized lamb and 60 ml for a big lamb. As soon as the injection has been completed, the lamb should be warmed up to a core body temperature of 102 °F.

Injury to the central nervous system (CNS) at birth

This should not occur as a physical injury with the correct lambing techniques. However, lack of oxygen can readily occur during parturition, particularly in lambs presented in a posterior presentation.

Myodystrophia foetalis deformans

The lambs affected by this condition are often called stiffed-limbed lambs. There are often difficulties at parturition. The condition is mainly found in Welsh mountain breeds. It is caused by a lethal recessive gene.

Swayback

This condition is normally congenital although delayed swayback can occur. With congenital swayback, the severity of the symptoms varies from mild hind limb ataxia to severe brain damage and death soon after birth. The blood of either the lamb or its mother will show low copper levels, and the copper content of the lamb's liver will give a definitive diagnosis. There is no treatment, as the demyelination that has occurred is irreversible, but if the lambs somehow manage to reach up and suck they can survive. Nevertheless, mildly ataxic animals will live and fatten. The condition occurs in primary copper deficient areas or, more commonly, in areas with high molybdenum or sulfate which bind up the copper so that it is unavailable. It can be prevented by giving copper to the ewes between the tenth and sixteenth week of pregnancy. Excess of copper is toxic to sheep and so it cannot be supplied by mineral blocks or licks. Before treatment of a flock, it is advisable to take some blood samples from a test sample of the ewes to confirm the need for treatment.

Neurological diseases of unweaned lambs

Delayed swayback

This is rare. It should only be suspected if there have been other cases of swayback earlier. It will have a gradual onset. The lamb will be mentally normal and slowly become ataxic. There will be no pyrexia. There is no treatment.

Listeriosis

This can occur in young lambs. It is caused by the bacterium *Listeria monocytogenes*. The lambs will be mentally abnormal and have a very high rectal temperature. They will also have a stiff neck which may lead to opisthotonos. However, in young lambs *L. monocytogenes* is more likely just to cause septicaemia. In theory, the bacteria should be sensitive to penicillin, although in the author's experience oxytetracyclines are more likely to bring about a cure. Dexamethazone is useful if given at a high dosage rate of 1 mg/kg daily in the morning, either iv or im, every 48 h. See also below under 'Neurological diseases of adult sheep', 'Neurological diseases of goats' and 'Eye conditions of older sheep and goats'.

Meningitis/encephalitis

This does not occur in isolation but is normally associated with other conditions, e.g. navel infections, septicaemia, enteritis or polyarthritis. All of these conditions result from poor hygiene at lambing. These conditions should be corrected. Shepherds should not rely on prophylactic broad-spectrum antibiotics. Polyarthritis can be caused by *Pasteurella multocida* (Petridou *et al.*, 2011).

Spinal abscess

Atlanto-occipital infection is very common in young lambs and should always be considered in the ataxic 2–4 week old lamb. The lambs are mentally normal. Spinal abscesses may occur as a result of tail docking or infections originating in the navel or in the tonsil. Symptoms are progressive, beginning with slight ataxia, which deteriorates over a few days to complete hind limb paralysis. There is

quite a good response to antibiotic treatment if it is started early enough. NSAIDs should be given for pain relief.

Tetanus

This disease should always be suspected if a lamb is stiff, hyperaesthetic and showing spasms. The vaccination history should be checked as the organism is likely to have gained entry at castration or at tail docking. High doses of penicillin may allow the lamb to survive, but welfare must always be considered. See above under 'Diseases of the Gastroenteric Tract', 'Enteric diseases caused by bacteria and their treatment' for more information.

Tick pyaemia

Tick pyaemia will obviously only be seen in tick areas. The lambs will be mentally normal but may show some degree of ataxia. There will be multiple abscesses caused by *Staphylococcus aureus*. Normally, this bacterium is not resistant to penicillin so a penicillin/streptomycin mixture given by injection daily is the treatment of choice.

Neurological diseases of growing lambs

Cerebrocortical necrosis (CCN)

This condition has a sudden onset with no pyrexia. Any lamb which is recumbent, blind, and showing strabismus and opisthotonos is likely to have CCN. Response to iv thiamine is the best pointer to a correct early diagnosis. A heparinized blood sample can be taken for transketolase estimation, which is a specific test for CCN. The pathognomic sign at postmortem is that macroscopically the cerebral hemispheres will show a yellow discoloration and fluoresce under ultraviolet light. See also below under 'Neurological diseases of goats'.

Gid

Affected lambs will show visual and postural deficits, which have a slow onset. They may circle and show head aversion on account of a space-occupying lesion in the cerebral cortex. The cause is the cyst of the tapeworm *Taenia multiceps* (*Coenurus cerebralis*). Diagnosis will be difficult because softening of the skull as in classical cases of 'gid' only occurs in very advanced cases. The cyst may be seen on radiographs. Drainage of the cyst may be attempted as a surgical treatment.

Lead poisoning

Chronic lead poisoning occurs in areas of high soil lead content. The animals will be ataxic and often have fractures on account of osteoporosis. Acute lead poisoning could occur in lambs of this age group which have licked paint off old gates. Treatment using calcium edetate (EDTA) iv is often successful.

Louping ill

This disease is caused by a *Flavivirus* transmitted by ixodid ticks. The virus has been isolated in Norway, Spain, Turkey, Bulgaria and the UK. The clinical signs are considerably worse in the presence of the rickettsia *Anaplasma phagocytophilum*. It causes a diffuse, non-suppurative meningoencephalomyelitis. This is shown as a sudden onset incoordination, progressing to paralysis in 24 h and followed by coma and death in a further 24 h. Diagnosis is by virus isolation from heparinized blood or cerebrospinal fluid (CSF). There is a vaccine.

Plant poisoning

In the UK, the following plants may cause neurological signs if ingested: aconite (*Aconitum napilus*), blind grass (*Stypandra glauca*), bracken (*Pteridium aquilinum*), branched onion weed (*Trachyandra divaricata*, originally from south-west Australia), fool's parsley (*Aesthusa cynapium*), goldenrod (*Haplopappus heterophyllus*, originally from the USA), hemlock (*Conium maculatum*), laburnum (*Laburnum anagyroides*), lupins (*Lupinus* spp.), male fern (*Dryopteris filixmas*), marijuana (*Cannabis sativa*), mare's tails (*Equisetum* spp.), marshmallow (*Malva parviflora*), poison morning glory (*Ipomoea muelleri*), rushes (*Juncus* spp.), tobacco (*Nicotiana*

tabacum), water dropwort (*Oenanthe crocata*) and water hemlock (*Cicuta virosa*).

Ryegrass staggers

The signs are caused by a toxin produced by a fungus living in ryegrass (*Lolium* spp.) seeds. Animals will show tremors and knuckling of the joints. They may even collapse, but will recover after rest.

Sarcocystosis

All ages of the flock may be affected by sarcocystosis but this is primarily a neurological disease of fattening lambs. The disease is caused in the UK by two microcystic species: *Sarcocystis arieticanis* and *S. tenella*. These are obligate two-host parasites. The sheep is the intermediate host and the dog is the main final host, although the fox may take on this role. There are also macrocystic species, but these appear not to be pathogenic.

Microcystic cysts are very common, with at least 85% of sheep showing them either in the myocardium or in striated muscle. However, clinical signs are very rare. Affected sheep show muscle weakness and ataxia of variable severity, and hind limb paresis may sometimes progress to recumbency (Jeffrey, 1993). Some sheep may die without premonitory signs. Sheep with nervous signs are usually still bright, alert and appetent. Less severely affected sheep may recover with supportive therapy. Diagnosis is extremely difficult as most sheep show antibodies and the cysts are common at postmortem. If several sheep are affected by a strange neurological condition, this disease should be suspected. See also below under 'Diseases of the Reproductive System', 'Abortion and its causes'.

Spinal abscess

The lambs will slowly become ataxic. They will be mentally alert and have a raised white cell count (WCC). They may be pyrexic. Antibiotics may be helpful. Animals showing an increased level of protein in a CSF sample are not likely to recover and euthanasia is indicated.

Tetanus

This condition should be extremely rare as there are very good vaccines available. See above under 'Diseases of the Gastroenteric Tract', 'Enteric diseases caused by bacteria and their treatment' for more information.

Neurological diseases of adult sheep

Botulism

This condition has a worldwide distribution and is caused by *Cl. botulinum* types C or D. Several cases will be seen in a flock eating big-bale silage which has been badly made. The signs are muscular weakness, leading to flaccid paralysis; the signs are progressive and symmetrical – they involve cranial and peripheral nerves. Normally the condition begins with the hind legs and progresses cranially. There will be no rectal tone seen when taking the animal's temperature. The speed of the progression of the disease is dose related. It may cause sudden death, be peracute, acute or even chronic. Mortality can be as high as 90%. In the early stages, the animals will have an unusual stilted gait. Clinicians should note that pyrexia and a loss of sensibility are not features of the disease. Confirmation of the disease is difficult as demonstration of the toxin is difficult. There is no useful specific treatment.

Cervical injury

This will occur as a result of fighting in groups of adult rams. When mixing rams they should always be penned up in a tight bunch for 48 h so that they cannot reach a speed fast enough to cause severe trauma when head butting.

Fibronecrotizing pachymeningitis

This condition is rare and is normally caused by *Arcanobacterium pyogenes*. WCC and rectal temperature are raised. The treatment is with antibiotics and is often effective.

Heartwater

This condition is caused by *Rickettsia ruminantium*. It is transmitted by the larval or nymph stages of two species of tick, *Amblyomma hebraceum* in South Africa and *A. variegatum* in the rest of Africa south of the Sahara and the Caribbean. The incubation period is approximately 2 weeks. The sheep initially are lethargic with a fever before showing neurological signs. They bleat continuously and will be seen to be constantly moving their tongues. They will circle before collapsing into convulsions and death. Treatment with oxytetracyclines in large doses is often successful provided that the animal has not deteriorated into convulsions. See below under 'Diseases of the Circulatory System', 'Diseases of the cardiovascular system' for further information.

Listeriosis

This is mainly a disease of silage-fed sheep. However, clinicians should be aware that sheep will contract listeriosis if they graze grass contaminated by sheep which have been fed silage. Affected animals will show marked depression and may circle. They will often show a raised rectal temperature. As well as treatment with antibiotics, steroids are extremely useful. The latter should be given as dexamethasone at 1 mg/kg every other day in the morning im. See also above under 'Neurological diseases of unweaned lambs' and below under 'Neurological diseases of goats' and 'Eye conditions of older sheep and goats'.

Maedi-Visna (MV)

In sheep flocks, it is usually only when over 50% of the flock has become infected that clinical signs of this disease – caused by *Visna/ maedi virus*, a *Lentivirus* – become evident. The virus is spread through colostrum and milk from an infected ewe to its own lambs or to fostered lambs, particularly soon after birth. It can also spread from the respiratory tract in the form of aerosol droplets, but it only travels very short distances in the air so very close contact, i.e. nose to nose contact, is required between animals. It is likely that the disease is spread between ram and ewe as the virus has been found in the male reproductive tract. In milking sheep, the virus can be spread at milking with a machine by back flow. It can definitely be spread on contaminated needles. Trans-placental infection has been recorded but is extremely rare, so advantage of this can be taken to salvage unborn lambs from infected ewes. Infected ewes can be detected through blood testing before clinical signs are seen and, it is hoped, before the disease has spread. There is no treatment. Culling all animals with a positive result on blood testing is the way forward.

Scrapie

Scrapie is a primary spongiform encephalopathy of sheep and goats which has been recognized in the UK since the mid-18th century. In sheep and goats the disease has been notifiable in the UK since 1 January 1993, and was known then to be widespread. In endemically infected and genetically susceptible flocks it was also known to be an important cause of economic loss. The disease originated in Spanish Merino flocks, and spread widely in Europe and North America. Although it was on occasions introduced to Australia and New Zealand, prompt identification and slaughter of imported sheep has kept these countries scrapie free.

The disease will be manifest in individual animals over 2 years old. Clinical signs are non-specific and variable. Any adult animal showing neurological signs, particularly excessive scratching, should be a suspect case. The pathognomic sign is lip nibbling when the back is scratched. Some cases will show incoordination and abnormal behaviour which will get steadily worse over a period of weeks. In younger sheep, the clinical signs come on quicker. If euthanasia is carried out, it should be done chemically and not by shooting as the head and ultimately the brain are required for histological confirmation of the disease.

Blood samples in EDTA (normally a purple top Vacutainer) for genetic examination may point to the disease, particularly in pedigree flocks with familial relationships to other cases. In the UK, the blood samples should be sent to the Virology Department of the Central Veterinary Laboratory in Surrey. The scrapie monitoring scheme in the UK is moving rapidly towards eradication of the disease.

It is now known, for example, that the incubation period of scrapie is controlled by one major gene with two alleles. Recent research has also shown that scrapie prions can be demonstrated in sheep saliva up to at least 20 months before clinical disease is seen in sheep. This is likely to be the same in goats. Prions can be detected in the milk of sheep long before clinical signs are seen. This also is likely to be the same in goats. So although the monitoring scheme is working well in the UK, it may have to be adjusted to reflect this recent research.

There is an increased incidence of scrapie in the offspring of affected ewes which may in part be due to the transmission of infection from mother to offspring. A breeding policy which aims to decrease the genetic susceptibility of the population should decrease the incidence of scrapie and removing the offspring of scrapie-affected animals from affected flocks could contribute to the control of the disease as well (Hoinville *et al.*, 2010). Furthermore, scrapie control policies based on selecting animals with a scrapie-resistant genotype (*ARR/ARR*) for breeding can be used without the loss of genetic polymorphisms from sheep breeds (Nodelijk *et al.*, 2011).

Within the past decade, other scrapie-like conditions in sheep – Nor98, or atypical scrapie – have been reported in many parts of the world (Dawson *et al.*, 2008). In the UK, the vast majority of such cases have been identified by active surveillance via the abattoir and surveys of fallen stock following the introduction of sensitive immunoassays for prion protein (PrP) detection. Compared with classical scrapie, atypical cases have a different pattern of brain PrP deposition. Sheep are also older in atypical cases. Both types of scrapie show a change of temperament, but with classical scrapie the cases show a fine body tremor which is not seen in atypical cases. There is ataxia with both types of scrapie, but atypical cases sometimes show circling. Loss of condition is shown by both types of scrapie too, but classical cases commonly show pruritus, usually with a scratch reflex, whereas this is not a consistent sign with atypical scrapie.

Spinal abscess

Affected sheep slowly become ataxic. They are mentally alert and have a raised WCC. If they are pyrexic, antibiotics may be helpful. Animals showing an increased level of protein in a CSF sample are not likely to recover and euthanasia is indicated.

Neurological diseases of goats

Border disease

Congenital border disease is seen in kids born alive following *in utero* infection. The kids will show the typical nervous tremor but the hairy coat seen in affected lambs is not a feature (see above under 'Neurological diseases of neonatal lambs').

Caprine arthritis encephalitis (CAE)

This disease is caused by a retrovirus (*Caprine arthritis encephalitis virus*) which is part of the *Lentivirus* family. It is a slow virus with a long incubation period and is very similar to the virus that causes MV in sheep. In fact, there is compelling evidence that there is cross-species transmission. CAE is primarily a disease of dairy goats. It is not a large problem in fibre-producing goats and certainly is not a problem in meat-producing goats. Clinically, the arthritis manifestation of the disease is seen in adults and is the most common and important aspect of the disease. The virus causes severe neurological signs in kids between 2 and 4 months of age and these are progressive. The kids are ataxic with hind-limb placing deficits which progress to paralysis, with the forelimbs also involved. There is marked depression with a head tilt progressing to opisthotonos, torticollis and paddling. Euthanasia is the only course of action.

The virus is spread through colostrum and milk from an infected doe to its kid or to fostered kids, particularly soon after birth. It can also spread via the respiratory tract in the form of aerosol droplets, but it only travels very short distances in the air so very close contact – probably nose to nose – is required. Venereal spread is a possibility. In milking goats the virus can be spread at milking with a machine by back flow. Trans-placental infection has been recorded but this is extremely rare. Adult goats can develop a progressive interstitial pneumonitis, which will be manifest as a chronic respiratory disease with weight loss. The animals appear alert and are not anorexic. Mastitis may be the most important clinical manifestation of the disease. Infected goats can be detected through blood testing before clinical signs are seen and before the disease has spread.

Cerebrocortical necrosis (CCN)

This condition, which is of obscure aetiology, causes progressive neurological signs. It can occur in all ages of goat but is more common in growing kids. The aetiology is considered to be usually associated with the proliferation of excess populations of rumen bacteria which produce thiaminase, an enzyme which destroys thiamine (vitamin B_1), and thereby reduces its availability to the goat. The conditions that favour thiaminase-producing bacteria are unclear and it is likely that the various feeds affect rumen flora differently. Outbreaks occur more commonly in housed animals fed concentrates, but can also arise at pasture. Recently weaned kids are particularly at risk.

Affected goats eventually become recumbent with opisthotonos. Even at this stage, effective treatment is possible with iv injections of vitamin B_1 (thiamine). These injections, together with supportive therapy, may have to be continued for several days. Sometimes goats will lose their sight. However, even this may be restored with treatment. See also above under 'Neurological diseases of growing lambs'.

Listeriosis

The most common sign is encephalitis. It is seen early in the course of the disease. The head is turned and tilted to one side, with the neck held stiffly. The goat becomes more incoordinate and will start circling. All the muscles of the head and neck will be flaccid so that the eyelids and ears will droop. The tongue will protrude and so saliva and rumen contents will drool out as swallowing is impaired. This will be followed by recumbency, opisthotonos, convulsions and death. Abortions will occur in what appear to be healthy goats. They will also occur in cases of encephalitis and septicaemia. Vaginal discharge from metritis after abortion is common. Keratoconjunctivitis may occur in animals which appear healthy in all other respects.

Treatment needs to be carried out early in the course of the disease. The drug of choice would be trimethoprim/sulfadiazine given in high doses iv. High doses of tetracyclines given iv may be equally as effective. Supportive therapy should include NSAIDs and, if severe, intravenous fluids. The keratoconjunctivitis should be treated with sub-conjunctival injections of 20 mg dexamethasone and atropine sulfate in each eye. The disease in goats is nearly always associated with feeding spoilt grass or maize silage.

See also above under 'Neurological diseases of unweaned lambs' and 'Neurological diseasess of adult sheep', and below under 'Eye conditions of older sheep and goats'.

Scrapie

Classical scrapie but not atypical scrapie is seen in goats (see above under 'Neurological diseases of adult sheep', 'Scrapie').

Swayback

This is often called enzootic ataxia and may not be directly comparable with swayback in lambs (see above under 'Neurological diseases of neonatal lambs'), although both the congenital form and delayed swayback (see above under 'Neurological diseases of unweaned lambs') may occur. Kids may be born normally and show no clinical signs for 6 months. Forelimb weakness and anaemia may suddenly be seen. Very low copper levels will be found in the blood and in liver samples at post-mortem. The typical histological signs of lack of myelination of the CNS will also be found at post-mortem. Angora goats seem to be particularly susceptible.

There is no treatment for swayback. Kids may survive if they are not severely affected.

Copper deficiency may be actual deficiency or may be brought on by an excess of molybdenum or sulfur. Black goats will show bleached hair, as in cattle when they are copper deficient. They will also show harsh coats and angora goats will show the classic 'steely' coat as seen in sheep. In addition, copper-deficient goats will have diarrhoea. Blood tests on these animals will show a marked anaemia as well as low plasma copper levels.

Conditions associated with the eye of neonatal lambs and kids

Congenital cataracts

These can occur from a genetic defect in both lambs and kids. They can be as a result of border disease infection. There is no treatment. Often just one of a twin may be affected with genetic cataracts and the condition will not be recognized until weaning as the semi-to-totally blind animal manages to use its twin as its eyes.

Microphthalmia

This is usually a genetic defect. It has been recorded in Kerry Hill sheep, South Down sheep and Texels. It can occur in older sheep and goats as a result of a vitamin A deficiency.

Split eyelid syndrome

This is seen in the upper eyelid. It is a genetic defect linked to the four-horned gene. It is seen in Jacob and Jacob cross Suffolk sheep, and also in Hebridean and Manx Loghtan sheep. The syndrome is rarely seen in Norfolk horned sheep and Soay sheep. It is extremely rare in four-horned goats.

Trauma

This occurs at parturition when a lamb or kid with its head back has been handled roughly at delivery. It may occur when there is a 'hung lamb', i.e. a lamb which has only its head out of the vulva and the ewe has been in labour for some time in brambles or some other thicket. The eyes should be bathed and antibiotic eye ointment should be applied.

See also 'Entropion' under 'Surgical Conditions of the Neurological System' (Chapter 6).

Eye conditions of older sheep and goats

Blindness without obvious ocular involvement

There are many conditions which could be included in this classification e.g. pregnancy toxaemia, CCN and a space-occupying lesion in the brain. It is also reasonable to include progressive retinal atrophy (PRA) which is often termed 'bright blindness'. In reality, PRA does affect the eye as the retinal damage can be seen with an ophthalmoscope. It is a symptom of bracken poisoning. Affected sheep have a high head carriage and high stepping gait. The condition is irreversible. There is no treatment. It is not seen in sheep less than 2 years of age.

Excess lachrymation without ocular disease

This occurs with fly irritation. Foreign bodies should always be suspected in the individual case with a single eye affected. Clinicians should bear in mind that if there is poor husbandry, e.g. poor placement of hay racks, there may be more than one animal affected. If the eye has only recently been affected, it should be irrigated with a human eyewash preparation; these are supplied in polythene bottles so some pressure can be applied. If the lesion is long standing any foreign body will have become incorporated into the inflammatory reaction. In this case, the eye should be anaesthetized with local anaesthetic solution and the foreign body should be removed very carefully with fine forceps. Antibiotics should be instilled into the eye.

Tumours of the eyelids are quite common. They normally are squamous cell carcinomas of the third eyelid. These have a good prognosis if they can be removed before the tumour has invaded the conjunctiva. Surgery is straightforward as the eyelid can be removed with a pair of scissors under anaesthesia.

Haemorrhage is minimal and suturing is not required. A haemangioma of the third eyelid may occur but these are rare. Papillomas of viral origin will occur on the eyelids as well. These should not be treated as they will regress spontaneously.

Excess lachrymation with ocular disease

INFECTIOUS KERATOCONJUNCTIVITIS　This is the most common infectious ocular disease of sheep. It is called 'pink eye' in the UK and 'contagious ophthalmia' in other parts of the world. The cause can be either *Mycoplasma conjunctivae* or *Chlamydophila psittaci*, or it may be a combination of both. Sheep can get ocular disease in outbreaks of abortion caused by *C. psittaci*. Equally, *C. psittaci* can be isolated as a cause of the abortion and there is no ocular disease. There is no doubt that there is a crossover infection between sheep and goats as *C. psittaci* occurs in wild sheep and goats which act as a reservoir for the infection throughout the world. It is possible that deer may be the reservoir in the UK. Other bacteria causing the disease may be opportunist pathogens; these include *E. coli*, *Branhamella ovis* and *S. aureus*.

Regardless of the cause of the disease, it always shows a sequential pathogenesis. As many animals are likely to be affected, the clinician will see all the phases at one time. Initially there will be inflammation of the sclera, blepharospasm and an increase in lachrymation. This will lead to corneal inflammation and opacity. There may or may not be corneal vascularization. Lastly, there will be corneal ulceration. Treatment is with antibiotic eye ointment. It is important that corticosteroids are not instilled at the same time. Antibiotics may also be given parenterally. Oxytetracyclines are ideal as they appear in the tears and have long-acting formulations. To help reduce the pain and the inflammation, NSAIDs can be given parenterally.

LISTERIOSIS　This condition can affect the eyes and cause conjunctivitis with excess lachrymation when animals are suffering from systemic disease. It will also cause the specific ocular disease of uveitis. This is commonly called 'silage eye', as it is linked with the feeding of silage in round bale feeders. Careful examination with an ophthalmoscope will reveal a uveitis. The best treatment is a sub-conjunctival injection of 0.5 ml of 2% dexamethasone and 0.5 ml of atropine. If treatment is going to be carried out by shepherds, both of these drugs can be given as eye drops. In this case, treatment should be carried out daily for 3 days. See also above under 'Neurological diseases of unweaned lambs', 'Neurological diseases of adult sheep' and 'Neurological diseases of goats'.

TRAUMA This is likely to be self-mutilation from an irritant condition such as sheep scab, facial eczema or photosensitization. Obviously, it is important to treat the underlying cause as well as the ocular condition.

YERSINIOSIS *Yersinia pseudotuberculosis* is a significant cause of ocular disease in goats (Wessels, 2010). It will present as a sudden-onset mucopurulent ocular discharge, blepharospasm, moderate-to-marked chemosis and conjunctival hyperaemia, with corneal opacity and neovascularization. Diagnosis is by direct culture of swabs. Treatment is with parenteral tetracyclines.

Metabolic Diseases

The predominant signs

- Recumbency
- Anorexia
- Rumen stasis
- Neurological signs

Diagnosis

The age of the animal is important, as metabolic diseases normally affect adults. The history taken needs to include the state of pregnancy (if any), particularly the eminence of parturition. Any change in nutrition or other cause of stress should also be noted. The clinical signs should be observed and a blood sample should be taken before treatment. This can be stored if the clinician is certain of the diagnosis and only analysed if treatment is not successful.

Hypocalcaemia

In sheep, even in dairy sheep, this is a disease of late pregnancy prior to parturition and seems to follow a stressful experience. In goats, it is a disease which occurs after parturition. The rectal temperature will be low. By definition the blood calcium levels will be low. Obviously, samples should be taken before treatment. However, treatment should not be delayed by waiting for results as a positive response to treatment with calcium borogluconate is diagnostic. Ideally, a 50 kg animal should receive 3 g iv. This will be accomplished by injecting 75 ml of a 20% solution. The effect will be rapid, with the animal returning to normality within a couple of hours. Treatment by sub cut injection will be effective but will take longer, i.e. 12 h or overnight.

Hypocalcaemia can occur as a result of the ingestion of certain plants. In plants that contain oxalates, the oxalates rapidly bind the blood calcium and cause hypocalcaemia with the normal signs as described above. Plants that do this in the UK include fat hen (*Chenopodium album*), rhubarb (*Rheum rhaponticum*) and sugarbeet (*Beta vulgaris*) tops. In other parts of the world, plants that cause hypocalcaemia (with similar signs) include: in the tropics, buffel grass (*Cenchrus ciliaris*); in North America and Mexico, greasewood (*Sarcobatus vermiculatus*); and in Australia, soft roly-poly (*Salsola kali*).

Hypomagnesaemia

This condition is rare in sheep and very rare in goats. Magnesium, which is readily available in most feeds, needs to be both ingested daily and absorbed daily. If the transit time is too rapid through the bowel then there will be insufficient absorption. Although lush green grass is a very good source of magnesium, it causes a rapid transit time of ingesta through the bowel and so can provoke hypomagnesaemia. If blood levels of magnesium are low then any stress will cause the signs, which are neurological. Sternal recumbency is rapidly followed by lateral recumbency and convulsions. The heart rate is raised and so is the rectal temperature. There is frothing at the mouth and rapid eye movement. The legs will paddle.

The sex of the animal is not relevant, although it is possible that the condition is more common in entire adult males. Certainly the condition can occur in pregnant and lactating animals. In temperate climates, it is a condition of the spring and autumn. This is due to the likelihood of lush grass at these times and the very changeable weather, which may act as a trigger. Diagnosis can be made based on clinical signs and confirmed by low magnesium blood levels. In the dead animal, a presumptive diagnosis can be made by low magnesium levels in the aqueous humour.

Treatment is rarely successful if the animals are convulsing. Although blood magnesium levels can be restored to normal, there is usually irreparable brain damage. Treatment can be attempted. It should consist of a *sub cut* injection of 50 ml of 25% magnesium sulfate (up to 100 ml can be given to a large animal). It is important that this drug is given sub cut as it will cause death if given iv. It is prudent to give other supportive treatment, e.g. a mixture of 20% calcium borogluconate, 5% magnesium hypophosphite and 20% glucose given sub cut, coupled with NSAIDs.

Ketosis

This is commonly called twin lamb disease in sheep, or pregnancy toxaemia. It occurs during the last weeks of pregnancy and is often related to a twin pregnancy, as the name suggests. It is the most important metabolic disease in sheep, but is rare in goats. The trouble actually starts before tupping. In the UK, ewes are given access to good grass after weaning and become too fat. They are unable to use this fat, and it is deposited in the liver and causes ketosis. A raised level of ketones will be found in the serum. If the ewes undergo a stress – even just having multiple lambs *in utero* may be sufficient, they will develop pregnancy toxaemia. They will be anorexic and depressed, and this will quickly lead to recumbency, bruxism and the classic star gazing carriage of the head.

Treatment is often unrewarding unless instituted immediately the first signs are seen. It should consist of iv injections of 50 ml of 40% glucose solutions three times daily and oral high energy drenches. Injections of NSAIDs iv are beneficial. Some authorities advise inducing parturition with injections of dexamethazone. In the author's experience, this is rarely good therapy as it often results in the deaths of both the ewe and the lambs, as these are often not viable.

The more common form of ketosis seen in goats is 2–3 weeks after kidding. This is equivalent to acetonaemia in dairy cows, and is more common in dairy goats. If ketone levels are very high the goats will show neurological signs. These are relatively mild, with the goat walking with its head excessively raised and with starry eyes. The animals rarely become recumbent but will certainly be hyperaesthetic. Treatment is straightforward as dexamethazone can be given at 1 mg/kg in non-pregnant does. High-percentage glucose drinks will also be helpful.

Diseases of the Respiratory System

Non-infectious conditions of the upper respiratory tract

Chondritis of the larynx

This condition is mainly seen in rams, particularly Texels. The main signs are respiratory distress and a loud snoring noise. The rectal temperature will remain normal. The lungs are difficult to auscultate. The animals remain quiet and normal.

Prompt treatment with antibiotics, e.g. oxytetracyclines and dexamethasone, will cure the disease. Ideally, a long-acting preparation of oxytetracycline and dexamethazone should be injected every second day for five treatments. If treatment is delayed, the inflammation of the larynx can be reduced but the noise will continue. Certain cases may be caused by *Actinobacillus* sp. These should be treated with twice daily injections of streptomycin for 5 days. Even when they are making a loud snoring noise, the rams can still serve normally.

Collar trauma

This is seen in tethered goats if they are attacked by carnivores. Normally the collar trauma is the least of the goat's problems. Clinicians should examine the neck carefully for bite wounds.

Nasal foreign bodies

These are extremely rare and are normally grass seeds. If they are in a rostral position they will cause a unilateral nasal discharge. If they are in a more caudal position they will cause a bilateral nasal discharge. Removal is extremely difficult.

Nasal tumours

These are very rare. The most common are polyps or adenopapillomas. These can be removed if they are large and near the nasal orifice. If they cannot really be visualized and cause a nasal discharge, that will cause a problem with diagnosis. A pragmatic approach would be to treat the sheep for nasal myiasis (see below under 'Infectious diseases of the upper respiratory tract') and antibiotics. If the tumour is a squamous cell carcinoma the condition will deteriorate rapidly and euthanasia will be the only option.

Infectious conditions of the upper respiratory tract

Enzootic nasal adenocarcinoma

This condition is caused by a retrovirus. The tumours form on the mucosa covering the turbinates. The condition is not found in the UK or in Australia and New Zealand. It is principally found in South Africa and also has been seen by the author in Kenya. Diagnosis is mainly on clinical signs of a chronic seromucous nasal discharge. There is a PCR available which can be used on the discharge but not on serum. There is no treatment or vaccine available.

Nasal leeches

These are found in northern India. The causative species is *Dinobdella ferox*. These leeches invade the nostrils causing sneezing and a bloody nasal discharge. Systemic ivermectins are ineffective, although if instilled up the nose they are said to effective and the leeches are expelled within a few hours.

Nasal myiasis

This is caused by the sheep bot fly, *Oestrus ovis*, which attacks sheep and goats. The adult fly deposits larvae around the nostrils. These invade the nasal cavity and develop into second-stage instars which invade the sinuses in the head. The mature larvae are sneezed out up to a year later. The infestation is easily treated with ivermectins and rarely causes problems.

Retropharyngeal lymph node abscesses

These abscesses are caused by *Corynebacterium pseudotuberculosis*. Owing to the proximity to the carotid artery, euthanasia is advised.

Rhinitis

This is a rare relatively mild condition which occurs in weaned lambs. The causative bacterium is *Salmonella arizonae*. There is a transitory nasal discharge. The condition is self-limiting and it is probably better not to give antibiotics. In goats, the condition can be caused by *Caprine herpesvirus* and there will be a purulent nasal discharge leading to more severe systemic signs. This is rare in North America and is not found in the UK. Bacterial rhinitis can occur in goats but is normally linked with *Pasteurella multocida* pneumonia.

Non-infectious conditions of the lower respiratory tract

Aspiration pneumonia

This is also called inhalation pneumonia. It may be seen in several animals in flocks which have been drenched by an inexperienced shepherd.

Ruptured diaphragm

This is an exceptionally rare diagnosis but the condition can occur. In theory, a diagnosis can be made in the live sheep with ultrasonography and surgery could be performed.

Squamous cell carcinoma

These are seen in goats as secondaries in the lungs. The clinical picture will be similar to tuberculosis (TB). Euthanasia should be carried out.

Thymomas

These cause diverse clinical signs which include respiratory distress, ventral oedema and a marked visible jugular pulse. In some animals, the only sign will be wasting. There is no treatment.

Winter cough

This is a rare condition seen in goats that is caused by an allergic response to fungal spores in hay and straw. In acute cases, treatment can be attempted with clenbutorol injections given iv. Further treatment can be given orally at 0.5 g/10 kg. The only real cure is for the goat to be kept outside permanently and never given hay or straw. If the goat is inside, dust-free environments using shavings and silage might be successful with dedicated management.

Infectious conditions of the lower respiratory tract caused by viruses

Ovine parainfluenza 3 (OPI3)

OPI3 virus infects 10–12 week old lambs. The clinical signs are mild with a short duration of pyrexia and a serous nasal discharge. The ewes are normally asymptomatic but will show mild interstitial pneumonia.

Ovine pulmonary adenomatosis or Jaagsiekte

This is a bronchoalveolar carcinoma caused by a retrovirus. It is seen clinically in sheep from 2 years of age. Animals will appear not to thrive. They remain bright and continue feeding even though they become hyperpnoeic and lag behind the rest of the flock. Fluid progressively accumulates in the lungs and can be heard on auscultation. There is often secondary *M. haemolytica* infection which may well kill the animals. Diagnosis can be made earlier by the 'wheelbarrow' test. The hind legs of the sheep are raised and then fluid will pour out of the sheep's nose (Fig. 5.2). There is also a reliable PCR diagnostic method. There is no treatment.

Infectious conditions of the lower respiratory tract caused by bacteria

Contagious caprine pleuropneumonia (CCPP)

This notifiable disease in the UK is still seen in Africa and the Middle East. The disease causes 100% morbidity and often over 75% mortality. It is caused by *Mycoplasma capricolum* subsp. *capri-pneumoniae*. The disease is species specific and only occurs in goats.

Histophilus somni

This can be found as a sole pathogen in sheep and goat pneumonia. It may also cause other problems, namely epididymo-orchitis, metritis, meningoencephalitis and mastitis.

Mannheimia haemolytica

This is a major cause of bacterial pneumonia, either as a primary or secondary infection. In the majority of combined infections, it is presumed that the other respiratory pathogens involved disrupt the lung's protective mechanisms and predispose the animals to a secondary *M. haemolytica* infection. The source of the infection is usually carrier adults, although the organism can survive in the environment, on grass or bedding, and in water. Outbreaks normally occur in fattening lambs, but indoor lambing ewes can be affected.

Often, the trigger factor can be difficult to pinpoint as it takes up to a month for the outbreak to occur. Housing is obviously one of the main predisposing causes, but movement from a hill environment to a fattening lowland situation can be the trigger. Weather changes

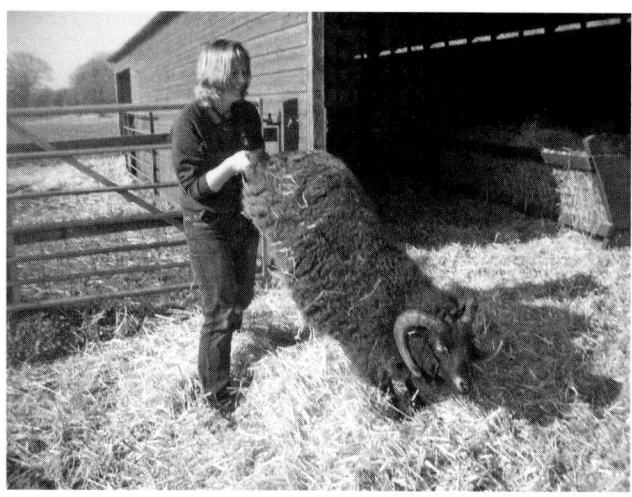

Fig. 5.2. The 'wheelbarrow' test in a sheep.

may play a part too. The chill factor is very important. On hills with rocks and deep heather the lambs can get shelter. On arable land, when fenced away from the hedgerows there is a marked chill factor. Animals may be found dead or vigilant shepherds may pick them out in the early stages of the disease when they have a high temperature and a nasal discharge. Coughing and an ocular discharge can also be a feature.

Treatment with antibiotics, especially more modern ones developed for cattle, can be rewarding if the disease is caught early enough. Morbidity can reach 40%, with a figure of half that for mortality, so blanket antibiotic treatment should definitely be considered. NSAIDs will help affected animals and will also decrease the number of chronically affected animals. Vaccination with two doses of vaccine must be carried out before possible outbreaks but the logistics of this are difficult for shepherds with hill lambs. *M. haemolytica* infection may occur secondarily to a mycoplasmal infection.

Mycoplasmas

Mycoplasmas are found in sheep throughout the world, but they alone do not seem to be able to cause pneumonia. The most common is *Mycoplasma ovipneumoniae*, but *M. argininii* and even *M. bovis* may also be found. These may cause severe respiratory disease in goats (Rifatbegović *et al.*, 2011). They all appear to cause subclinical disease and require the presence of *Mannheimia haemolytica* to cause clinical disease. In turn, a trigger factor, e.g. transport, mixing or markets, is required. It should not be forgotten that mycoplasmas have a definite role in other syndromes such as keratoconjunctivitis, polyarthritis and mastitis. The mastitis maybe linked with 'contagious agalactia', which is a notifiable disease in the UK.

Pasteurella multocida

This bacterium can cause pneumonia in fattening lambs and young goats. Treatment is the same as for *M. haemolytica*. *Pasteurella* vaccines do not confer immunity in goats. In contrast, vaccinating goats against clostridial diseases is very important. It is just the 'P' combinations that should be avoided (i.e. clostridial vaccines to which a component has been added for the control of *Pasteurella* pneumonia). Angora goats seem particularly prone to *Pasteurella* pneumonia.

Tuberculosis (TB)

TB is rare in sheep and is usually an incidental finding at slaughter or at post-mortem examination. An outbreak in the UK with clinical signs has been described by one author (van der Burgt, 2010). There was chronic weight loss seen in 10% of a flock of 220 Lleyn sheep. *Mycobacterium bovis* was isolated from three carcasses. As a diagnosis of chronic wasting disease with possible respiratory signs in sheep, TB should not be overlooked.

Goats also get TB (Quintas *et al.*, 2010). The most commonly affected organs are the lungs, so goats will show respiratory signs. Normally these signs will be chronic, as well as chronic weight loss. The respiratory signs may turn into acute respiratory distress if a tubercle bursts in the lungs. Goats can be infected with cattle TB (*M. bovis*) and human TB (*M. tuberculosis*), and have recently been 'awarded' their own TB (*M. caprae*). It is also possible that caseous lymphadenitis (CLA; see below under 'Diseases of the Integument', 'Bacterial skin diseases', 'Caseous lymphadenitis (CLA') may make goats more susceptible to TB (Sharpe *et al.*, 2010), so practitioners should be careful not to miss dual infections.

TB in sheep and goats is a notifiable disease in the UK.

Infectious conditions of the lower respiratory tract caused by parasites

Parasitic pneumonia

This can be caused by the lungworm *Dictyocaulus filaria* (a parasitic nematode) in young sheep and goats, normally in the autumn. Severe signs and deaths are very rare. There is a strong immunity generated so that *D. filaria* is rare in adult animals. The lungworms are effectively killed by ivermectins. Two other lungworms, namely *Protostrongylus rufescens* and *Muellerius capillaris*, are seen normally as an incidental finding at slaughter or post-mortem. They can cause respiratory distress and weight loss in lambs and are sensitive to ivermectins. Lungworm larvae may be seen using the Baermann technique. The intermediate stages of the tapeworm, *Echinococcus granulosus*, will occur as 'hydatid cysts' in sheep lungs. These are normally asymptomatic.

Diseases of the Circulatory System

Diseases of the cardiovascular system

Heartwater

This disease is caused by the rickettsia *Ehrlichia ruminantium*. It occurs in sheep and goats in Africa south of the Sahara. It also occurs in the Caribbean, and in the tropical areas of North and Central America. It is a tick-borne disease and so its distribution is linked to suitable vectors, which are *Amblyomma* spp. On the whole, acute heartwater occurs 2–4 weeks after new sheep or goats move into a tick-infested area. They will show a high fever and acute respiratory signs, which may be due to the cardiac symptoms. Pericarditis may be heard on auscultation. Convulsions then precede inevitable death, with mortality as high as 90%. However, there may be a less acute form of the disease with a fever from which animals will recover without developing neurological signs. Diagnosis is difficult in the living animal.

Treatment is tetracyclines ideally given iv initially, followed by im injections at 10 mg/kg. It is advisable to inject long-acting tetracycline preparations at 20 mg/kg to all the animals that have been exposed to the infected ticks. Naturally, all the animals should be treated to remove ticks and prevent reinfestation.

Poisonous plants

Foxgloves (*Digitalis* spp.) and oleander (*Nerium oleander*) are the most common poisonous plants to cause cardiac signs in the UK. Different plant species are responsible in other countries.

Rupture of the aorta

This occurs in sheep and goats that harbour the nematode *Spirocerca lupi*, which is found in tropical areas of Asia. The parasite lives in nodules in the aorta. On rare occasions, the blood vessel will be weakened so that it ruptures. A similar parasite, *Onchocerca armillata*, has been found in India. This extremely rarely causes rupture but it is often associated with chronic blood loss and anaemia. Injections of ivermectins are an effective treatment.

Schistosomiasis

This is caused by a trematode parasite that lives in blood vessels; as such, they cause a variety of different signs and symptoms. These parasites occur throughout the tropics but are also found in central Asia, the Middle East and the Mediterranean. They mainly live in the mesenteric and portal veins and so they cause diarrhoea, dysentery, anaemia, emaciation and death. The pulmonary form on infestation causes respiratory signs. Oral praziquantel at 25 mg/kg is an effective treatment if repeated at weekly intervals for a minimum of 5 weeks.

Vegetative endocarditis

This occurs in small ruminants. If the tricuspid valve is affected the condition is called right-sided heart failure. There will be ascites, peripheral oedema and a marked jugular pulse. If the bicuspid valve is affected the condition is called left-sided heart failure. There will be oedema of the lungs which will show as a dull area in the ventral thorax. The animal will have a cough and a raised resting pulse rate. Clinicians should remember that dropped beats are normal in sheep and goats. Animals should be treated for at least 2 weeks with antibiotics, which may be effective.

Diseases affecting the haemopoietic and lymphatic systems

Babesiosis

This is caused in the UK by a tick-transmitted protozoal parasite of the red blood cells called *Babesia motasi*. The main sign is haematuria. Diagnosis can be confirmed by identification of the parasite in Giemsa-stained red blood smears.

Theileriosis

Theileria ovis and *T. recondite* cause this disease. These are tick-borne protozoa which initially infect the lymphocytes, followed by the erythrocytes. They have been isolated from sheep in Wales, UK, but have not been associated with disease.

Tick-borne fever

This is a sheep tick-borne disease caused by infection of white blood cells (WBCs) with the rickettsial organism *Anaplasma phagocytophilum*. Goats can harbour the infection but very rarely show any signs. Sheep will show pyrexia and malaise within 24 h of infection. This will last for 3 weeks and renders the animals more susceptible to concurrent secondary viral and bacterial infections. There are antigenic variations, so often no immunity is established. Lambs cannot be protected by colostral antibodies. Naive pregnant ewes moved into infected areas may abort and rams may be infertile.

The disease can be avoided by bringing the ewes out of the tick-borne area to lamb. The ewes and lambs can then be returned after being treated with an effective pour-on to prevent tick infestation/reinfestation. Diagnosis can be made by seeing the *A. phagocytophilum* inclusion bodies in the cytoplasmic vacuoles of monocytes and neutrophils in Giemsa-stained blood smears. PCR and ELISA tests will be available soon.

Diseases of the Urinary System

Medical conditions of the urinary tract

Nephritis

This can occur in sheep and goats. The presenting sign will be general malaise and low-grade abdominal pain. It is rarely painful enough to be termed colic.

Nephrosis

This is a distinct clinical entity in young lambs 2–4 weeks of age. They will stop sucking and yet appear to be thirsty as they will stand over the water supply. The cause is unknown. There is no treatment.

Tumours of the urinary system

The most common tumours found in sheep and goats are in the bladder and are related to eating bracken. Highly malignant adenocarcinomas are very rarely seen in the kidneys of sheep and goats.

Diseases of the Reproductive System

Abortion and its causes

Clinicians should advise their clients to isolate and mark animals which abort. Then either the clients should submit fresh placentae and aborted fetuses, or clinicians should submit abdominal fluid and abomasal fluid in a sterile manner to a laboratory to obtain a diagnosis of the cause. Owners should adopt the following procedure when dealing with an abortion:

1. Immediately isolate an aborting animal.
2. Ear tag and record which animals have aborted on which date to help with possible blood sampling for serology later on.
3. Remove all cleansings and fetuses.
4. Contact their practitioner to discuss which samples to collect for laboratory diagnosis.
5. Not foster female neonates on to aborted mothers.
6. Not allow any pregnant women anywhere near the aborting animal, the products of abortion or owners' overalls.

Akabane

This condition is caused by an *Orthobunyavirus* (*Akabane virus*) which is insect transmitted and causes congenital abnormalities in the CNS of sheep and goats. It is spread by biting midges in Australia, Japan, Kenya and Bahrain. The lambs and kids will show pulmonary hypoplasia and hypoplasia of the spinal cord. A presumptive diagnosis can be made on the basis of these gross pathological signs and can be confirmed by testing the sera of unsuckled affected offspring and their dams for serum-neutralizing antibodies. There is no specific treatment for affected animals. There is a vaccine available in Japan.

Border disease

This disease is caused by a *Pestivirus* very similar to that causing bovine viral diarrhoea (BVD). It can occur at any stage of pregnancy. The disease should be suspected if live lambs are born showing the pathognomic signs of a hairy coat and trembling. Shepherds call the lambs 'hairy shakers'. These signs are not shown by infected kids. Other than abortion, the ewes and does show no other signs. A precolostral blood sample taken from an affected neonate is the diagnostic sample of choice. Affected neonates may be BVDV antigen positive, or BVDV antibody positive and antigen negative. BVD vaccines have been used but there is no evidence of their effectiveness in sheep or goats.

Brucellosis

The main *Brucella* species to cause abortion in sheep and goats is *B. melitensis*. *B. ovis* is the species that is linked to sheep and causes infertility in rams but is not associated with abortion. Both species occur in East and southern Africa, as well as in the Middle East. There is a vaccine available against *B. melitensis* but it is not licensed in the UK.

Cache valley virus

The disease caused by this mosquito-transmitted bunyavirus causes infertility, abortions and stillbirths in sheep in Mexico, the USA and Canada. By the time the sheep has aborted it is no longer infective. The disease occurs as abortion storms and then appears to die down for several years. Diagnosis is by paired blood samples which show a rising titre. There is no vaccine or treatment available.

Campylobacteriosis

Campylobacter usually enters a group of sheep or goats through a carrier animal which could be another mammal or a wild bird. The mothers pick up the infection from aborted fetuses, placentas or birth fluids. Abortion occurs 1–3 weeks after infection, often in large numbers. Once an animal is infected, she will develop a lifelong immunity to the disease and an abortion storm is very unlikely to recur in the same group in the following year. There is a vaccine available to protect against campylobacteriosis but it is not very effective and so farmers have to rely on strict hygiene and biosecurity when dealing with aborting animals. Oxytetracycline injections help reduce the abortion rates in does but not in ewes.

Caprine herpesvirus

This virus not only causes abortion but also vulvovaginitis and balanoposthitis. It is spread venereally but only to goats (not sheep). It is a virus of growing importance in southern Europe as it links with *M. haemolytica* and causes fatal respiratory disease in young kids. In adults, the main signs are related to the vulva. There is swelling and there are also erosions of the mucosa. A bloody discharge turns in 2 days to a pus-containing discharge. Bucks show erosions on the prepuce and a discharge. Abortions tend to occur in the first year that a herd has become infected. There is now a reverse transcriptase PCR (RT-PCR) test to help with diagnosis.

Concurrent disease

Any disease which causes a high temperature is likely to cause an abortion. Multiple abortions will occur in any group which is infected with a highly contagious or infectious disease, e.g. FMD or BTV.

Enzootic abortion of ewes (EAE)

Enzootic abortion of ewes is caused by ovine strains of the zoonotic microorganism *Chlamydophila abortus* (formerly *Chlamydia psittaci*) which exhibits a predilection for placental tissue. It also causes abortion storms in goats. The infection is most commonly introduced into a clean flock by an animal carrying an asymptomatic enteric infection. Normally, abortion occurs in the last 3 weeks of pregnancy. There will also be stillborn full term and weak neonates born. Dead fetuses will appear to be normal but there will be necrosis and thickening of the cotyledons and the rest of the placenta. Diagnosis is relatively straightforward from impression smears from affected areas of the placenta.

The main period for the mother to become infected is in the eleventh to fourteenth week of pregnancy; the animals then abort 5–6 weeks later. The numbers of abortions can be greatly reduced if the mothers can be given long-acting tetracycline injections at 20 mg/kg every 2 weeks during this period. The best method of control is vaccination a month before mating. The risk of human infection is real for pregnant women and so hygienic precautions should be taken.

Leptospirosis

The only really specific pathogen causing this disease is *Leptospira interrogans* although many other *Leptospira* spp. have been found in aborted fetuses or placentas as opportunist pathogens. Goats are affected by the cattle bacterium *Leptospira* serovar Hardjo.

Listeriosis

This is primarily a neurological disease. However, the causative organism, *Listeria monocytogenes*, can cause abortion at any time during pregnancy. Abortion will usually occur approximately 7 days after infection. The organism can be found in the placenta or the fetus.

Neosporosis

The causative organism of this disease is *Neospora caninum*, which is very similar to the causative organism of toxoplasmosis (*Toxoplasma gondii*). It is primarily a condition of cattle and dogs rather than sheep and goats. *N. caninum* can be differentiated from *T. gondii* by FAT.

Nutritional causes

Certain mineral deficiencies, e.g. of iodine or selenium, will definitely cause abortion, but general malnourishment does not.

Q fever

Q fever is caused by the obligate intracellular rickettsial organism: *Coxiella burnetii*. It is distributed worldwide. The disease is a zoonosis and is much more common in goats than in sheep. It is not common in the UK but there was a recent severe outbreak in goats in the Netherlands. When an animal becomes infected, Q fever can be shed via a variety of secretions, including faeces, urine and uterine fluids in particular, and in milk. Once an animal is infected, the organism can be shed for several weeks or months, and shedding can occur at two successive parturitions. There is a vaccine available but this is not licensed in the UK.

Rift Valley fever (RVF)

Rift Valley fever virus is spread by *Aedes* spp. mosquitoes, which are not found in the UK but causes abortion in sheep and goats in Africa, mainly south of the Sahara, and in Egypt. There are massive abortions storms approaching 100% when the virus hits a naive pregnant flock or herd. It also causes deaths in lambs and kids, which may die within hours. The main sign is haemorrhages and congestion in all the mucous membranes. Some orifices may even drip blood. Diagnosis in the live animal can be confirmed by virus isolation, agar gel immunodiffusion (AGID), the complement fixation test (CFT) and quantitative real time RT-PCR (qRT-PCR). Control is carried out by vaccination.

Salmonellosis

In sheep this is caused by a specific *Salmonella* serotype: *S. abortus ovis*. This pathogen has been found in other places in northern Europe but not in the rest of the world. Abortions in sheep, and in goats, can be caused by other *Salmonella* species/serovars as well, namely *S. arizonae*, *Salmonella* serovar Dublin, *Salmonella* serovar Montevideo and *S. typhimurium*. These abortions occur worldwide. These bacteria may be the actual cause of the abortion, i.e. the organism will be found in the aborted placenta or fetus, or they may cause abortion by the associated pyrexia. The abortions may also cause deaths and morbidity may be high. Abortions caused by *S. abortus ovis* rarely cause clinical disease. There is no specific treatment or vaccination available. *Salmonella* spp. are zoonotic organisms.

Sarcocystosis

There are various *Sarcocystis* spp. found in sheep throughout the world, of which the most commonly reported is *S. tenella*. The most commonly reported species in goats is *S. capricanis*. *Sarcocystis* is a cyst-forming coccidian in carnivores, mainly in dogs, which are the definitive host. The sheep and goat are intermediate hosts. The role of the organism in abortion in sheep and goats is far from clear. Massive infections will cause severe illness with a high fever and abortion. Death may follow, but most infections are low and cause no clinical signs.

Schmallenburg virus (SBV)

The disease caused by SBV is an *Orthobunyavirus* which does not normally cause abortions but rather deformed lambs and kids at birth. Often, one of a twin will be normal with the other having gross deformities. SBV is thought to be spread by midges but there is a possibility of spread from animal to animal.

Sporadic abortions

The two most likely causes of sporadic abortions are *Bacillus licheniformis* and *A. pyogenes*. Rare isolates of *Staphylococcus* and *Streptococcus* spp. are also found in aborted fetuses. Extremely rarely found are *Yersinia* spp., *F. necrophorum*, *E. coli* (Vero toxin producing) and *Pasteurella* spp. Lastly, a variety of fungal organisms have been found but their significance is often in doubt.

Streptococcus pluranimalium

This organism has been isolated from the placenta of an aborted lamb (Foster *et al.*, 2010) and from a full-term lamb dead from a dystocia problem. The inference is that the organism may have been responsible for the abortion as no other pathogen was isolated. It has been isolated from the tonsil of a goat but has not previously been associated with abortions in small ruminants.

Stress

The part played by stress in causing abortions is very confusing. Clinicians should be very careful in blaming stress for an abortion storm in a flock of sheep. An infectious cause is very much more likely and strenuous efforts should be made to take adequate samples from the aborted lambs and their placentas so that a confirmed diagnosis is made. Stress from vaccinating heavily pregnant animals for clostridial disease is possible. Heat stress may cause abortion, and is likely to occur in late pregnancy in housed animals which are over-fat. It does not seem to be a problem in the tropics in animals that are native to the area.

Thogoto virus

Thogoto virus is an orthomyxovirus and was first reported to cause abortion in sheep in Kenya. The virus is spread by the 'brown ear tick', *Rhipicephalus appendicularis*. It is only found in areas where this tick occurs in East Africa.

Tick-borne fever (TBF)

TBF is a rickettsial disease spread by hard ticks. It is not itself the direct cause of the abortion which follows exposure of the susceptible pregnant animal to the infection, but is the result of the biphasic pyrexia alone.

Toxoplasmosis

This zoonotic disease is of major economic importance. It is caused by the obligate intracellular protozoan parasite *T. gondii*, which has a two-stage asexual life cycle which can take place in warm-blooded animals, and a coccidian-type sexual cycle which is confined to the intestine of members of the cat family. It is the domestic cat which is the real zoonotic danger to man. The disease is relevant to sheep and goats in that wild rodents and birds can harbour bradyzoites in tissue cysts within the brain and muscle. In addition, infection in mice can also be passed vertically from generation to generation without causing significant illness, thus helping to maintain a long-lasting reservoir of infection for susceptible cats (Buxton, 1989). The cat is also the main danger to sheep and goats, as cats spread the disease in their faeces as very resistant oocysts which contaminate animal concentrates, fodder and bedding. Infection of the placenta and conceptus occurs only when the initial infection establishes in susceptible pregnant animals, following the ingestion of oocysts. The oocysts encyst in the digestive tract and the released sporozoites penetrate the cells lining the gut so that tachyzoites eventually reach and infect the placenta and fetus.

If this infection occurs before 2 months of the pregnancy the fetus will be resorbed and the animal will appear barren. If the infection occurs between 2 and 4 months then the animal will either abort, or have a stillborn fetus or a very weak neonate. Ewes infected in the last month of pregnancy often have normal full-term lambs. Diagnosis of the condition can be carried out by histopathological examination of the cotyledons.

Once infected, animals have a lifelong immunity. There is a good vaccine available which should be injected into the animals at least 2 weeks before service. If a clinician is faced with a confirmed outbreak, decoquinate can be given orally; to be fully effective it needs to be fed for the last 14 weeks of pregnancy. The most practical manner to get decoquinate into the animals is to have it in a palatable lick; 14 kg tubs are prepared with 4400 mg/kg decoquinate. One tub per seven females will cover a 14 week period.

Congenital and hereditary conditions in goats

Hermaphroditism

True hermaphroditism, when the goat has both ovarian and testicular tissue, is extremely rare, but pseudo-hermaphroditism is relatively common. It is linked with the poll gene in the following goat breeds: Alpine, Saanen, Shami and Toggenburg. Freemartins – when a female which is twin to a male is unfertile – have been recorded but are very rare.

Contagious agalactia

This is found in goats in countries around the Mediterranean and is caused by *Mycoplasma mycoides* subsp. *capri*. As the name suggests, it is a disease of the mammary gland, but it will also cause polyarthritis in kids (Agnello *et al.*, 2012).

It is has not been recorded and is notifiable in the UK.

Mastitis

The most common causative organism of mastitis in both sheep and goats is *S. aureus* which can cause peracute gangrenous life-threatening mastitis as well as subacute and chronic forms. *Streptococcus* spp. are uncommon in mastitis in goats and rare in sheep. *Mycoplasma* spp. are found in goats with mastitis and *M. haemolytica* is found in sheep. *E. coli* and *A. pyogenes* are both found in sheep and in goats. No treatment with either parenteral antibiotics or intra-mammary antibiotics is very effective. In fact, in the author's experience the latter is contraindicated on account of possible teat damage. The normal outcome is the loss of the affected mammary gland. NSAIDs do help in severe cases.

Reproductive disorders in goats

Clostridium septicum *metritis in goats*

This bacterium causes a very serious metritis in goats, which is likely to be fatal. High doses of penicillin should be given iv. The goat should be supported by NSAIDs also given iv. The uterus should be washed out with warm isotonic saline containing crystalline penicillin and then the goat should receive 30 IU oxytocin iv. Goats should be protected by vaccination but care should be taken as some of the polyvalent vaccines do not contain cover for this disease.

False pregnancy in goats

False pregnancy or hydrometra is a unique condition to the goat and is not seen in sheep. It is called a 'cloud burst' and is relatively common, occurring in about 5–10% of females. It can be differentiated from pregnancy by ultrasonography or a blood test for oestrone sulfate after 50 days. There is a persistent corpus luteum, so treatment relies on its regression, which is encouraged by prostaglandin injections. Dairy goat owners do not worry about this condition as the doe will have a rise in daily milk yield without any problems of parturition. On many dairy goat farms there is a surplus of kids, particularly male kids, and therefore kids are not desired.

Maiden milkers

Many young goats from heavy-milking breeds may show udder development and milk production, particularly when they are on a high plane of nutrition. These animals should not be milked unless a maiden lactation is desired. This condition may be self-limiting, particularly if the plane of nutrition is reduced.

Problems with oestrus

Goats are seasonal breeders and come into oestrus when the day length starts reducing. Out-of-season breeding can be encouraged by the injection of pregnant mare serum gonadotropin (PMSG). The expression of oestrus can be quite intense in goats and is often mistaken by owners as pain. Animals will visibly shake and may be very vocal. They make take aggressive action towards humans or other goats of both sexes.

Tumours of the reproductive system

These are extremely rare. Most are benign ovarian stromal tumours. Adenocarcinomas, which are highly malignant, are seen starting in the uterus. The presenting sign will be a foul-smelling necrotic/haemorrhagic discharge. Adenomas will occur extremely rarely in the udder. Granulomatous tissue is common in the udder, but is normally refractive to treatment.

Diseases of the Integument

Inherited skin diseases

'Redfoot'

This condition is restricted to 'Blackface' sheep and their crosses. It occurs in the first few weeks of life. The progressive signs of ulceration of the oral mucous membranes and corneal opacity accompany the loss of hoof horn. Death of the lambs is inevitable and euthanasia is recommended.

Sticky goat syndrome

This is restricted to Golden Guernsey goats. It only occurs in pure-breds not crossbreds. Euthanasia is recommended.

Viral skin diseases

Caprine herpesvirus

The disease of goats caused by *Caprine herpesvirus* might cause confusion as there are lesions on the feet as well as on the lips which look like those of FMD. Both conditions produce vesicles and have a very low mortality. However, unlike FMD, the disease caused by *Caprine herpesvirus* has a very low morbidity. The main problem with this virus is that it can cause a venereal disease by. affecting the vulva and the penis. The main signs in the individual animal disappear in 20 weeks unless there is a secondary infection. Antibiotic treatment is helpful. The disease probably occurs worldwide. It has not been found in the UK but is definitely present on mainland Europe. There is no vaccine.

Caprine viral dermatitis

This condition, which is caused by a poxvirus is rare and restricted to central Asia. The lesions are deep ulcers seen all over the body and are slow to heal. Antibiotics by injection and local creams are used in treatment.

Contagious pustular dermatitis

This is primarily a disease of sheep although it will affect goats. It is perhaps the most important viral skin disease of sheep and is called 'orf'. It is highly contagious and is found worldwide. It is caused by a *Parapoxvirus*. The lesions most commonly occur on the commissures of the lips and muzzle, and occasionally on the feet and genitalia. The initial lesion consists of a number of red papules within which vesicles develop, rupture and form a thick scab. Proliferative changes may then occur resulting in papillomatous lesions. Secondary bacterial infection is common, and in ewes with infected lambs, mastitis may occur. Diagnosis should be clinically straightforward and can be confirmed by virus isolation.

Although the disease is caused by a virus, antibiotics are useful. A blanket dose of a penicillin/streptomycin injection is very helpful. Really bad lesions should be treated with oily creams. Antibiotic aerosols should be avoided as they tend to cause the scabs to harden. When the scabs are knocked off there are large eroded areas underneath. There is a live vaccine available for sheep, but this should not be used in goats as very bad reactions have been reported.

Goat pox

This is caused by *Goatpox virus*, a *Capripoxvirus*. A similar disease (sheep pox) occurs in sheep which is caused by another *Capripoxvirus*, *Sheeppox virus*. Goat pox occurs in Eastern Europe, the Middle East, Central Asia and Africa. It is not just a skin disease and causes a high mortality in young animals. There is a high fever and pneumonia. The skin lesions of pus-filled papules are mainly seen around the mouth and nose. The lymph nodes show painful swellings. There is a vaccine available which is very useful in preventing the spread of the disease. It is possible that there is an insect vector.

Venereal orf

This is a rare condition, which is caused by two viruses. They are the viruses causing contagious pustular dermatitis and ulcerative dermatosis. It is not entirely clear whether the presence of both viruses is required to give signs of the disease. The presence of the bacterium *Fusiformis necrophorus* certainly makes the lesions more severe. Lesions are seen on the vulva and perineum of the ewe and the prepuce and penis of the ram. The disease is called 'pissile-rot' by shepherds in the UK. It appears at mating time and is spread by mating. It can result in a failure to mate, with resultant late service or failure in conception, entailing many barren ewes and a drawn-out lambing period. Often the first sign of venereal orf is when a ram newly put out with the ewes is seen to be off colour. On examination, it will be seen to have proliferative and crusted lesions on the penis and prepuce. When further rams are caught and examined they will be found to have similar lesions but to a lesser extent. All the rams should be withdrawn and examined.

Affected rams should immediately be separated and treated with daily injections of a mixture of penicillin and streptomycin. An initial injection of a NSAID will be helpful. The penis and prepuce should be treated daily using a topical oily cream (a mixture containing benzene hexachloride (BHC) and acriflavin is ideal). The ewes also should be examined and the affected ewes should be separated. Any badly affected ewes should be treated daily with injections of penicillin and streptomycin and topically with oily creams. This process should be repeated in 7 days. The clean rams may then be admitted to the clean ewes. The affected ewes can be allowed to run with affected rams.

Vesicular stomatitis

This is only seen in goats and is caused by a very rare rhabdovirus. It is really only of relevance as it may cause confusion with FMD. There are small vesicular lesions in the mouth causing excess salivation, but no foot lesions. The disease is self-limiting.

Bacterial skin diseases

Actinobacillosis

This will occur in small ruminants. It is normally associated with the head and neck but has been reported on the body in Norfolk in the UK. It is characterized by thickening of the skin with multiple granulomatous swellings often associated with the lymphatics. These swellings are unrewarding to lance as the pus is only in small pockets. The causative organism is *Actinobacillosis lignieresii*. Treatment is daily dosing with streptomycin at 10 mg/kg for 10 days.

Actinomycetic mycetoma

This is a very rare condition found in sheep and goats in Central Asia. There have been two organisms isolated: *Actinomadura madurae* and *A. pelletieri*. The lesions are very similar to those caused by *Actinobacillosis lignieresii* and treatment is also similar Diagnosis is by culture.

Caseous lymphadenitis (CLA)

This is caused by *Corynebacterium pseudotuberculosis*. It occurs in sheep and goats throughout the world. It was first isolated in the UK in 1990 (Baird, 2003) from an importation from Germany. Studies have revealed that all cases in the UK have come directly from that case. Rams tend to show a much higher prevalence of clinical disease than ewes, although there is no evidence to suggest that males are more susceptible to infection than females. Abscesses usually develop in the lymph nodes under the skin but can also occur in internal organs, most commonly in the lungs. Swollen abscessed lymph nodes are easy to see. In sheep, if incised, they take on an onion-like appearance with concentric rings of fibrous tissue and inspissated pus. In goats, they are just filled with soft pasty pus.

The flock or herd can contract the disease through importation of infected animals but can also obtain the disease from contaminated fomites, e.g. clipper blades, sheep hurdles, lorries, etc. Diagnosis can be made on clinical grounds and is confirmed by culture of the organism from an abscess. There is a useful ELISA blood test in sheep. This has not yet been validated in goats. Culling is the only course of action as there is no effective treatment. Total eradication can be achieved (Baird and Malone, 2010). There is a vaccine available but it is not licensed in the UK.

Clostridial cellulitis

This is called malignant oedema and can occur in sheep and goats. However, it is most common in rams as a result of fighting wounds, and has been called 'big head disease'. A variety of *Clostridium* spp. have been isolated from cases, namely *Cl. chauvoei*,

Cl. oedematiens, *Cl. perfringens*, *Cl. septicum* and *Cl. sordellii*. All these organisms are now covered by a licensed vaccine for sheep, which can also be used in goats. The area of swelling is initially hot and painful with crepitus. This then turns cold and gangrenous. Initially the animal has a fever, but this rapidly abates before death.

Diagnosis should be made on clinical grounds and on the basis of smears using fluorescent antibody techniques (FAT). Treatment may be attempted if the disease is caught in the febrile stage. High doses of crystalline penicillin should be given iv together with NSAIDs.

Dermatophilosis

This is called mycotic dermatitis, which is a misnomer as it is caused by the bacterium *Dermatophilus congolensis*. In sheep, the disease is also called 'lumpy wool', and when found on the lower limbs it is called 'strawberry footrot' (see under 'Lameness in adult sheep and goats' in Chapter 6). The condition is manifest as an exudative dermatitis affecting the ears, face and lower limbs of lambs and the back and flanks of adult sheep. In rams, the scrotum may be affected and in ewes the udder. The disease is progressive. It starts with exudation which then crusts and scabs. The initial penetration is facilitated by prolonged wetting of the fleece during periods of protracted wet weather.

Diagnosis may be made on clinical grounds and confirmed by Giemsa stain of the scabs. Treatment in severe cases is with parenteral antibiotics and antibiotic cream on the raw areas.

Fleece rot

This is caused by *Pseudomonas aeruginosa*. Its correct name is necrotic dermatitis. It appears to follow prolonged rainy conditions, particularly within 6 weeks of shearing. Animals can become very ill if the area of the skin affected is large. The diagnosis can be confirmed on culture.

Morel's disease

This is clinically very similar to CLA. The causal organism is *S. aureus* subsp. *aerobius*. It has a shorter incubation period than CLA – 3 weeks, rather than months. The abscesses are not as closely related to the lymphatics as in CLA. The disease has not been seen in sheep but only in goats in Europe (Poland, Germany and France). It has also been seen in Africa and Asia. Antibiotic treatment appears to be ineffective.

Nocardiosis

This disease was first reported in Cambridge, UK (Jackson, 1986). It is very rare in the UK, though it seems to be widespread in Central Asia. The signs are rows of pus-filled nodules linked with the lymphatics.

Periorbital eczema

This is thought to be a bacterial disease and is likely to be caused by a *Staphylococcus*. The condition characteristically affects the ewe in the final 4–8 weeks of pregnancy. It also occurs in trough-fed goats. The early lesion is seen as a small inflamed and scabbed area on one or other of the bony prominences of the face or, less commonly, on the nose. This usually extends around the eye, hence the name, to give an alarming scabbed, discharging sore. Most cases are self-limiting and do not require treatment, although severe cases may require aggressive antibiotic treatment.

Scald

This is also called benign foot rot in lambs, although all age groups are vulnerable. It mainly occurs in warm moist conditions with animals on lush pastures. The interdigital skin becomes inflamed and painful. Normally there is no separation of the horn or suppuration. Certain strains of *Dichelobacter* (formerly *Bacteriodes*) *nodosus* are probably involved, along with *F. necrophorum* and penicillin-resistant *S. aureus*. Individual cases respond well to antibiotic aerosols. If large numbers of animals are affected then foot bathing in 0.5% zinc sulfate is helpful. This condition, along with various other foot infections, causes lameness (see Chapter 6).

Staphylococcal dermatitis

This may actually be the same condition as periorbital eczema, as it occurs on the face and nasal bones in sheep and goats.

However, it also occurs on the limbs, vulva and prepuce. It is a suppurative condition which takes 4–6 weeks to resolve. The causal organism is a beta-haemolytic *S. aureus*.

Staphylococcal folliculitis

This is a benign condition which affects young lambs and kids. Occasionally, it will affect the udders of ewes and does. The clinical signs are normally mild with small pustules on the lips, muzzle and nostrils. Diagnosis should be made on clinical grounds and can be confirmed on the isolation of a beta-haemolytic *S. aureus*, or histologically as a pyogenic folliculitis with ulceration of the epidermis. The condition will normally resolve without treatment in a few days.

Fungal skin diseases

Aspergillosis

This is a rare disease of goats caused by *Aspergillus fumigatus*. It is found sporadically in East Africa. Sheep running with the goats do not seem to become infected. The condition shows the form of ulcerating nodules in the groin. It is refractive to treatment. As the disease may be contagious, slaughter should be advised. The disease may be diagnosed by culture but false negatives will occur. Histopathology is a safer method of diagnosis.

Cryptococcosis

This is an extremely rare skin disease of goats caused by *Cryptococcus neoformans*. Nodules are seen on the head and they may become ulcerated. The disease is seen in Central Asia.

Malassezia *dermatitis*

This is a confusing condition as *Malassezia* spp. may be isolated from the skins of normal sheep and goats, and can be seen on impression smears stained with a modified Wright's stain such as 'Diff-Quik'. If very large numbers of 'peanut-shaped' yeast organisms are found on diseased skin they may well be significant. The clinical signs will include erythema, scale, hyperpigmentation and malodour. Workers

(Uzal *et al.*, 2007) have reported infection with *M. slooffiae* which was associated with generalized trunk alopecia.

Various baths seem effective, e.g. chlorhexidine, enilconazole, miconazole or selenium sulfide can be used twice weekly for a minimum of 3 weeks and then regularly at weekly intervals until the condition resolves. If there is a trigger factor involved, this will need to be treated at the same time.

Phaeohyphomycosis

This is rarely seen in goats and is caused by a free-living fungus, *Peyronellaea glomerata*. The disease has been recorded in Central Asia but not in the UK. It forms papules and aural plaques on the ears. It appears to be self-limiting.

Pythiosis

This is a rare fungal disease seen in South America in wool sheep. It seems that the causal organism, *Pythium insidiosum*, can only affect the skin of wool animals which are exposed to total immersion in water for some hours. The ulcerated plaques will heal if the animals can be kept dry for 3–4 weeks.

Ringworm

This is a rare condition in wool sheep and fibre goats. It is normally seen on the non-fibre covered areas. On hair sheep and goats it may be found all over the body. The most common causative organism is *Trichophyton verrucosum*, which is normally caught from cattle. Another organism, caught from another animal, is *Microsporum canis* from dogs. The species actually linked to sheep and goats is *Trichophyton mentagrophytes*. In normal animals, the infection is self-limiting in a few months. If treatment is required for special animals, e.g. showing animals, there are tropical fungicides such as natamycin.

Protozoal skin diseases

Besnoitosis

This is a disease of goats in South America. It does not seem to affect sheep. It is caused by the protozoan *Besnoitia caprae*. Diagnosis can only be made from skin biopsies. The condition is refractory to treatment. Euthanasia is advised.

Leishmaniasis

This is seen in sheep in South Africa. It occurs as crusty lesions all over the head. The causative organism (*Leishmania donovani*) can be seen on Giemsa-stained deep skin scrapings. The condition is refractory to treatment and slaughter is recommended.

Sarcocystosis

This is caused by *Sarcocystis capricanis*. It has been reported in Central Asia although in fact it occurs throughout the world. Diagnosis can only be made from skin biopsies. See also under 'Diseases of the Neurological System', 'Neurological diseases of unweaned lambs' above.

Parasitic skin diseases of sheep and goats

Mites

CHORIOPTES CAPRAE   There is some doubt as to whether this mite is a different species from the cattle mite *C. bovis*. Pygmy goats seem to be particularly sensitive to infestations. The mite tends to affect the feet, perineum, udder and scrotum with alopecia, erythema and crusting. Some individual goats are particularly susceptible to infestation and develop a severe hypersensitivity response leading to significant self-trauma and clinical signs. Injectable doramectin or ivermectins do not seem to be very effective. Regular topical treatment with fipronil or pour-on ivermectins painted on to affected areas seems to be the treatment of choice.

DEMODEX CAPRAE   This infestation of goats is very rare but when it does occur it is difficult to cure. It often occurs in immune-incompetent individuals. The mite affects the hair follicles and sebaceous glands. There is alopecia on the face, ears, neck and legs. There is secondary bacterial infection. Treatment should

include antibiotics by injection for several days and topical treatment with amitraz. Amitraz can be toxic so it may be prudent to treat only a quarter of the goat's body on the first day, and then treat the next quarter and so on a 4 day cycle until there is some resolution. A skin biopsy may be required to make a definitive diagnosis.

PSOROPTES CAPRAE   This mite mainly lives in the ears of goats and causes chronic irritation which may lead to aural haematomata in floppy-eared species. The mites are very sensitive to doramectin.

PSOROPTES OVIS   This highly contagious ectoparasitic disease of sheep is called sheep scab. It is highly pruritic and will cause serous exudation and severe debilitation. It is primarily a condition of wool sheep but will occur in hair sheep and goats. Diagnosis can be made from skin scrapings from the edge of the lesions which are examined under low power microscopy. Recently, an ELISA test has been developed so that sheep scab can be detected before signs of infection are shown by the sheep. It is vital that treatment of the whole flock is carried out, together with disinfection of sheep handling equipment. The drug of choice is a single injection of doramectin im at 33 mg/kg. This mite can also occur in goats.

RAILLIETIA CAPRAE   These mites are found in the ears of goats in Turkmenistan. They can be seen with the naked eye as small pinhead-sized dots. However, they are much more clearly visible with a magnifying glass. They do not appear to cause much irritation. Treatment is with injectable doramectin or ivermectin.

SARCOPTES SCABIEI   This mite causes very serious mange in goats. There is acute irritation and formation of papules which turn into crusts. As well as affecting the skin generally, there are excoriations affecting the eyelids, prepuce and vulva. Ivermectin is a more effective antiparasitic treatment than doramectin. Injections should be repeated at weekly intervals for 4 weeks. Antibiotics may need to be injected in serious cases, together with cream containing acriflavin and BHC applied daily to the sore areas.

TROMBICULA AUTUMNALIS These free-living mites attack the legs, the ventral abdomen, the face and the ears in the autumn and cause irritation in both sheep and goats. There are three other genera of free-living mites, namely *Cheyletiella*, *Dermanyssus* and *Tyroglyphus*, which have all been recorded as causing dermatitis in goats.

Flies and other insects

CULICOIDES SPP. Together with *Culex* spp., *Culicoides* spp. will attack sheep and goats in the UK. Apart from causing severe irritation and the risk of self-trauma, they may cause a hypersensitivity reaction. They also spread diseases. Most repellents are not very effective. Diethyl-meta-toluamide (DEET) is effective but only lasts for 6 h.

CUTANEOUS MYIASIS This is often called fly strike and is a debilitating and sometimes fatal condition caused by the feeding and development of fly larvae on the host's dead or living tissues, usually at the skin surface or a body orifice. In the UK, the primary fly involved is *Lucilia sericata* (the greenbottle, a blowfly). Diagnosis is usually very easy following a thorough clinical examination. Maggots may not be obvious on a brief inspection if they have burrowed into the skin. The sheep are restless in the early stages, and then become separated from the rest of the flock. In later stages of the infestation animals become toxaemic, depressed and recumbent. Death soon follows.

If more than a third of the skin area is involved the prognosis is hopeless. To treat the condition, the area around the lesion should be clipped to gain access to the wound. The margins of these areas often contain clusters of unhatched yellow eggs, which should be removed. The clipping will disturb the maggots which can then be scraped away. BHC and acriflavin cream is then applied. Deltamethrin should be applied to the other areas of the fleece. Broad-spectrum antibiotics and NSAIDs should be given and continued for 3–5 days as necessary. The hydration status of the patient should be considered too; oral fluids may be required. If the animal is recumbent and toxic, the prognosis is hopeless so euthanasia is necessary on welfare grounds.

The condition should be prevented by good farm management, which is just as important as the use of chemicals in the prevention of strike. Blowfly strike in meat and dairy goats is not as common as in wool sheep. It is very common in angora goats and other fibre-producing goats. It is vital, therefore, in these breeds that preventive measures as described for wool sheep are carried out. Fly strike will normally occur in goats when there is a wound. However primary strike has been reported in temperate countries and commonly occurs with screw worms in tropical and subtropical countries.

LICE Sheep can be infested with biting lice, *Damalinia ovis*, and with sucking lice, *Linognathus ovillus* and *L. pedalis*. Biting lice are more commonly found on the fleece areas. Sucking lice are usually confined to the hairy areas and are more commonly found in hair sheep. The goat biting louse *Bovicola caprae* is very common in all goats worldwide. It is host specific and causes pruritus and major hair loss.

Infested animals should be washed in synthetic pyrethrins, e.g. deltamethrin, cypermethrin or permethrin. Modern 'louse powders' are rarely effective unless applied weekly for several applications. Angora goats are affected by *B. limbata* and *B. crassiceps*. These biting lice cause severe fleece damage and are very common. Goats also suffer from infestations of sucking lice; *L. stenopsis* is found in temperate areas and *L. africanus* in Africa and other tropical areas. Sucking lice suck blood and in large numbers can cause severe anaemia. They are easily controlled with injectable ivermectins.

MELOPHAGUS OVINUS *M. ovinus*, or sheep keds, are wingless flies 5–7 mm long with six legs. They cause irritation in a similar manner to lice. They should be treated with synthetic pyrethrins.

PRZHEVALSKIANA SILENUS This is the goat warble fly. It only attacks goats and not sheep. It is found in Central Asia but is no longer common as it is sensitive to ivermectins. The eggs are laid on the legs of goats. The larvae hatch and when still very small, burrow into the skin. They migrate through the goat increasing in size to pop out through the skin on the back.

PULEX IRRITANS   This flea attacks humans in the UK. When humans live in very close proximity to goats this flea can be a problem, not only to man but also to goats. It can cause severe anaemia in goats, with chronic hair loss. Goats can develop a flea sensitivity. The fleas should be removed from the goat using synthetic pyrethrins, and the goat treated with antibiotics by injection and, if the skin is very inflamed, by corticosteroid injections. The skin should be treated with cream containing acriflavin and BHC to aid healing and prevent fly strike.

TICKS   In the UK, ticks only occur on sheep in certain areas, but there are concerns that their numbers are increasing and that their distribution and competency to transmit disease are changing, partly as a result of changes in climate and in land management (Sargison and Edwards, 2009). Only three species of tick readily infest sheep in the UK and they are all hard ticks: *Ixodes ricinus* found in many heath and hill areas; *Haemaphysalis punctata*, found in southern England and coastal Wales; and *Dermacentor reticulatus*, found in coastal southern England and throughout Wales. In sheep, the ticks usually attach to the head, particularly the ears, neck, axillae and groin. Many thousand may attach themselves to one sheep and cause anaemia. Worldwide, there are many species of hard and soft ticks that will infest both sheep and goats.

Tick control depends on the use of acaricides to prevent infestation. Organophosphate dips are very effective and are used throughout the world, but they are banned in the UK. Diazinon as a plunge dip is licensed in the UK and affords 3–6 weeks protection. Synthetic pyrethrins can be used as pour-ons.

Nematodes

ELAPHOSTROGYLUS RANGIFERI   This worm will affect goats kept in close proximity to reindeer. It is spread by tabanid flies, and causes chronic irritation. Neurological signs have been reported, particularly after ivermectin treatment. The animals normally recover.

PARELAPHOSTRONGYLUS TENUIS   This worm requires the goat to ingest an infected slug or snail, which are intermediate hosts. The main primary host in North America is the white-tailed deer. The deer passes the larvae out in its faeces and these are eaten by snails. Goats may show neurological signs as well as linear crusty lesions in the thorax or abdomen. The skin lesions are cleared with avermectins but the neurological signs are normally fatal.

STEPHANOFILARIA SPP.   These helminths are spread by biting flies and cause a pruritic crusting dermatitis on the face and necks of goats. They are very rare. *S. kaeli* is reported in Malaysia, *S. assamensis* in India and *S. dedoesi* in Indonesia. Ivermectins by injection are effective treatments.

Vitamin- and mineral-related skin diseases

Cobalt deficiency

Animals will have a rough, brittle hair coat or wool.

Copper deficiency

Animals will show ill thrift, diarrhoea, general malaise and even death. Black sheep and goats will have a lack of pigment, and fibre animals will show a lack of crimp.

Iodism

Excess iodine will cause alopecia and scaling in sheep and goats if they are fed foods very rich in iodine, e.g. seaweed over long periods of time.

Sulfur deficiency

This is extremely rare but it has been reported in sheep and goats. It is more marked in fleece animals as fleece biting and alopecia occur.

Vitamin A deficiency

This is extremely rare in sheep and goats. The coat will show a generalized seborrhoea. The main sign is an irreversible retinal atrophy, causing blindness.

Vitamin E deficiency

This is not a real deficiency but rather a vitamin E/selenium-responsive dermatosis. The animals appear healthy and are non-pruritic but are losing their hair.

Zinc deficiency

This is really a zinc-responsive condition. There is marked scaling and crusting. Clinicians should remember that any blood samples for zinc levels must be taken into bottles without rubber stoppers or erroneous results will be obtained.

See also 'White muscle disease' under 'Lameness in lambs and kids' (Chapter 6).

Physical causes of skin disease

Frostbite

This will occur in sheep and goats when they are outside in extreme weather conditions. It is normally the ears which are affected. The skin will slough. The animals should be given antibiotics to prevent secondary bacterial infection and NSAIDs to lessen the pain. Obviously, they should be brought inside until the weather improves.

Photosensitization

This occurs because of the presence of photodynamic substances in the skin capable of causing severe dermatitis in the presence of sunlight. Such agents release energy obtained from the light in hyperoxidative processes harmful to the skin. This may be primary, as a result of a photodynamic agent, e.g. a plant such as St John's wort (*Hypericum perforatum*) or a photosensitizing drug such as phenothiazine, or secondary, owing to impairment of liver function which results in failure to denature chlorophyll and build-up of the photodynamic agent phylloerythrin in tissues. The plant bog asphodel (*Narthrecium ossifragum*) has been implicated in this secondary type of photosensitization.

The clinical signs typically occur in non-pigmented areas of the animals free from wool in sheep and anywhere on hair sheep and goats. Animals should be housed and any severely affected areas treated with oily creams.

Sunburn

This is caused by the harmful effects of ultraviolet radiation from direct sunlight. It can cause problems in newly shorn sheep or shorn fibre goats, particularly in areas where there is no shade. Encrustment of the non-pigmented skin will ultimately cause necrosis of the epidermis, upper dermis and superficial sebaceous glands. Animals should be housed and oily creams applied to the affected areas. Antibiotics and NSAIDs may be required in severe cases.

Trauma

Airgun pellets will cause abscesses, normally on the flank. The pellets may be found when the abscesses are lanced or confirmed quite simply with a rectal linear scanner. Tethered goats will develop tether galls or bell-strap galls. Chronic foot lameness in the front legs will result in excessive kneeling and the formation of hygromas on the carpi. Burn cases will often result in keloids and crusty nodules. There are some more unusual forms of trauma, e.g. attacks by magpies. Shearing wounds are, sadly, rather common.

Toxic causes of skin diseases

Hyalomma *toxicosis*

This occurs sporadically in East Africa. The tick *Hyalomma truncatum* produces a toxin which causes a systemic disease in wool sheep. All the wool falls off, leaving a thickened, reddened skin. Sheep will recover if kept out of the sunlight and given antibiotics parenterally to prevent secondary infection. The sheep should have all the sore areas covered with oily cream before dipping.

Milk toxicity

This will develop in lambs in a manner similar to photosensitization when they are suckling on ewes that are suffering from hepatic toxicity as a result of eating certain poisonous plants, e.g. sacahuista or beargrass (*Nolina* sp.).

Neoplastic conditions

Benign cysts

These occur in the wattles or in the salivary glands.

Malignant tumours

These may occur in the skin anywhere on the body. Histiocytomas, lymphosarcomas, malignant melanomas and squamous cell carcinomas have all been recorded. The latter occur in the conjunctiva, on the third eyelid, on the penis and on the vulva. Melanomas are not restricted to white sheep or goats. They can occur in animals of other colours. They are particularly malignant in the pigmented areas of Suffolk sheep.

Tetragenic dental cysts

These are seen on the faces of goats.

Thymomas

These will occur in goatlings and are normally benign.

Thyroid gland tumours

These are benign and have no relationship to iodine deficiency.

Tumours of the skeletal system

Bone tumours are exceptionally rare in sheep and goats. They may be seen as a metastasis of a melanoma. Tumours of the cartilage of the ribs are not that unusual. Subcutaneous fibromas and fibrosarcomas may occur in rams around the horns or even in polled animals.

Skin diseases of uncertain aetiology

Pemphigus foliaceus

This causes a diagnostic challenge for the clinician. It is an autoimmune-mediated disease. Bacteria, fungi and even parasites may well be found as secondary invaders. If the skin condition persists after treatment for these conditions, the practitioner should suspect pemphigus. It can be confirmed by a biopsy. Pemphigus is very common in pygmy goats. The main presenting signs include a generalized severe pustular eruption involving most of the body.

Treatment is difficult as all of the secondary bacteria, fungi and parasites have to be removed before regular steroid treatment is carried out. In theory, dexamethazone should not be effective if given orally but that has not been the author's experience. The dose is 2 mg/kg of dexamethazone given orally every other morning throughout the summer in temperate countries. Normally, the condition calms down during the winter months only to flare up again in the spring.

Wool slip

This condition is associated with winter shearing. It seems to affect animals in poor condition. There may be a link with either low copper levels or secondary low copper as a result of high molybdenum levels. This alopecia is non-pruritic and the underlying skin appears normal. There is no treatment. The condition can be prevented by raising the nutritional level at times of stress, i.e. changing the time of shearing/housing.

Common Causes for Sheep and Goats to be Found Dead

Iatrogenic causes of sudden death

Sudden death is a misnomer. In reality, sudden death usually means that death has occurred since the animal was last seen. The owner will very rarely see an animal die. It is even rarer for the clinician to see death. Sadly, when such deaths do occur it is usually at the time of veterinary treatment. The likely causes of these iatrogenic deaths in sheep and goats are shown in Table 5.1.

Table 5.1. A list of possible iatrogenic causes of sudden death in sheep and goats.

Anaphylaxis from administration of medicines
General anaesthesia
Lumbar/sacral collection of cerebrospinal fluid or administration of epidural
Massive haemorrhage (this could occur at parturition where there is no human involvement)
Intra-arterial injection
Intravenous (iv) injection
Sedation (particularly iv xylazine injection)

Reasons for animals to be found dead

True sudden deaths are very rare. Possible causes of such deaths in sheep and goats are shown in Table 5.2.

Table 5.2. A list of the causes of sudden death in sheep and goats.

Cast on the back
Chemical poisons
Clostridial disease
Drowning (may occur at dipping or in deep water)
Electrocution (shearing when wet)
Hypomagnesaemia
Lightning strike
Poisonous plants
Ruptured uterine artery
Snake bite
Trauma (mainly fighting in rams, rare with fighting billy goats)

6

Sheep and Goat Surgery

_____

Introduction

The chapter starts with a discussion of the basic procedures used for analgesia, sedation and anaesthesia in sheep and goats. This is followed by an account of surgical conditions and procedures which is organized by system, highlighting any differences between sheep and goats. The first three systems covered are the gastroenteric tract, the neurological system and the urinary system. The reproductive system is then discussed in two separate sections: the first is devoted to the female reproductive system, and includes accounts of parturition, dystocia and associated conditions and surgical procedures; the second looks at the male reproductive system. The locomotory system and the integument are covered next. Lastly, there is a brief section on euthanasia.

Analgesia and Sedation

Sheep and goats are very sensitive to xylazine although this is the sedative of choice. Butorphanol is a good analgesic and can be given at 0.1 mg/kg. Longer term analgesia can be maintained with nonsteroidal anti-inflammatory drugs (NSAIDs), although there are none of these licensed for sheep or goats in the UK. However, NSAIDs licensed

for cattle can be used under the cascade principle (see Chapter 2). With good restraint, analgesia and accurate local nerve blocks, sedation can be avoided. Caesarean sections and other emergency reproductive surgical procedures are certainly best performed without sedation. Goats are very sensitive to lidocaine hydrochloride, normally in a 2% solution, and the maximum dose of 6 mg/kg should not be exceeded, i.e. 30 ml for a 100 kg goat. This is a much smaller dose than used in sheep. Great care with placement of the local block should be taken to give local anaesthesia without overdosing.

Anaesthesia

General anaesthesia

General anaesthesia (GA) in adult sheep and goats is not a safe procedure. There are dangers of regurgitation of rumen contents and resulting inhalation. There is also a risk of bloat, either during anaesthesia or during recovery. The safest method is to premedicate with 0.1 mg/kg of xylazine im. After 10 min, ketamine can be given at 0.2 mg/kg iv. This will give approximately 20 min of anaesthesia. The sheep or goat should be kept in sternal recumbency. The author has never had need of longer anaesthesia in emergency situations in either sheep or goats. With all ages of goat, practitioners should be aware of the danger of hypothermia in anaesthetized goats, and an assistant should constantly monitor rectal temperature. The safest method to warm a goat is to use hot water bottles under dry blankets.

Regional anaesthesia

Epidural anaesthesia

The normal site used by practitioners for the administration of an epidural is the sacrococcygeal space. A 3 cm 20 G needle should be used at a very shallow angle and 1 ml of 2% lignocaine should be injected; 0.1 ml of 2% xylazine may be added to lengthen the duration of the anaesthesia. This anaesthetic is very useful for replacing uterine or cervical prolapses.

Lumbosacral epidural anaesthesia should only be attempted after suitable training (Fig. 6.1). It gives sufficient anaesthesia for a variety of surgical procedures, e.g. Caesarean sections (where it is particularly useful if there are uterine adhesions from a previous Caesarean), fracture repair of the hind limbs and joint flushing. The downside of lumbosacral epidural anaesthesia is that hind limb paralysis may last for 4 h.

Regional anaesthesia of the lower limb

A tourniquet is applied immediately above the carpal or tarsal joint. Two small rolls of bandage should be inserted either side of the

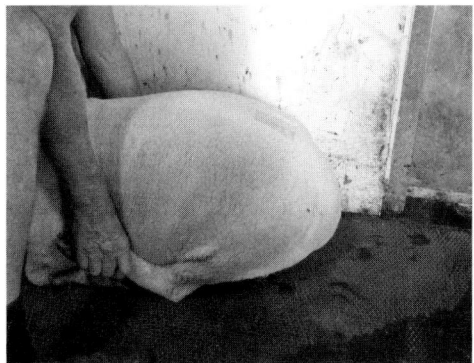

Fig. 6.1. Site clipped for lumbosacral epidural anaesthesia in a sheep.

Achilles tendon when applying the tourniquet to the hind leg. The mid area of the metacarpus or metatarsus should be clipped and surgically cleaned. A suitable superficial vein should be selected. Using a 2 cm 21 G needle, 5–10 ml (depending on the size of the animal) of 2% lignocaine should be injected extremely slowly into the vein. Full regional anaesthesia will be achieved within 5 min and will last for over an hour. Anaesthesia will cease as soon as the tourniquet is removed.

Surgical Conditions of the Gastroenteric Tract

Atresia ani

Atresia ani is a congenital condition that may be inherited, but this has not been proven. Normally, the condition is not seen until sometime after birth. The place where the anus should be located will be bulging out and full of meconium. This area should be cleaned and a skin bleb of local anaesthetic should be injected. A small cruciate incision should be then made with a scalpel. No suturing is required. The tetanus status of the lamb or kid should be checked and it should be examined in 48 h to check that patency has been maintained.

Atresia recti

Unlike atresia ani, this condition is often not readily seen and its surgical correction is extremely difficult. Euthanasia is likely to be the kindest and most economic course of action.

Cheek tooth removal

Radiographs should be taken to accurately pinpoint the diseased tooth. This is easier if there is external abscessation as a radio-opaque probe can be inserted into the fistula. If the roots of the upper molars, i.e. the caudal three cheek teeth, are involved there will be no external fistula as the roots lie in the maxillary sinus. In these cases, there will a unilateral malodorous nasal discharge. The clinician will have to study the roots very carefully on oblique radiographs to decide which tooth is diseased. If in doubt, referring the radiographs to a more experienced practitioner or to a human dentist is advisable. Before surgery, antibiotic cover should be given, usually a mixture of penicillin and streptomycin. NSAIDs should also be given and the tetanus state of the animal checked. The animal should be kept standing with a holder astride and holding the head in a normal position. If the animal is fractious, a very small dose of xylazine (0.05 mg/kg, i.e. 0.125 ml of a 2% solution per 50 kg) may be given im.

The tooth to be removed should be examined using a head torch and a gag (see Fig. 6.2). A very small equine dental pick should be used to elevate the gingival mucosa on both the lateral and medial aspects of the tooth. The dental pick should be forced between the tooth and the alveolar socket. Small molar separators should be placed rostral and caudal to the tooth to try to obtain some tooth movement. The tooth should be grasped with a pair of small right-angled molar extraction forceps. A careful, persistent medial/lateral rocking motion should be commenced, and when the tooth is loose it should be elevated using a long pair of artery forceps as a fulcrum. There is no need to pack the alveolar socket as in the author's experience these fill with granulation tissue extremely rapidly. The owner should be instructed to maintain antibiotic cover and pain relief for several days.

Colic

Colic is extremely rare in adult sheep and goats. Pain will be seen in bottle-fed lambs when there is too much gas in the abomasum. Treatment with a solution containing 4 mg butylscopolamine bromide and 500 mg/ml metamizole at a dose of 1 ml/20 kg iv is usually effective.

Fractures of the mandible

These are quite common as a result of vehicle accidents. Wiring under GA is very rewarding (Fig. 6.3).

Incisor removal

This is a relatively straightforward procedure if an incisor tooth is loose. It is quite easy to fracture the root so elevation is worthwhile. Local anaesthetic (1 ml 5% procaine hydrochloride) should be instilled under the mucosa rostral and caudal to the tooth. The clinician must use judgement on whether removal will be a help to the animal or not. Normally, incisors should be left unless they

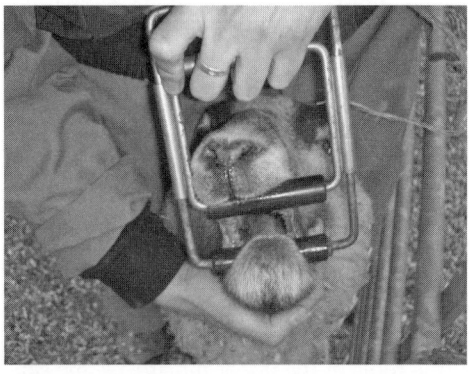

Fig. 6.2. A gag in place for examination (and extraction) of a sheep's cheek tooth.

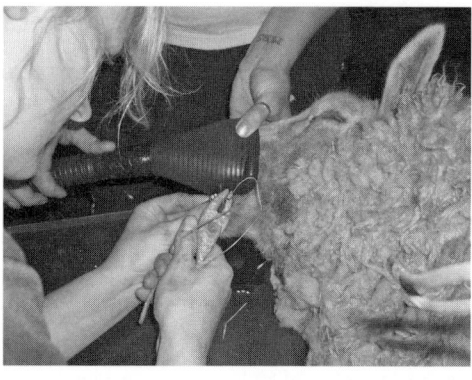

Fig. 6.3. Wiring a fractured mandible in a sheep.

are very loose or much displaced. Sheep can manage remarkably well with very worn incisors (Fig. 6.4).

Intussusception

This can occur in any age of sheep or goat. It is extremely rare. The author has only seen three cases, two in young lambs and one in a neonatal kid, and all of these cases were only seen on post-mortem. Another author (Scott, 2010) has reported two cases in neonatal Texel lambs. The clinical signs started with depression, inappetence/reluctance to suck, abdominal discomfort manifest as an arched back, increasing abdominal distension with gas over several days, and tenesmus with passage of scant mucus containing fresh blood which caused variable staining around the tail and perineum. Frequent painful vocalization alerted the shepherd to the illness. Euthanasia was performed on welfare grounds. The diagnosis was obvious on post-mortem, but would have been very difficult in life. Ultrasonography might have been helpful. Surgery, although possible, would not have been an economic option.

Prolapsed rectum

The causes of this very rare condition are obscure. It has been suggested that homosexual behaviour might be a cause, and it does appear to be more prevalent in rams. Severe coughing caused by lungworm or pneumonia has also been postulated as a cause. The animal should be given antibiotic and NSAID cover, and the tetanus status checked and fly control implemented. With the animal in the standing position, an epidural regional anaesthetic should be given. The perineal area should be cleaned before a purse-string suture is put in place. It is important that this is placed before replacement of the rectum; otherwise the rectum will re-prolapse while the suture is being placed. After replacement of the rectum using plenty of obstetrical lubricant, the purse-string suture should be drawn tight to only allow one finger in the orifice. The animal should be kept on a laxative diet and regularly checked. The suture should be removed in 10 days. In the majority of cases, the rectum will now remain *in situ*. If it re-prolapses, euthanasia is indicated.

Rumen cannularization

This will be required to treat cases of frothy bloat. The wool or hair is removed from the para-lumbar fossa on the left-hand side. A bleb of 2 ml of local anaesthetic is injected under the skin and into the muscles in the centre of the fossa. A 1 cm incision is made with a scalpel in the centre of the fossa. A 'red devil' trocar and cannula is pushed through the incision, through the muscles and into the rumen, all the time keeping the trocar within the cannula. When the phalange of the cannula is flush with the skin, the trocar is removed. Mineral oil can be injected through the cannula to disperse the froth.

Rumenotomy

The indications for this procedure are rare, but include poisoning cases and the ingestion of foreign bodies, e.g. pieces of cloth. The whole of the left flank caudal to the middle of the rib cage should be clipped and prepared for surgery. Using as little local anaesthetic as possible, a 15 cm line block is placed vertically in the para-lumbar fossa. A 15 cm vertical incision is made through the skin and musculature, including the peritoneum, taking

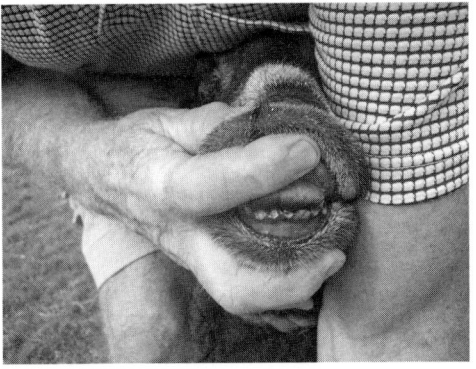

Fig. 6.4. Very worn incisors in a sheep.

care not to incise the rumen. A continuous layer of absorbable sutures are placed around the incision sealing the rumen to the peritoneum approximately 2 cm inside the original incision. A 10 cm incision can now be made into the rumen and the contents removed. The rumen can be closed with a continuous layer of absorbable inverting sutures and the wound closed in the normal manner.

Surgical Conditions of the Neurological System

Entropion

This is the most common eye problem in neonatal lambs. It may go unnoticed by inexperienced shepherds, who will imagine that it has developed slowly. They may think it is 'New Forest Eye'. In fact, it will be present at birth and set up a secondary keratitis, which then develops quite quickly. This is an inherited condition and causes severe welfare problems if it is not treated promptly. Every effort should be made to stop using sires that have the gene.

Often, if the condition is observed at birth, the curled-in eyelid can be immediately uncurled and an entropion will not develop. If the condition is missed, then treatment has to be initiated. Antibiotic eye ointment, provided that no steroid is included, will help but obviously will not influence the long-term disease. The turned-in eyelid needs to be turned out permanently. This can be accomplished in three ways:

1. The simplest method is to inject 0.5 ml of liquid paraffin, an inert oil, into the affected lids; normally there is only one affected lid but often the problem occurs in both eyes. The oil will remain *in situ* for 24–48 h and keep the outside woolly eyelid away from the cornea. If there is keratitis, it will allow the eye to heal and come back to its original size, which will keep the eyelid turned out in its correct position.
2. The second simple treatment is to put a bleb of local anaesthetic under the skin of the eyelid. Then a stitch can be put in to draw the eyelid back. This needs to be placed carefully or a cure will not be initiated. The suture needs to be removed in 48–72 h.

3. The final piece of surgery, which is the best treatment, but a little time-consuming, is to treat the lamb like a dog and carry out a 'cake slice op'. After putting in the local anaesthetic, the area around the eye needs to be clipped and prepared for surgery. A small slice of skin is then removed. The wound is then sutured with fine interrupted simple sutures. The eyelid is then permanently in the correct position. The sutures need to be removed in 10 days.

In kids, entropion is a very rare condition, but the treatment is the same.

Enucleation of the eye

In all cases where there is no chance of the eye condition in any disease or traumatic problem recovering, enucleation should be considered on welfare grounds (Fig. 6.5). This can be carried out under heavy sedation, normally with xylazine. Local anaesthetic should be instilled all around the orbit, not only under the skin but into the deeper tissues, by means of a single very deep injection of 5 ml behind the eye to block the optic nerve. The eyelids should then be sutured together and the whole area clipped and prepared aseptically. A careful incision is then made through the skin parallel to the upper eyelid margin but not entering the conjunctival sac. Using blunt dissection the eye muscles are sectioned around that half of the eye. The same procedure is then carried out to

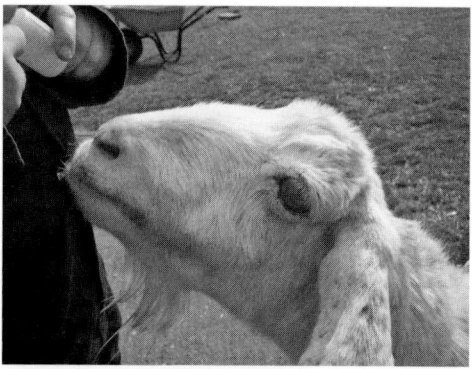

Fig. 6.5. Enucleation should be considered in any case where there is no chance of an eye condition or disease recovering.

the lower half. Eventually a pair of curved scissors can be used to section the optic nerve and the eye can be removed. The remaining socket can then be obliterated with sub-cuticular suturing with absorbable material and the remaining eyelids can be sutured with non-absorbable material. The animal should receive antibiotics and NSAIDs for a minimum of 5 days.

Surgical Conditions of the Urinary System

Congenital and hereditary conditions of the urinary system

Persistent patent urachus

This is usually a congenital condition, as the urachus fails to close at birth. If it occurs a few days after birth it is likely to be as a result of a septic omphalophlebitis. Differentiation is important as the treatment is likely to be different. If the urachus remains patent at birth, it can be ligated immediately. The animal should receive antibiotics for 10 days and its tetanus status should be ascertained. A careful check by the clinician should be carried out in 10 days. Fly control is important. In the event of the urachus not closing with this treatment, or if it has become patent some days after birth as a result of infection, more aggressive surgery needs to be carried out.

The neonate should be anaesthetized and surgically prepared. The practitioner should perform a laparotomy so that the urachus can be traced back to the bladder. It should be sectioned and the bladder closed with a double layer of continuous Lembert sutures of an absorbable material. The umbilical vessels should be ligated proximally to any infected and diseased tissue. This tissue should then be totally removed. The abdomen should be closed with interrupted sutures of monofilament nylon. These should all be laid individually before any are tightened in a 'vest over pants' configuration. When the practitioner is satisfied that there are enough sutures to close the abdomen and that no small intestine is trapped the sutures can be tightened. It is very important that no extra sutures are added after this on account of the danger of perforation of

the small intestine. A sub-cuticular layer of continuous sutures of an absorbable material should be laid before the skin is closed with interrupted horizontal mattress sutures of monofilament nylon. It is important that the animal receives aggressive antibiotic treatment until 10 days later when the sutures, if clean and dry, can be removed. If there is any doubt, they should be left in place and further antibiotic treatment should be given.

Surgical conditions of the male urinary tract

OBSTRUCTIVE UROLITHIASIS Retrograde flushing is impossible. Surgery must be performed as soon as possible to prevent bladder or urethral rupture. If the obstruction is seen in the vermiform appendage, this can be snipped off at its base with a pair of scissors. There are a large number of surgical options described if the obstruction is higher than the vermiform appendage. The author favours surgical tube cystostomy as described by workers in India (Fazili *et al.*, 2010). This is a minimally invasive technique through the left para-lumbar fossa which can be performed in lambs or kids. A catheter is placed in the bladder lumen through a metal cannula and fixed to the skin with a stay suture. The surgery can be performed either standing or in right lateral recumbency. On acidification of the urine, the (causative) urinary crystals are dissolved, leading to the restoration of full urethral patency in successfully treated animals within a few days. No hospitalization is required. The catheter is removed after normal urination occurs. No recurrence of the condition was noted by the workers in a 6 month follow-up.

URETHRAL OBSTRUCTION This may occur in male animals, whether castrated or entire, but it is much more common in the former. Surgical treatments have a poor success rate and have welfare implications, and so preventive measures are very important. Urethral obstruction will quickly turn to bladder or urethral rupture, renal failure and death. Early diagnosis is very important and can be aided by ultrasonography. Scott (2000) states that diagnostic-quality images of the abdomen and bladder of sheep can be readily obtained using a 5 MHz sector transducer connected to a real-time, B-mode ultrasound machine. Normally, the bladder is contained within the pelvis, and therefore cannot be visualized during ultrasonographic examination; a bladder that extends for up to 10 cm or more over the brim is considered an abnormal finding.

Surgical Conditions of the Reproductive System

Surgical conditions of females

Normal parturition in sheep

BIRTH INJURY AND PERINATAL LOSS IN LAMBS   Clinical disorders such as pregnancy toxaemia and, less commonly, hypocalcaemia, can lead to uterine inertia and consequent anoxia of the fetus, which frequently results in stillbirth (Wilsmore, 1989). As well as fetal oversize, malpresentation of the lamb, if it is not corrected carefully and professionally, results in birth injury. Congenital abnormalities such as arthrogryposis may make it impossible for the lamb to be presented in a normal posture for delivery and therefore these cases also suffer injury. Schmallenburg disease virus (SDV) will also cause fetal abnormalities. The amount of input from the shepherd supervising lambing and the level of expertise are also both major factors which influence the incidence of birthing injury.

Oedematous lesions, mainly of the head, are commonly seen following dystocia in cases of malpresentation, e.g. only the head presented with no legs. They are also seen in cases of relative fetal oversize. Oedema formed in this manner is colourless and should not be confused with accumulations of blood-stained extravasations of fluid under the skin and in the body cavities seen in autolytic lambs that die *in utero* before the birth process begins. In the latter cases, fluid escapes from blood vessels and cells whose walls become permeable after death of the tissues. Unlike the birth-injured lambs, all the tissues and the transudates of these latter fetuses display red staining by haemoglobin from lysed erythrocytes

(Wilsmore, 1989). The reasons for these deaths should be investigated by post-mortem and bacteriology. There is a simple method to see if a lamb was stillborn. A piece of lung is removed and dropped into water. If it sinks, this indicates that the lamb has never taken a breath. Conversely, if it floats, the lamb has at least taken a breath.

It is important that shepherds are supplied with all of the equipment listed below:

- arm-length sleeves
- lubricant
- lambing ropes
- a teat for feeding a lamb
- a lamb stomach tube and 60 ml syringe with catheter tip
- dried colostrum
- thermometer
- a marker spray
- 21 G × ½ in. needles for injecting lambs with antibiotics
- 19 G × 1 in. needles for injecting lambs ip and ewes sub cut
- an elastrator applicator and rubber rings
- a pair of sheep hoof trimmers
- a pair of dagging shears

In the UK, the medicines shown below should only be supplied if the farm has been visited within the last year:

- penicillin/streptomycin injectable suspension (see Chapter 2)
- long-acting penicillin injectable suspension (see Chapter 2)
- antibiotic aerosol spray
- 40% dextrose solution
- an injectable NSAID

Induction of parturition in sheep

This is not a common procedure. The major limitation to the technique in sheep is the poor survival of premature lambs and the frequent lack of precise information concerning the stage of gestation of ewes (Ingoldby and Jackson, 2001).

There are only three indications for the induction of parturition: to synchronize lambing in flocks where tupping has been synchronized and lambing dates are known; to aid survival of a pregnant ewe; and to aid the survival of unborn lambs. The most likely reason for the two latter reasons is in ewes with pregnancy toxaemia. Practitioners will have to use their clinical judgement. If the lambs are too premature their survival is unlikely. If the ewe is really sick, the delay of 36–48 h that is involved will result in her death as well as that of the lambs and so an elective Caesarean is a better option provided that the ewe is not more than 5 days from her due date. Dexamethazone given as far before surgery as possible will help dysmature lambs to survive. Corticosteroids are the only reliable medicine for inducing parturition in sheep; a dose of 16 mg of dexamethasone will bring about parturition in a mean of 42 h. Prostaglandins do not bring about parturition in the sheep, and oxytocin will only speed up parturition and not initiate it. Antibiotics should be given with the corticosteroids to lessen the danger of infection likely to be caused by the increased susceptibility to disease.

Dystocia in sheep

A careful history should be taken before any examination takes place, together with various preparations, which include taking account of the answers to the following questions:

- Is the fetus full term or is it an abortion?
- Is there a known infective agent in the flock causing abortions?
- Is the dystocia part of an abortion; if so, extra precautions need to be taken on account of the possible zoonotic problems.
- Is there sampling equipment ready to collect the placenta?
- Has the ewe been scanned for numbers of fetuses?
- Is she a maiden? If not, has she had problems before?
- What is the breed of the sire? This is important in cases of possible fetal oversize.
- Have the fetal membranes been seen? If so, how long ago were they first seen?
- Has there been any interference by the shepherd? If so, how much traction was applied?
- Have any medications been given to the ewe?

The ewe should be given a general examination to see what state she is in.

- Is the sheep bright, depressed, exhausted or suffering from any other condition, e.g. pregnancy toxaemia? It is very important at this stage for the clinician to carry out a risk analysis, as if the animal is very ill or depressed euthanasia must be carried out sooner rather than later on welfare grounds, apart from any economic considerations.
- The body condition score is important as overfat ewes are likely to have large lambs and the pelvis may be obstructed with fat deposits.
- The udder should be checked for the presence of colostrum or mastitis.
- If there is an absence of colostrum this will give an indication of an abortion.
- The perineum and the vulva should be examined for signs of bruising. This will give an indication of the extent of any interference by the shepherd.
- Obviously, any limbs or the head should be examined for signs of oedema. Whether the limbs are forelegs or back legs is important.
- Any ropes *in situ* should be noted.
- Any fetal membranes should be examined for evidence of autolysis.
- The presence of fresh blood, which gives evidence of trauma, should be noted.
- The presence of meconium staining will give an indication of any distress of the lambs.
- An unpleasant sweetish odour will suggest either an abortion or that the lambs have been dead for a few hours, but a putrid smell will indicated that they have been dead for longer than 24 h.

After the general examination described above, a vaginal examination should be carried out, preparatory to any delivery. The procedure is as follows:

- Before carrying out the vaginal examination, the perineum of the ewe should be cleaned. Antibiotics and NSAIDs should be given at this stage.
- Initially, the author uses a gloved hand and obstetric lubricant. However, if

manipulations are required, the glove is discarded and the exposed hand and arm are used after careful cleaning and scrubbing.

- The examination of the cervix is crucial.
- Lack of dilation can indicate that the ewe is not yet ready to lamb or that there is a 'ring womb'. Clinicians will usually be able to distinguish the latter as it will feel harder and show no elasticity. A Caesarean section is the only option in cases of 'ring womb'.
- If the cervix feels normal the ewe should be left for further signs to develop.
- If a rifling effect is felt then this will indicate a uterine torsion.
- If the cervix is dilated, the lamb or lambs will be felt.
- Joint flexion will inform the clinician whether a foreleg or a hind leg is being felt. If there is a combination of legs it is likely that they come from different lambs and twins should be anticipated. If the joints will not flex, this may indicate ankylosis, possibly a deformed lamb or Schmallenburg disease.
- If neither legs nor head can be felt then there is a possibility that a grossly deformed lamb is present. There may be two heads on one lamb or extra legs. There may also be hydrocephalus, anasarca or ascites.
- Schistoma reflexus lambs have been recorded. Clinicians should examine any small bowel presented to see if it is from a lamb or from the ewe.
- Experienced clinicians will be able to differentiate twins and will be able to relate legs to torsos, etc. They will also be aware that twins are much more common than monsters with multiple legs or two heads.
- Normally, if there twins or triplets, they will not be that large so that there is much less likelihood of relative fetal oversize. The latter condition is usually in first-time ewes with a single fetus.
- Occasionally, there may be damage to the pelvis of the ewe which reduces the size of the birth canal and so the fetus will appear to be oversized. A useful yardstick is that if traction cannot be accomplished

by one person pulling with thin ropes wrapped around their hands, then it is likely that there will be severe damage to the ewe.

- Hydrops allantois, or the similar condition hydrops amnion, will appear to be similar. The ewe will be very large in her abdomen but will have a low condition score. When the fetal membranes rupture there will be a massive amount of fluid expelled, up to 10 l. The lamb or lambs will generally be on the small size and be very far back in the uterus.
- Clinicians must always check the uterus after delivery is thought to have finished, to make certain that there is no damage to the birth canal and, more importantly, that there is no lamb left in the uterus.

The positioning of the ewe for parturition is very important:

- In nearly all situations, the ewe is most comfortable standing while an examination or a delivery is being carried out. In this position, pressure is taken off the underside of her spine.
- The ewe is better on her back if she has a ventral hernia or if the lamb's head is flexed under its chest.
- If the ewe is exhausted and is laying in ventral recumbency, it is best to roll her on to her side. This is particularly helpful if there is a leg back and then that can be uppermost. Equally, if the head is back that needs to be on the upper side.
- Certain repositioning procedures require repulsion. This is best carried out with the hindquarters raised. However, this is uncomfortable for the ewe and puts pressure on her diaphragm and so the length of time that she is in this position should be kept to the minimum.

Various factors should be considered in the drawing of the lambs/s:

- Obstetric lubricant is very important. With dead lambs which have become dry the insertion of some powdered 'J Lube' can be very helpful.
- With twins, it is often difficult to decide which lamb should be drawn first.

There are no hard and fast rules. Normally, unless it is very large, if there is a lamb in posterior presentation that should be drawn first.

- Clinicians would be well advised to put ropes on to the two hind legs before drawing the lamb as otherwise, if the lamb gets stuck in the pelvis, it will drown before ropes can be put on.
- If there is a lamb with its head back a small lambing rope should be placed over the head and into the mouth so that the head can be drawn up before there is traction on the legs. Traction should never be applied to the lower jaw of a lamb unless it is definitely dead.
- If the lambs are viable, clinicians should make a decision early as to whether a vaginal delivery is possible, as they will quickly become weak and die. So the decision to carry out a Caesarean must be made quickly.
- If the lambs are dead and putrid, a Caesarean is not an option. Welfare is extremely important and so if in any doubt the ewe should be destroyed.
- In certain instances, an embryotomy is appropriate. It should be remembered that there is no bony attachment of the front legs and so with a rotten lamb these can be removed individually. Then a noose can be put around the head and the rest of the whole lamb can be drawn.
- With viable lambs, it is important that they are revived as they are delivered. Ideally, this should be carried out by an assistant, this allowing the clinician to deliver the next lamb. The nose and mouth of the lamb should be cleared of all fetal fluids. This is easily performed with paper towel. The use of suction may be appropriate, or the lamb can be held upside down to allow drainage. Breathing can be stimulated by rubbing the chest or tickling the nose. Chemicals, e.g. doxapram, may be useful. Hygiene and zoonoses should be considered before mouth-to-mouth resuscitation is performed. There are small plastic pumps available for this purpose.
- After the clinician is 100% satisfied that all the lambs have been removed the ewe should be given 20 IU oxytocin im.

Caesarean section in sheep

The main indication for performing a Caesarean section is where there are live or freshly dead lambs. If there has been considerable manipulation carried out or if the lambs are dead and rotten the ewe should be destroyed on humane grounds unless an embryotomy can be completed without compromise to welfare considerations. Clinicians should be aware that if the ewe is aborting and not full term then there is not the urgency to remove the lambs. In that case, up to 48 h can be given for the cervix to dilate and for the macerated aborting lambs to be passed. Naturally, the ewe should receive antibiotic and NSAID cover. The main indications for a Caesarean section are:

1. failure of the cervix to dilate (so-called 'ring womb')
2. irreducible malpresentations
3. fetal oversize (particularly important if a large lamb is presented posteriorly)
4. fetal abnormalities
5. maternal abnormalities

Some clinicians administer an epidural before surgery to reduce straining. The author does not value this procedure as straining usually ceases as soon as the lambs are removed from the uterus and before stitching is started. Sedation is rarely necessary. The ewe should receive antibiotics and NSAIDs before surgery, and its tetanus status should be checked. It is placed on an operating table on its right side with its head held and its legs tied individually to the table. The wool is shorn from a large area off the left flank. The area is cleaned. Local anaesthesia is instilled in an inverted L block in the lower left paralumbar fossa.

The area then is prepared surgically. A 20–25 cm incision is made through the skin and the muscle layers, taking care not to incise the rumen. Having identified a limb of a lamb through the wall of the uterus, the uterus should be exteriorized, if possible, before it is incised, to lessen abdominal contamination.

The uterus should then be incised as far from the cervix as possible but also without coming near to the ovary. As a rule of thumb, the incision should be from the foot to the hock of the lamb in a hind leg or the equivalent in a foreleg. All the lambs should be drawn out and passed to assistants to be revived. It is vital that a thorough check is made in the uterus to make completely certain that all the lambs have been removed. If the afterbirth can easily be removed, this task should be carried out. If not, it can easily be left in the uterus to be expelled later *per vagina*.

The uterus should be closed with a single layer of uninterrupted inverting Lembert absorbable sutures, making sure that no pieces of placenta are left protruding or included in the suture layer. The ewe should be given 20 IU oxytocin after the uterus has been carefully replaced in the abdomen in its normal position; 5 mega units Crystapen (3 g benzylpenicillin) dissolved in 20 ml of sterile water should be instilled into the abdomen and along both sides of the muscle incision; note that Crystapen is not licensed for farm animals in general, only for horses, but it can be used under the cascade principle. The muscle layers should then be sutured in two layers starting with the peritoneum and the deeper layer of muscle. Closure should be accomplished with a layer of continuous, inverted mattress absorbable sutures making sure that the peritoneum is fully opposed from side to side. The same suturing method should be used for the outer layer of muscle. The skin is then closed with interrupted mattress sutures using a cutting needle and monofilament nylon. After cleaning, the area should be sprayed with antibiotic spray. The shepherd should be instructed to continue with NSAIDs and antibiotic cover for a minimum of 4 further days.

Lamb survival

After delivery of the lambs and their initial revival it is vital that they are looked after properly. The ewe should be treated with all the appropriate medicines and have her udder checked for mastitis, etc. Then she should be allowed to lick the lambs while some colostrum is prepared. Each lamb should be given 100–180 ml of colostrum depending on its weight and then put with the ewe in a warm pen with straw bedding. If the ewe is strong, she should be allowed to nurse her lambs. If a Caesarean or a lambing has been performed at a veterinary surgery, it is vital that the lambs are kept in a warm box until the shepherd takes them home. They should not be left on a cold concrete floor.

Retained placenta in sheep

This is quite a common condition. It is more likely to occur after a difficult parturition, an abortion or an induced parturition. The ewe should be given penicillin on account of its good uptake by the uterus. NSAIDs should also be given. The placenta should be left *in situ* to rot away on its own. If the ewe is pyrexic the uterus can be flushed with 1 l warm normal saline and the ewe can be given 20 IU oxytocin im.

Uterine torsion in sheep

This is an extremely rare condition. It is not actually torsion of the uterus but torsion of the anterior vagina. Normally, there is only a single lamb. Diagnosis is very simple as rifling will be felt on vaginal examination. One authority (Scott, 2011) thinks that diagnosis may not be easy for shepherds and that the condition may be more common than previously thought. He advises that ultrasonography may aid diagnosis, as in some cases the torsion will be a true uterine torsion, i.e. it will occur cranial to the cervix. In the normal presentation of a torsion of the anterior vagina, the history will be of a ewe looking as though she going to lamb but not getting on with parturition.

If there is only 180° torsion, the condition can usually be corrected via the vagina. If this fails, or there is a 360° torsion, the ewe will need to be rolled from a position of lateral recumbency in the direction of the twist. Two people are required to accomplish this manoeuvre. Further vaginal examination will reveal that the torsion has been corrected, but generally the cervix will then be only partially dilated. At that stage, it is not a 'ring womb' but will soon (in 30 min) become one. To avoid this, the cervix should be carefully dilated manually and the lamb should be drawn. Obviously, if the torsion cannot be corrected by rolling, a Caesarean section is indicated.

Normal parturition in goats

Goats will vocalize as the cervix opens during the first stage, and during the second stage as the fetus is delivered. The whole of the first and second stages lasts on average for 2 h. The third stage, expulsion of the fetal membranes, should be completed in less than 4 h. If the fetal membranes are not expelled, that is no cause for alarm if the doe is well, and the membranes can be left to macerate for several days. Antibiotics and NSAIDs should only be given if the doe is ill.

Induction of parturition in goats

Relative fetal oversize is more common in goats than in sheep and therefore induction is often demanded by goat owners who are concerned when gestation lengths have become extended. If an elective caesarean is contemplated induction should be carried out and surgery should be commenced at the start of cervical dilatation. The recommended induction method is a combination of corticosteroids e.g. dexamethazone at 3 mg/50 kg (as a lung surfactant) and prostaglandin at 250 micrograms per 50 kg (to help luteolysis).

Dystocia in goats

The general advice regarding dystocia in the ewe also applies in the doe. Kid survival, retained placenta and uterine torsion, should be addressed in a similar manner.

Caesarean section in goats

Although classically 'ring womb' is a condition of sheep, it also occurs in goats and, together with other birth canal obstructions, e.g. vaginal prolapse and pelvic injuries, it is the most frequent reason for Caesarean section. Relative fetal oversize is more common in goats than in sheep. Malpresentations can normally be corrected, as can uterine torsion.

Fetal monsters are more common in goats than in sheep. Schistoma reflexus has been recorded in goats.

Although some surgeons have used a mid-line approach in goats under GA, the author prefers a left-flank approach with the doe in right lateral recumbency. If possible, sedation should be avoided. Helpers should be warned of vocalization. Before surgery, the doe should be given antibiotics and NSAIDs, and the tetanus status checked. Relaxation of the uterus is not as marked as in the ewe and so the use of a uterine relaxant, e.g. clenbuterol, is indicated. Regional anaesthesia using an inverted L block should be carried out. There is a danger of using too big a volume of local anaesthetic solution, which will give toxic effects. This danger is particularly likely in pygmy goats. In these animals, diluting the anaesthetic solution with sterile water for injection is highly recommended. Goats are very sensitive to hypothermia and so if the procedure is carried out in a cold place extra warmth in the form of hot water bottles should be placed around the doe. The actual surgery is exactly the same as for ewes.

Embryotomy in sheep and goats

In cases where the fetuses are putrid and rotten they will be emphysematous, and the vagina will be dry and swollen. If they cannot be delivered *per vagina*, Caesarean section carries a very poor prognosis and therefore unless a decision is made to destroy the ewe or doe on welfare grounds, a simple embryotomy must be performed. First of all, the ewe or doe should be given antibiotics and NSAIDs and the tetanus status must be checked. If the lamb or kid is in anterior presentation, using a large amount of obstetric lubricant or 'J lube', a rope should be put around one carpus and it should be drawn out as far as possible, and an incision made with a scalpel on the medial side of the leg to allow insertion of a disposable embryotomy knife. The knife should be put up as far as possible to cut the skin up into the axilla and, if possible, over the shoulder joint up to the top of the scapula. With the open hand, all the attachments of the shoulder blade to the chest wall should be broken down while pulling the leg constantly. The whole front leg can then be removed after cutting the remaining skin. This process should be repeated on the opposite side. A rope is then placed on the head and the whole of the rest of the lamb or kid is removed.

In cases of a 'hung lamb', i.e. when the head is out and the legs cannot be felt, it is vital to make 100% certain that the lamb is dead. In these cases the head can be cut off as near to the body as possible to allow the fore-legs to be located and extended. The lamb or kid can then be drawn. If the lamb or kid is alive, it is usually possible to repel the head, after putting a rope over the poll and into the mouth, and locate the legs. It is best if both legs are extended before drawing the lamb or kid. If one leg is in extension and the other is totally back against the body it is normally possible to draw the lamb or kid. Also, if the lamb or kid is in posterior presentation, it can usually be drawn. However, if it is dead and emphyse-matous, an embryotomy may be required. The hocks should be brought caudally and sectioned with embryotomy wire just distal to the hocks. The ropes can then be attached to the hock joint and the lamb or kid can be drawn using a large amount of lubricant.

Prolapsed uterus in sheep and goats

Unlike a prolapsed vagina (see below) this is an emergency and occurs after parturition (see Plate 10). The animal should be secured and given sacrococcygeal epidural anaesthe-sia. The fetal membranes should only be removed if they come away easily. Otherwise, they should be left *in situ*. Antibiotic cover and NSAIDs should be given. If the animal is still standing, the uterus should be elevated and replaced. If the animal is down, an assist-ant is extremely helpful for raising the pelvis, which helps replacement enormously. After replacement, the lips of the vulva should be sutured with a single 'Buhner' suture of uter-ine tape. This is done by inserting a long Seaton needle into the skin at the ventral end of the vulva. The needle is pushed carefully in a dorsal direction subcutaneously and slightly laterally to emerge ventral to the anus. The tape is threaded and withdrawn. This is repeated for the other side of the vulva.

The two ends of the tape are tied with a bow so that only two fingers can be inserted into the vulva. The animal should receive 20 IU oxytocin im. The suture should be left *in situ* for 48 h. Antibiotic cover and NSAIDs should be given for a minimum of 3 days.

Prolapsed vagina in sheep and goats

There are thought to be many factors, e.g. obesity, old age, bulky feeds, steep or hilly ground, hormonal imbalances and mineral imbalances, that raise intra-abdominal pres-sure or increase the laxity of the vagina and its supporting structures, thereby causing this condition. Vaginal prolapse is a condition of the last 2 months of pregnancy (see Plate 11), with most cases occurring in the last 3 weeks of the pregnancy.

All vaginal prolapses should be treated. This may be done in ewes by the shepherd who uses a vaginal spoon, a plastic or stain-less steel T-shaped device. The tongue is inserted into the vagina and the sides of the T are tied to a long piece of baler twine tied around the ewe just in front of the udder. If the case is treated early enough this device is often successful, particularly if it is linked to a leather or webbing harness.

In long-standing cases and in goats vet-erinary intervention is required. With the ani-mal standing, a sacrococcygeal epidural anaesthetic should be administered. After replacing the vagina and cervix the lips of the vulva should be sutured with a single Buhner suture of uterine tape (see above) tied in a bow. The keeper is advised to untie the bow but not remove the suture if the animal is thought to be parturient. If this is the case, the parturition can be completed and the suture removed as the condition should not recur in the non-pregnant ewe. However, if the cervix is closed and the ewe is not lambing then the suture should be retied as the condition will recur until parturition has occurred. Animals should be marked and culled as the condition will occur at any subsequent pregnancy.

Removal of supernumerary teats

This seems only to be a problem in goats. The author has never found them in milking sheep. They should not be removed in goats unless they interfere with milking. In that case, a small amount of local anaesthetic should be injected into the base of the teat to be removed. Practitioners would be well advised to check with the owners to make 100% certain that they are removing the required teat. A pair of small Burdizzo forceps is placed at the bottom of the spare teat and clamped shut. After 30 s they are removed and the spare teat is removed by cutting with a pair of curved scissors along the clamp line. The tetanus status of the animal should be checked and fly control should be implemented.

Reproductive ultrasonography

Ewes and does can be scanned for pregnancy and numbers of fetuses from 45 days onwards. Using calipers, the age of the fetus can be judged fairly accurately. The easiest method is with the animal standing and the probe on the right flank above the udder, using isopropyl alcohol as wetting agent.

Surgical conditions of males

Castration (and tail docking)

There are three basic methods of castration, which also apply to tail docking: surgical; ischaemic by application of a rubber ring; and ischaemic by application of a Burdizzo clamp (Fig. 6.6). All three methods require the use of

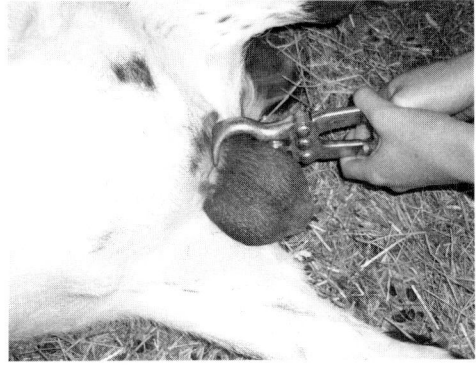

Fig. 6.6. Castration of a goat using a Burdizzo clamp.

local anaesthetic: if the animal is over 7 days old for the rubber ring method, and if over 3 months old for the other two methods.

The normal method of surgical castration is an open method. The tip of the scrotum is removed or two lateral incisions are made to the tip, so that there is good drainage. The tunics are incised and the testicles drawn out with twisting traction for total removal. Oily antiseptic cream containing acriflavin and benzene hexachloride (BHC) is applied to the wounds.

Surgical tail docking can be carried out in lambs by cutting the tail with a scalpel after local anaesthesia. The surgeon should try to cut between the coccygeal vertebrae and leave some skin in excess of the bone. The wound can be cauterized with a hot iron but this is not actually necessary as the haemorrhage will soon cease. Obviously, in pet sheep the procedure can be carried out in a correct surgical manner and the skin sutured after the tail has been removed, making sure there is adequate covering of the bone. This is particularly important in older animals when the tail is removed because of damage.

The ischaemic method of castration using a rubber ring is by far the most common method. It is very important that both testicles are distal to the rubber elastator ring. The ischaemic method of tail docking using a rubber ring is also by far the most common method. Here it is important that rubber ring is not placed too high up the tail. The tail should be long enough to cover the vulva in a female lamb and a similar length should be left in males. The ischaemic method of castration using a Burdizzo clamp can be used in rams and bucks. It is important that only one cord is crushed at one time. The other cord should then be crushed at a second crushing. The crushing lines of the second testicle should not be continuous with those of the first. The animals should be examined in 2 months after the Burdizzo method of castration to confirm that the testicles have regressed.

If the Burdizzo clamp is used for tail docking the clamp should be applied first and then the tail cut off. See also 'Surgical conditions of the Integument', 'Tail docking of adult sheep'.

Castration of animals with a retained testicle

These are extremely rarely true 'rigs', i.e. animals with abdominal testicles. The common presentation is when the elastrator ring has been put on distal to one or both testicles. It is unlikely that such an animal will be fertile as the testicles, being close to the body, will be too hot to produce live sperm. Hence the prudent and welfare friendly approach is to fatten these animals as quickly as possible and send them to slaughter before they reach sexual maturity.

However, in the case of pet animals, surgery may be demanded. After cleaning the area, local anaesthetic should be infiltrated where the scrotum should have been and in the spermatic cord near to the inguinal ring. The animal should be given antibiotics and NSAIDs for 7 days, and its tetanus status checked. The whole area should be carefully examined to see whether there is a single testicle or whether both are present, as obviously in the latter case both will need to be removed. The testicle should be pushed as caudally as possible before an incision is made over it. It is then twisted and pulled. The procedure is then repeated with the second testicle if one is present. Fly control is essential.

As already noted, true rigs are very rare, and in these cases surgery is not easy and a general anaesthetic may be recommended. Often the testicle can be retrieved from the inguinal ring under heavy sedation with xylazine.

Surgical Conditions of the Locomotory System

Conditions of the hooves

Lameness in adult sheep and goats

CHORIOPTIC MANGE This is caused by sheep-adapted *Chorioptes bovis*, which can cause lesions on the lower limbs of sheep and cause lameness. There is intense pruritus like there is with *Psoroptes ovis* infestation. It is difficult to differentiate the two conditions clinically but a diagnosis can be made from a skin scrape examined microscopically under low power, as psoroptic mites are twice as large as

chorioptic mites. Sarcoptic mites (*Sarcoptes* spp.) have also been reported on sheep but they are very rare. These mites are an intermediate size between the other two species. Treatment is with injections of moxidectin repeated at 3 weekly intervals.

CONTAGIOUS OVINE DIGITAL DERMATITIS (CODD) A spirochaete has been implicated in this disease. CODD infection differs from scald and foot rot (see below) in that the infection usually begins at the top of the hoof, in the area of the coronary band, rather than between the toes. It starts as small, ulcerated areas which quickly merge as the infection penetrates under the horn and spreads down towards the toe. As the infection spreads, the underlying tissues anchoring the horn to the toe break down, and it is not uncommon for the horn to separate completely leaving a raw stump. As the coronary band has been damaged, any regrowth of horn is weak and deformed, giving the foot a claw-like appearance. Treatment with oxytetracycline seems to be beneficial, particularly with zinc sulfate solution applied topically. For flock treatment, antibiotic footbaths are required. A combination of lincomycin and spectinomycin is good. Erythromycin has also been used successfully. There is no vaccine available.

EXCESS GRANULATION TISSUE FORMING FROM A SOLAR ABSCESS Care must be taken when draining these abscesses not to remove too much horn tissue. If the granulation tissue bubbles out from the hole, the hard horn tissue cannot grow over the top. The granulation tissue, which is very vascular but free of nerve endings, needs to be paired back and the whole foot bandaged. This should be changed twice weekly for at least 2 weeks.

FOOT ABSCESSES These are normally caused by *Arcanobacterium pyogenes*. Poulticing with magnesium sulfate paste on cotton gauze, kept in place with waterproof gutter tape, is a useful treatment, together with a sub cut injection of tilmicosin. In the UK, this is only licensed for veterinary administration and must not be used by non-veterinarians. If the owner is going to treat the animal, injections of either tylosin sulfate or lincomycin hydro-chloride can be used.

'FOOT ROT' This is caused by *Dichelobacter* (formerly *Bacteriodes*) *nodosus*. Treatment is with injectable preparations of penicillin and streptomycin. There is a good vaccine available.

INTERDIGITAL HYPERPLASIA This condition is seen in older rams. It does not seem to cause lameness unless there is an accompanying infection. Usually, if this can be controlled, the lameness will disappear so that the need for radical surgery is avoided. In the author's experience, surgery for this condition is not worthwhile as the rams seem even more susceptible to infections after it has been done than before.

SCALD This is a painful condition of the skin between the digits, possibly caused by three different bacteria: *Fusobacterium necrophorum*, penicillin-resistant *Staphylococcus aureus* or *D. nodosus*. All age groups are vulnerable but it is common in lambs and will appear as outbreaks, mainly in warm moist conditions with animals on lush pastures. There is usually no separation of the horn or suppuration. Treatment will vary according to the organism involved. *F. necrophorum* is the most common, so the starting treatment should be a 3 day course of an injectable preparation of a penicillin and streptomycin mixture and topical oxytetracycline spray. Should there be a poor response, then it is likely that there is a. *S. aureus* infection, which is resistant to penicillin. If that occurs, clinicians should change to a 3 day course of amoxicillin with clavulanic acid.

SOIL BALLING This occurs when sheep are kept on a sea of mud during severe wet weather and then there is a drying wind (Fig. 6.7). The soil will harden between the two claws.

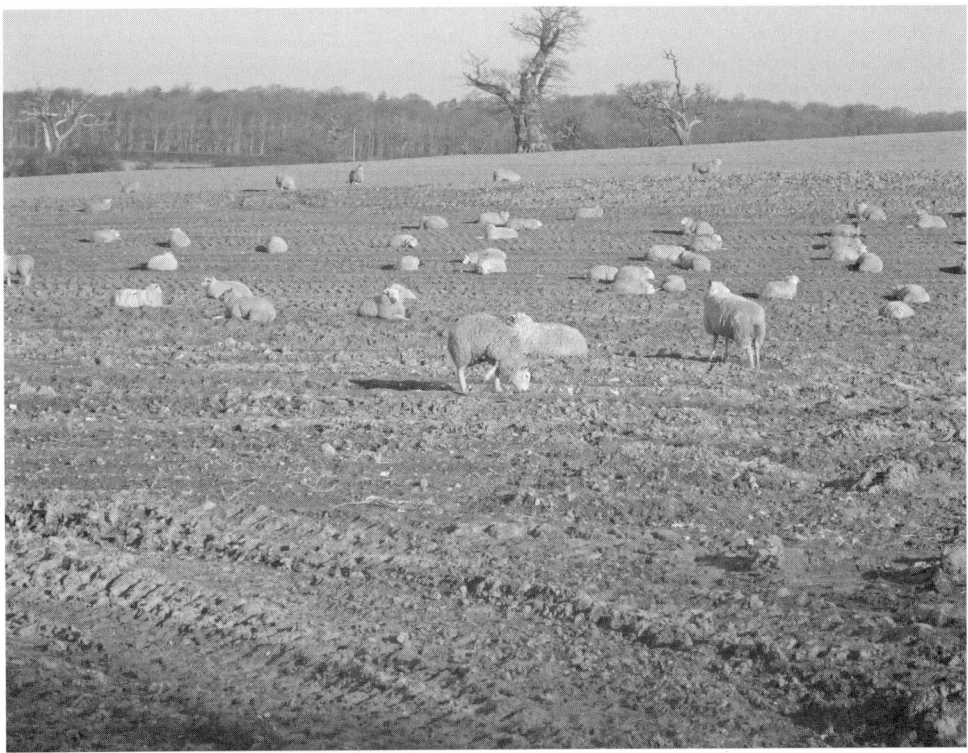

Fig. 6.7. Soil balling is likely when sheep are kept on mud during wet weather and then there is a drying wind.

Treatment is straightforward and should be carried out immediately or there will be a welfare issue.

STRAWBERRY FOOT ROT   This is a crusty condition of the skin around the pastern which is caused by an infection with *Dermatophilus* spp. The condition is made worse by grazing in long grass and is spread more rapidly if there are thistles or brambles in the pasture.

WHITE LINE ABSCESSES   These are often a sequel to foot rot. The underrunning infection needs to be exposed but as much horn should be saved on the wall as possible. Lincomycin hydro-chloride injections for 5 days help to remove any bacterial problems. Topical spraying with oxytetracycline spray is useful.

Lameness in lambs and kids

The causes of lameness in adult sheep and goats will also cause problems in lambs and kids, particularly if they are older, but lameness is very rare in very young animals. Conditions other than those already described that may cause lameness in lambs and kids include the following.

JOINT ILL   This infection is common in young lambs and kids, particularly if they do not receive enough good-quality colostrum. The most common causative organism is *Pasteurella haemolytica*, although *P. multocida* has been reported in an outbreak in Greece (Petridou *et al.*, 2011). It should be remembered that the organism can enter the body through the tonsil as well as the navel. Joint ill is also much more prevalent if the lambing pens are dirty. Treating the navels with iodine or oxytetracycline rarely stops the disease if the ewe's udders are dirty. Treatment should be carried out with penicillin and streptomycin combination injections daily for a minimum of 5 days. NSAIDs should also be given.

LAMINITIS   This has been reported in very fast growing older lambs, although it is extremely rare as very large numbers of lambs are fed ad lib creep feed with no ill effects. Further,

ram lambs and shearlings are also given large quantities of food to get them ready for sale, this too without ill effects.

POST-DIPPING SEPTIC ARTHRITIS   This is a condition of older lambs and is seen 2–5 days after dipping in a contaminated dip solution. The organism involved is *Erysipelothrix rhusiopathiae*. This is sensitive to penicillin.

SWAYBACK   This condition occurs if ewes or does are deficient in copper. It may be a true deficiency, which is rare, and is more commonly is brought on by an excess of molybdenum or sulfur in the diet. It can be controlled by treating the ewes with copper between weeks 10 and 16 of pregnancy. It is an easy disease to diagnose clinically, as the incoordination behind in an otherwise bright lamb or kid is pathognomic. If the lambs that are born like this somehow manage to reach up and suck, they can survive. Delayed swayback has been reported; this is extremely rare in lambs but is more common in kids. The aetiology is difficult to understand, as if the myelin is damaged in the womb the lamb or kid would be affected at birth, so maybe suspect cases are missed at birth? Blood sampling the ewes and does is useful in prevention. See also Chapter 5.

TETANUS   The root of infection in young animals is the navel, the site of docking or the site of castration. The vaccine is very inexpensive and effective. Treatment is possible if the disease is caught early enough. A large dose of tetanus antitoxin (TAT), e.g. 6000 IU, should be given immediately sub cut. Penicillin should be given daily.

WHITE MUSCLE DISEASE   This is not an uncommon condition. The lambs and kids are like rag dolls. They are weak and do not appear bright like swayback lambs. The actual aetiology is confusing. It is suspected that there are actually two forms: selenium deficient and vitamin E deficient. The treatment is, however, the same with commercial injection containing both selenium and vitamin E. If several cases are seen, it is justifiable to inject each lamb or kid as a preventive as soon after birth as possible.

Conditions of the limbs

Flying scapula

This is a very rare condition which may occur in sheep and goats, normally after weaning but before maturity. The muscles securing the scapula to the ribcage become weak and rupture to some extent so that the ribcage drops. The spine is then lower in the thoracic area than in the lumbar–sacral area. The animal is still mobile, but the condition is irreversible.

Fractures

Practitioners should always be on the lookout for fractures in small ruminants. In growing lambs, these can often be splinted (Fig. 6.8).

There several conditions that will increase the risk of fractures:

1. Severe copper deficiency has been reported to cause fractures as copper is needed for the development of a normal framework within the bone.
2. Long-standing parasitic infections, particularly of intestinal nematodes, also predisposes to fractures because damage to the gut wall prevents the young animal from absorbing enough phosphorus.
3. Where animals are kept in areas of old lead mining, the continual daily intake of small amounts of lead as they graze makes the bones liable to fracture.
4. Problems with rickets can occur in hill lambs that are away wintered on dairy farms. Following the move from the hill to lush grass, the lambs, including their bones, grow quickly. Vitamin D is required for new bone to calcify properly and become strong. Unfortunately, in the UK, and particularly in Scotland, sunlight only provides sufficient vitamin D between mid March and mid September. Affected lambs appear stiff or lame and will walk on their toes. There can be obvious bowing of the front legs, and the worst affected lambs will not recover enough to be kept as replacements. Rickets can be prevented by injecting or drenching lambs with vitamin D before they go to wintering.

Surgical removal of the digit of small ruminants

Septic pedal arthritis does occur in small ruminants but it is rare. Antibiotic treatment, even if prolonged, is rarely successful. Welfare must always be considered, and euthanasia is certainly an option for relieving further suffering. Full drainage of the distal phalangeal joint, with subsequent arthrodesis, may be considered, but this will result in a long period of severe pain.

Surgical removal of the digit is a more humane option (Fig. 6.9). It is vital that this surgery is not attempted if there is sepsis in the proximal joints, as pain will then persist. If clinicians are in any doubt, radiography should be carried out. Regional anaesthesia can be used. The distal limb can be cleaned but full asepsis is not required. A length of

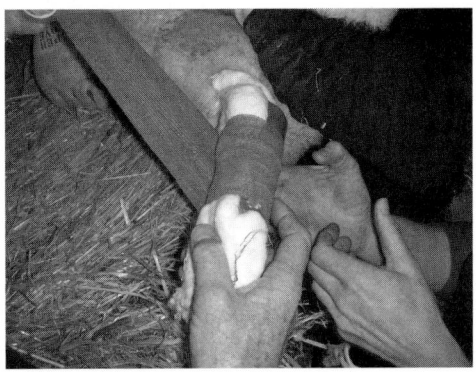

Fig. 6.8. Splinting a fracture in a lamb.

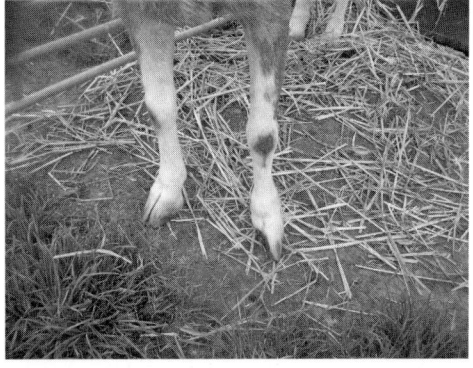

Fig. 6.9. A goat with a digit removed.

embryotomy wire is placed between the digits. The sawing direction should be at an angle of 45° above the horizontal. The skin, soft tissue and half the second phalanx should be removed. The foot then should be bandaged before removal of the tourniquet. The animal should be given antibiotic and NSAID cover for a minimum of a week. The bandage should be removed every third day until clean granulation tissue is seen.

Surgical Conditions of the Integument

Dehorning in goats and sheep

Disbudding of kids

This must be performed during the first week of life, but after only the kids have received adequate colostrum. Great care should be taken with the surgery and the anaesthetic. The surgery should take place in a warm environment. The kid is masked down using a halothane or isoflurane and oxygen mixture (Fig. 6.10.). The hair is clipped around the base of both horns. The kid should receive a sub cut injection of 1500 IU TAT, together with im injections of antibiotics and NSAIDs. The horn bud is removed with a scalpel. A specially prepared disbudding iron with a wide aperture is heated to red heat and applied to the horn after the oxygen has been turned off. The iron may have to be removed if the kid shows signs of movement so that the mask with the

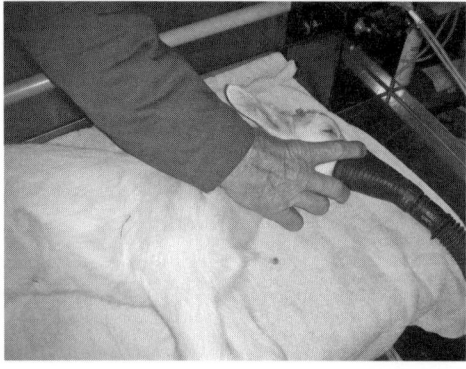

Fig. 6.10. A kid is masked down before disbudding.

anaesthetic mixture can be reapplied. It is vital that the iron is extremely hot and therefore will only need to be applied for bursts of 15 s. It is also important that all the horn-producing tissue is destroyed.

Animals with rudimentary horn stubs

These small horns are best left alone unless they get caught in wire, etc. and start haemorrhaging. Normally, there is no underlying bone tissue involved. The area can be anaesthetized with local anaesthetic and the horn, including a circumference of skin, can be removed. The area must be treated with a cream containing acriflavin and BHC, and allowed to heal by secondary intention. Special attention must be paid to the control of flies as well as tetanus immunization.

Removal of adult horns

This is major surgery and should only be undertaken after due consideration. It should not be performed for cosmetic reasons. If an adult horn has been fractured it needs to be removed. There is no reason why the good horn cannot be left *in situ*. If there is an ingrowing horn, the tip can be removed at regular intervals with a hacksaw or embryotomy wire. Provided that only the tip is removed and the deeper structures are not involved, there is no pain and an anaesthetic is not required. Certain individuals become aggressive to other animals or to humans and then, after due thought, dehorning can be undertaken.

The goat or sheep should be given a combination of xylazine 0.1 mg/kg and butorphanol 0.1 mg/kg iv as a premedication after being starved for 12 h. This is followed 5 min later by iv ketamine 0.2 mg/kg, which can be topped up if required, but with proper preparation and speed of action this can be avoided. The horn, including an area of skin at the base, is removed with embryotomy wire.

There will be considerable haemorrhage, which should initially, until both horns are removed, be controlled by pressure. Any arteries that can then be picked up should be ligated.

Two pads of folded gamgee covered with a cream containing acriflavin and BHC should be placed on the base of the horn. A pressure bandage is then applied in a figure of eight around the ears. If possible, the animal should be hospitalized or at least kept under careful observation for a minimum of 6 h. Some bandage will have to be cut away so that the animal can see. The dressing needs to be replaced every 2 days. Great care should be taken with bandaging so that the larynx and the trachea are not constricted. It should be stressed that the goat or sheep should be fully immunized against tetanus. Antibiotics should be given daily by injection, together with NSAIDs for pain relief, for a minimum of 10 days. Flies must be controlled. The goat or sheep should be separated from other animals to prevent head butting.

Tail docking of an adult sheep

This is only required when a tail has been injured. Repair is fairly straightforward provided that suitable aftercare is carried out. The sheep should be given preoperative antibiotic and NSAID cover and the tetanus status should be checked. The tail should be anaesthetized in the standing sheep with an epidural anaesthetic, and then should be clipped out and surgically prepared. The surgeon should aim to remove at least one coccygeal vertebra above the injured section. Some skin needs to be left to effect a good closure so the actual bony tissue should be removed by blunt dissection and the connective tissue of the tail cut through in between the vertebrae. The skin should be closed with several individual vertical mattress sutures of monofilament nylon. The tail must then be protected by bandaging. The bandage should be kept in place by securing it to a single piece of bandage around the circumference of the sheep in front of the udder or scrotum. The bandage should be replaced at regular intervals for at least a week after suture removal.

See also 'Surgical Conditions Male Reproductive System', 'Castration (and tail docking)'.

Euthanasia

Use of a firearm with a free bullet

This is a very satisfactory method of euthanasia in adult sheep and goats. In the UK, the operator must either be a veterinary surgeon with a current firearms licence for the weapon concerned or a licensed slaughterman with a similar firearms licence. The only exception to this is for the veterinary surgeon or the licensed slaughterman to use a shotgun (a smooth-bored gun, which is differentiated from a firearm proper) with permission of the owner of this gun.

There is no hard and fast rule on the size of the bullet or the bore of the shotgun. With a large old horned ram or buck a .310 or .320 calibre would be suitable. With a ewe or a doe or a younger animal, a .22 calibre would be safer and adequate. A twelve-bore shot gun would be suitable for a ram or buck, whereas a 4.10 shot gun should be used for a ewe or doe.

It must be remembered when using a shotgun that the end of the barrel needs to be a minimum of 6 in. from the skull and can be up to 3 ft away. The location of the position is the same for a firearm or a shotgun. It is a point in the middle of a cross made between the ears and the eyes on the opposite side of the face. The position of any horns should be disregarded. It should be stressed that the animal's head should be adequately restrained and no personnel should be behind the animal. With either of these methods, the animal should die instantaneously. There is no need to sever the carotids. Methods using firearms are not suitable for young lambs or kids.

Use of a captive bolt pistol

This used to be the standard method of euthanasia in slaughterhouses. A captive bolt .22 pistol is fired into the brain by directing the shot into the middle of a cross made by two lines from the animal's ears to its eyes. The animal is immediately bled out by severing all the major vessels in the neck. This method can be used for adult animals. It should not be used for young lambs or kids. No firearms licence is required. Farmers and shepherds should be given a short training course if this method is going to be used on the farm.

Chemical euthanasia

This is likely to be the method of choice for pet animals. Veterinarians must obviously not only be 100% welfare conscious but must also be mindful of the owner's concerns. For chemical euthanasia, good advice would be to sedate first using im xylazine with a 1½ in. needle (2 ml 2% solution for an adult animal). The client should be warned that the animal might make a moaning noise. This is not from pain but from the effect of the drug. When the animal is in lateral recumbency, completion of euthanasia can be carried out by injecting 20 ml of triple-strength barbiturate into the jugular vein (Fig. 6.11). The reasoning for this approach is firstly because larger doses of triple-strength barbiturate will be required without prior sedation and second because it is not easy to inject large volumes iv into a standing sheep or goat. It might be argued that a small dose of a solution containing 400 mg/ml quinalbarbitone and 25 mg/ml cinchocaine hydrochloride would be adequate, but this fluid is very viscous, and a large-gauge needle will be required. Also, the practitioner will be left with a part-used bottle of a solution containing the drugs as the

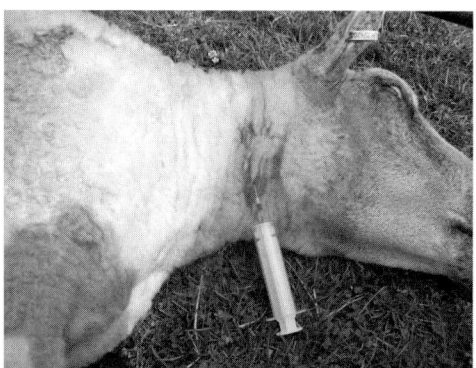

Fig. 6.11. Sheep in lateral recumbency for chemical euthanasia.

smallest bottles of this solution available are 25 ml. Care is also required for animals with long horns. When they are in lateral recumbency, the jugular is not that easy to visualize, so the use of a small pillow under the neck is helpful.

Chemical euthanasia is the method of choice for small lambs or kids. They should be held across the handler's chest, with the head restrained. The veterinarian can then raise the jugular and inject 5 ml of a triple-strength barbiturate solution using a 1 in. 21 G needle. If very large numbers of small lambs need to be destroyed, e.g. when affected or at risk from a highly contagious notifiable disease, then the triple-strength barbiturate solution can be injected using a 1 in. 19 G needle directly into the heart. The lamb should be held in a similar manner, across the handler's chest.

7

South American Camelid (SAC) Medicine

Introduction

The chapter starts with an account of the animal husbandry of SACs, which includes an explanation of the differences between SACs and ruminants, and provides some important behavioural notes. This is followed by a brief section on clinical examination of and history taking in SACs. The rest of the chapter describes SAC medical practice and is organized by system, with sections on diseases of the gastroenteric system, diseases of the neurological system, metabolic diseases (which can also be viewed as a category of neurological diseases), diseases of the respiratory system, diseases of the circulatory system, diseases of the urinary system, diseases of the reproductive system and diseases of the integument. The last section briefly covers common reasons for SACs to be found dead.

Animal Husbandry

Classification

SACs are normally classified into four types: llamas, alpacas, guanacos and vicuñas. The first three of these are placed in the same genus, *Lama*, as the species *L. glama*, *L. pacos* and *L. guanicoe*. Vicuñas are placed in a separate genus and species, *Vicugna vicugna*, which is subdivided into two subspecies, *V. vicugna mensalis* from Peru, and *V. vicugna vicugna* from Argentina. All four species are all classified in the tribe Lamini, which is part of the family Camelidae. The Camelidae family is part of the suborder Tylopoda which, with the suborders Cetruminantia (which includes cattle, sheep, goats, water buffalo, giraffes, deer, antelopes and bison) and Suinia (which includes pigs and peccaries) make up the order Artiodactyla. SACs are grouped with camels, both the dromedary and the bactrian, in the suborder Tylopoda. This suborder has some important differences from ruminants of the suborder Cetruminantia.

Ruminants have red bloods cells (RBCs) which are round and 10 µm in diameter; SACs have elliptical RBCs which are only 6.5 µm in diameter. Ruminants have feet which have hooves, consisting of a horn wall and a sole; SACs have toenails and a soft pad. The second and third phalanges are horizontal in camelids but in ruminants they are nearly vertical. However, both ruminants and tylopods are foregut fermenters, with regurgitation, re-chewing and reswallowing. Tylopods though have only three stomach compartments (C1, C2, C3) and are resistant to bloat, while ruminants have four stomach compartments and suffer from bloat.

The teeth in SACs cause real confusion, whereas in ruminants they are fairly straightforward. Ruminants have no upper incisors or upper canines. On each lower hemi-mandible they have three incisors and a canine. This canine has migrated rostrally and resembles an incisor. They therefore appear to have four lower incisors on each side. In contrast, SACs have on each upper hemi-maxilla one canine, and one upper incisor which has migrated caudally and resembles a canine. So they appear to have two upper canines on each side. On each hemi-mandible they have three incisors and one canine. There are also differences with the cheek teeth. Ruminants have three upper and lower premolars on each side. SACs have one, and maybe a second, upper and lower premolar on each side. Both SACs and ruminants have three upper and lower molars on each side.

It is perhaps in the reproductive system where ruminants are most at variance from SACs. Ruminants have an oestrus cycle, with spontaneous ovulation and no follicular wave cycle. SACs do not have an oestrus cycle and are induced ovulators, but they do have a follicular wave cycle. Ruminants copulate in the standing position with ejaculation short and intense. SACs copulate in the prone position and have prolonged ejaculation. The male SAC has a cartilaginous projection on the tip of his penis. This is absent in ruminants. SACs have a diffuse placenta and the fetus is surrounded by an epidermal membrane. Ruminant fetuses do not have such a membrane but have placental cotyledons.

SACs are primarily nasal breathers with an elongated soft palate, and mouth breathing in SACs is an extremely serious sign. Ruminants have a short soft palate and can breathe nasally or orally. The kidneys of SACs are smooth and elliptical. Some ruminants have smooth kidneys, e.g. the sheep, and some lobed kidneys, e.g. the ox. The female SAC has a sub-urethral diverticulum at the external urethral orifice. Ruminants have no such diverticulum. SACs have not only unique internal parasites and protozoa, but also share other species of parasite with cattle, sheep and goats. The picture with external parasites is confusing. SACs certainly have unique lice, and they may also have unique mange mites, but the classification is not yet confirmed.

Normal behaviour

SACs, even in the wild tend to defaecate in a pile. This is used by the male to smell for strangers and for receptive females. The faecal pile is also useful as it is a natural way to reduce intestinal parasites. Overcrowding should be avoided at all costs, as all types of disease will flourish. Also, disease control, particularly the control of internal and external parasites, will be very difficult, if there is overstocking. Heat stress is a real problem for SACs. Temperatures of over 26°C and humidity of over 80% need to be avoided, so fans, shade and ponds need to be provided in hot climates. However, the liver fluke is becoming a major parasite in the UK, so ponds should be avoided. SACs will also defaecate in water and so pollute it and increase the risk of coccidiosis. They are also excellent swimmers and so ditches, dykes and rivers will not contain them.

Vocalization by humming is the most common sound made by SACs. It is probably used to confirm contact as it will become louder on separation. A lack of humming may be a cause for concern. Groaning or bruxism are a real cause for alarm for the keeper as they indicates pain. Veterinary attention should be sought. Snorting denotes mild aggression. This will turn to screeching in males if they are being handled or meeting other males. The position of the ears and tail denotes status. Males may spit and kick, and may even charge and bite. Submission will be shown by a drooping of the upper eyelid and imitation mouth breathing. Males make a sound called ogling before and during mating.

Behavioural problems

The two most common 'vices' of SACs are splitting at people and the berserk male syndrome (this syndrome is not actually exclusively in males) in which SACs respond aggressively to people. Such animals become highly dangerous and should be destroyed.

Clinical Examination, Including History Taking

The rectal temperature in SACs can vary from 99.0 to 101.0°F (37.4–38.3°C). The thermoregulatory ability of the neonate is so poor that there can be a much wider range. Although SACs have evolved in harsh cool climates, the insulation ability of their fleeces allows a certain tolerance to the sort of heat extremes encountered in the UK and other countries where SACs are kept outside South America, and the fleece-free underside acts as an area for heat dissipation.

The resting heart rate of an adult SAC varies from 60 to 90/min and is best ascertained by auscultation caudal to the triceps in the fleece-free area medial to the elbow. Very few respiratory sounds will be heard either here or anywhere else unless there is some pathology. Borborygmi (rumblings) are much quieter than in sheep and goats, and mostly come from the major fermentation chamber C1. This first compartment contracts between three and five times a minute, depending on feeding.

Diseases of the Gastroenteric System

Problems affecting the head

Ptyalism and pseudoptyalism

Owners will complain of cud staining caused by ulcerative stomatitis, lingual paresis, malposition of the parotid ducts, early mega-oesophagus or choke. Passive regurgitation during sleep is a relatively common problem in young SACs aged 6–18 months. It tends to be self-limiting and stops after the age of 18 months.

Swellings of the soft tissue

These are unlikely to be tooth related and are usually abscesses, although they could be insect or reptile bites. Any fibre should be trimmed away and the area cleaned before an 18G needle is inserted. Pus will be seen in the needle and then the abscess may be lanced. Digital exploration should be carried out into the abscess to make sure there is no foreign body, e.g. a slither of wood or an airgun pellet. Antibiotics should be given and the tetanus status checked. If the swelling is unrelated to the underlying bone and not rapidly enlarging it is likely to be an *Actinobacillus lignieresii* infection, when lancing will be unrewarding. Treatment with daily injections of streptomycin for a minimum of 2 weeks should be carried out. Lymphomas will cause soft tissue swellings. Cud retention is likely to be tooth related, e.g. to a loose tooth or a displaced tooth.

Congenital and hereditary conditions

Atresia coli

These cases require euthanasia.

Mega-oesophagus

This is an extremely rare condition. The main sign is repeated regurgitation. Animals will show multiple non-specific signs such as weight loss, ptyalism, choke and halitosis. The cause can be a persistent right aortic arch or trauma to the vagus from jugular vein punctures. There is no worthwhile treatment but cases can usually be managed by only feeding the animal from an elevated position, with regular small feeds of highly digestible well-soaked food.

See also Atresia ani (Chapter 8).

Enteric diseases caused by viruses and their treatment

Bluetongue disease

The causative organism, *Bluetongue virus* (BTV), is an *Orbivirus* is that is borne by species of *Culicoides* biting midges. Endothelial damage and disseminated intravascular coagulation (DIC) cause the clinical signs. The incubation period is 6–9 days. The lesions are common in areas subject to mechanical trauma and abrasion, e.g. feet, mouth and eyes. There is fever up to 42°C. There are respiratory signs and abortion. The diagnosis is confirmed by PCR for viral RNA. There is no specific treatment for BTV. Antibiotics and nonsteroidal anti-inflammatory drugs (NSAIDs) are helpful. Nursing should include offering water and mushy food, and providing deep bedding out of the sun and heat. The vaccines available are inactivated (dead) vaccines against specific serotypes. See also below under 'Diseases of the Integument'.

Bovine viral diarrhoea (BVD)

Crias will show weight loss and diarrhoea. Some crias will be stillborn or show congenital neurological signs. Ill thrift and weight loss will be shown in adults, but diarrhoea in adults is rare. The virus (*Bovine viral diarrhoea virus*, BVDV) will cause abortion. Persistent infection (PI) has been demonstrated when SACs are infected in early pregnancy i.e. at 32–133 days. Most of these will be lighter than normal at birth, then grow slowly and will die before they reach 30 months of age. Both type 1 and type 2 viruses have been isolated in Chile, but only type 1 has been found in the UK. There is no treatment and animals with PI should be culled. See also below under 'Diseases of the Reproductive System', 'Abortion and its causes'.

Coronavirus

Coronaviruses are a relatively common finding in scouring crias. With careful hygiene and the use of electrolytes they are fairly easily controlled as crias will self-cure. There is rarely a need for antibiotic support or NSAIDs.

Foot-and-mouth disease (FMD)

FMD, which is caused by an *Aphthovirus*, is definitely contracted by SACs. They may only be carriers for a few days but they do spread the disease. The main signs are lameness and a reluctance to move. Excess salivation is invariably seen at some stage of the disease. A thorough examination of the whole SAC herd will reveal the typical erosions and ulcers on the mouths and feet of a considerable number of animals.

Malignant catarrhal fever (MCF)

MCF, which is caused by a herpesvirus, is a very serious disease in SACs with a high mortality but an extremely low morbidity. Animals will show pyrexia and mouth lesions. There is no treatment or vaccine available. See also below under 'Diseases of the Integument'.

Rotavirus

Rotavirus has been isolated from SACs, and will definitely cause diarrhoea, but often there is another pathogen isolated at the same time. This may be a bacterium, e.g. *Escherichia coli*, or a protozoan, e.g. a coccidian. Clinicians cannot treat the virus so attention should be drawn to the other pathogens.

Enteric diseases caused by bacteria and their treatment

Clostridial diseases

These are very important in SACs. The most common is enterotoxaemia, which is caused by *Clostridium (Cl.) perfringens* type D. This disease is normally manifest by sudden death although observant keepers will see sick lifeless, cold, moribund animals. There is no treatment. Malignant oedema is caused by several clostridial organisms, namely *Cl. septicum*, *Cl. chauvoei*, *Cl. perfringens* and *Cl. novyi*. Animals can be found dead or *in extremis*. They show swellings, which are often gaseous. The disease may follow wounds obtained by males fighting. Aggressive treatment with penicillin and NSAIDs may be successful if started promptly.

Sordellii abomasitis is caused by *Cl. sordellii*. In young crias over 3 weeks old it will cause acute inflammation of C3. In adults, it will cause sudden death or damage to C3 that leads to death, often from ulceration and peritonitis. There is now a vaccine available which is highly recommended in SACs. As the same vaccine is prepared for cattle it

1

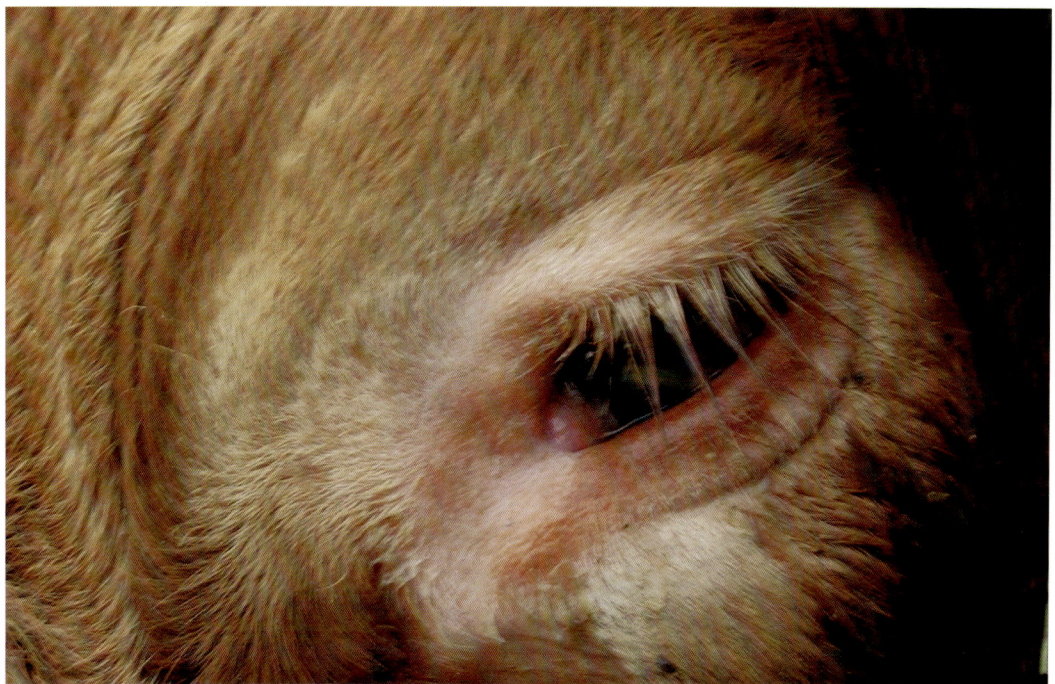

2

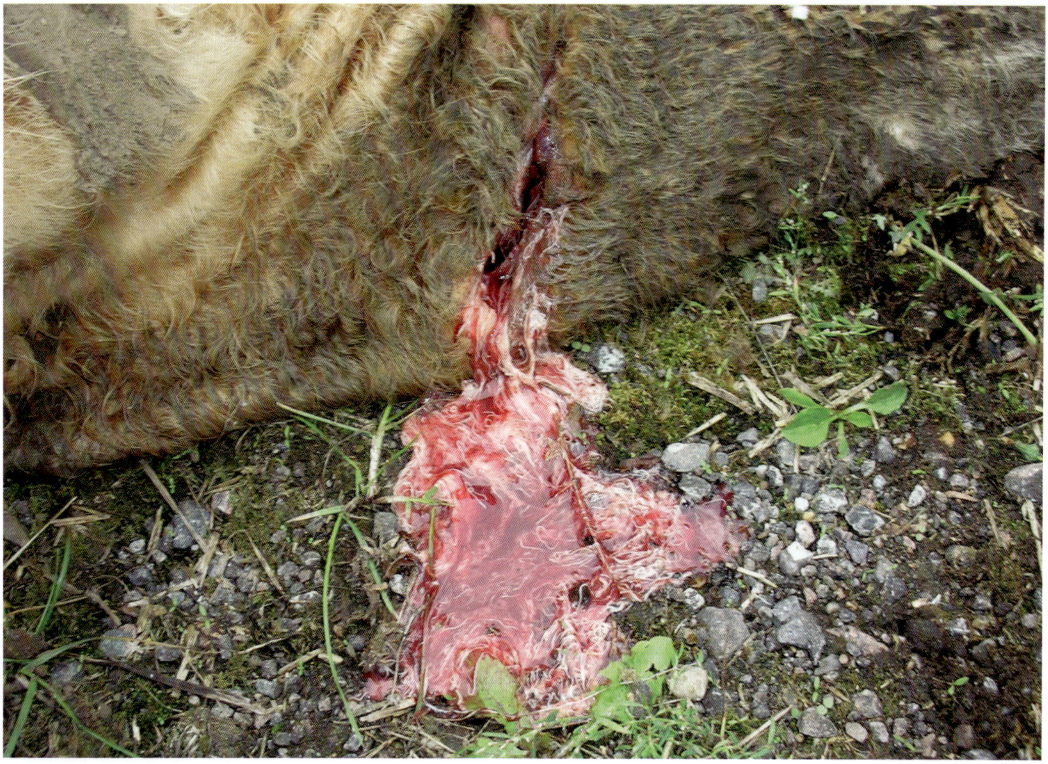

Plate 1. Oat flight on the cornea in a cow.
Plate 2. Lung worms in large numbers in the trachea of a cow.

3

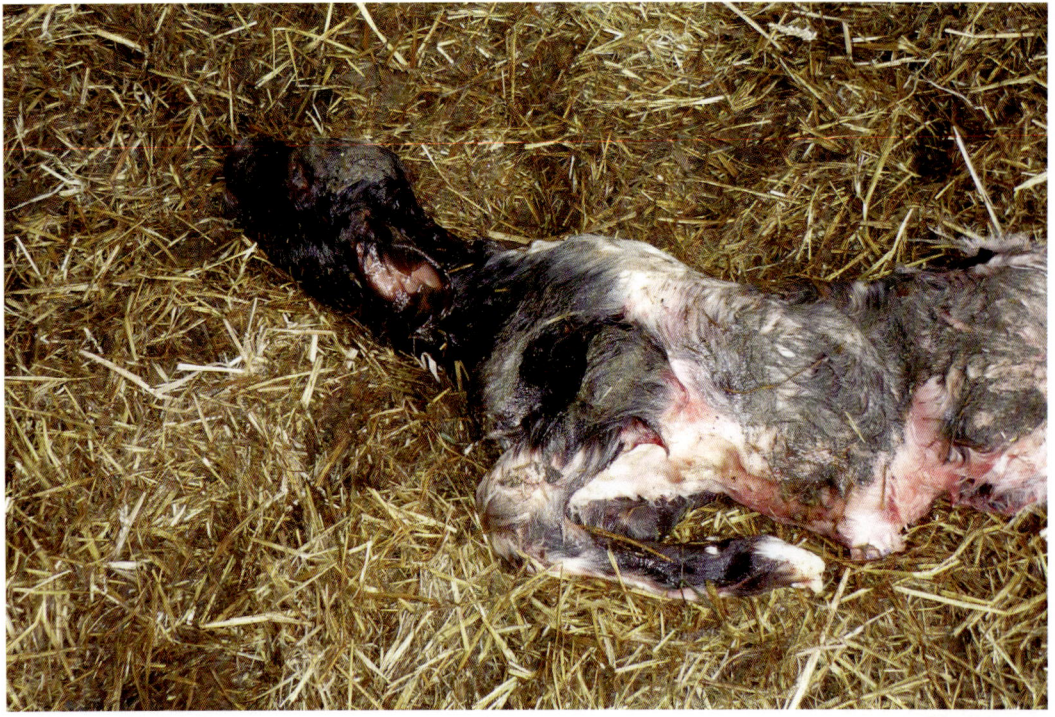

4

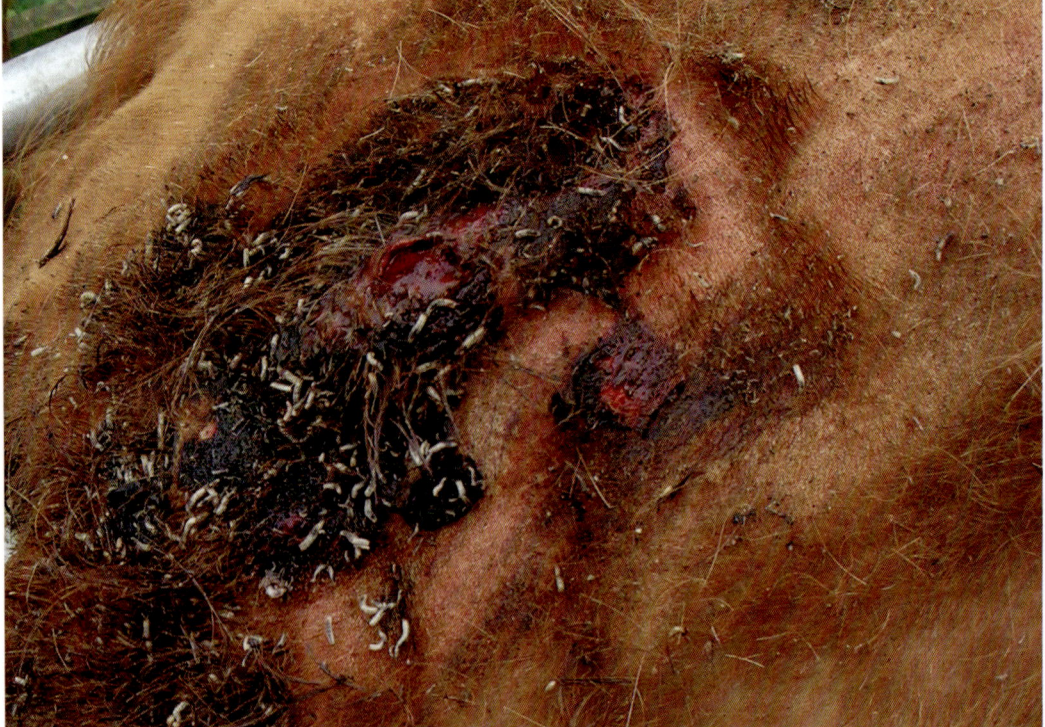

Plate 3. Limb abnormalities in a calf affected by Schmallenburg virus (SBV).
Plate 4. Fly strike on the wounded tail head of a cow.

5

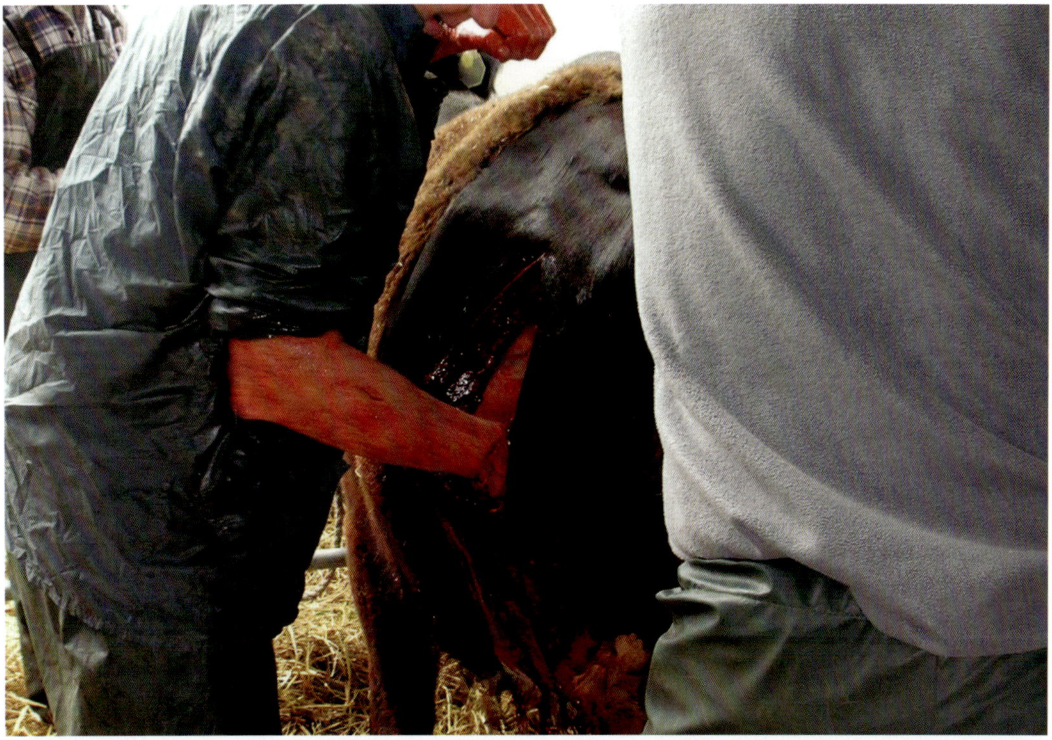

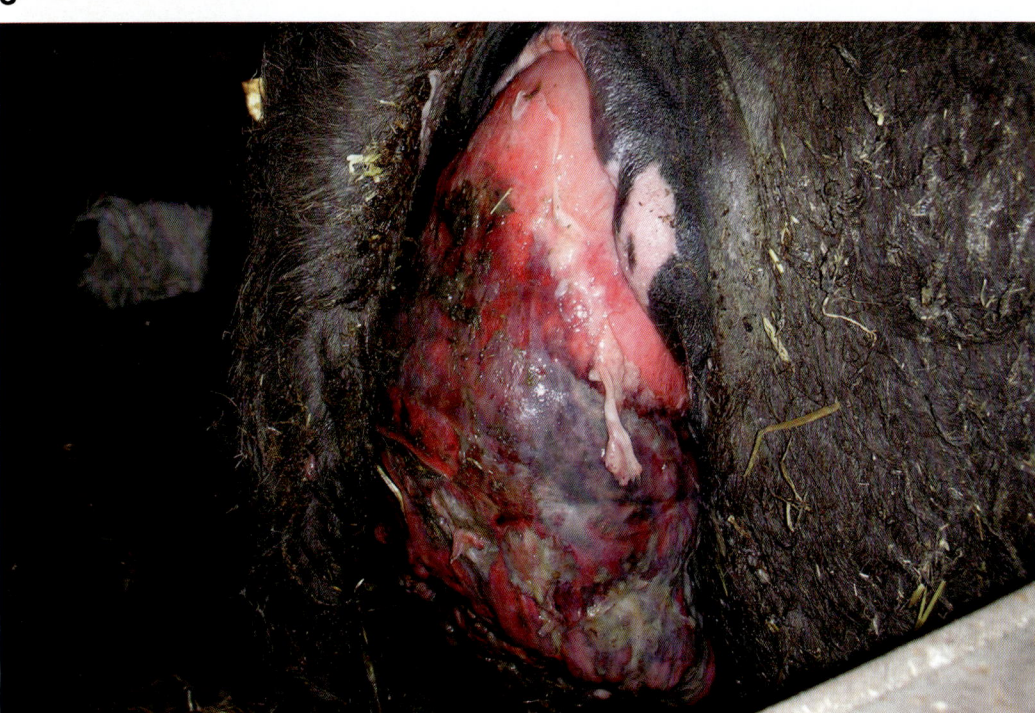

6

Plate 5. Caesarean section: elevating the calf to the skin incision is not easy.
Plate 6. Prolapsed cervix in a cow.

7

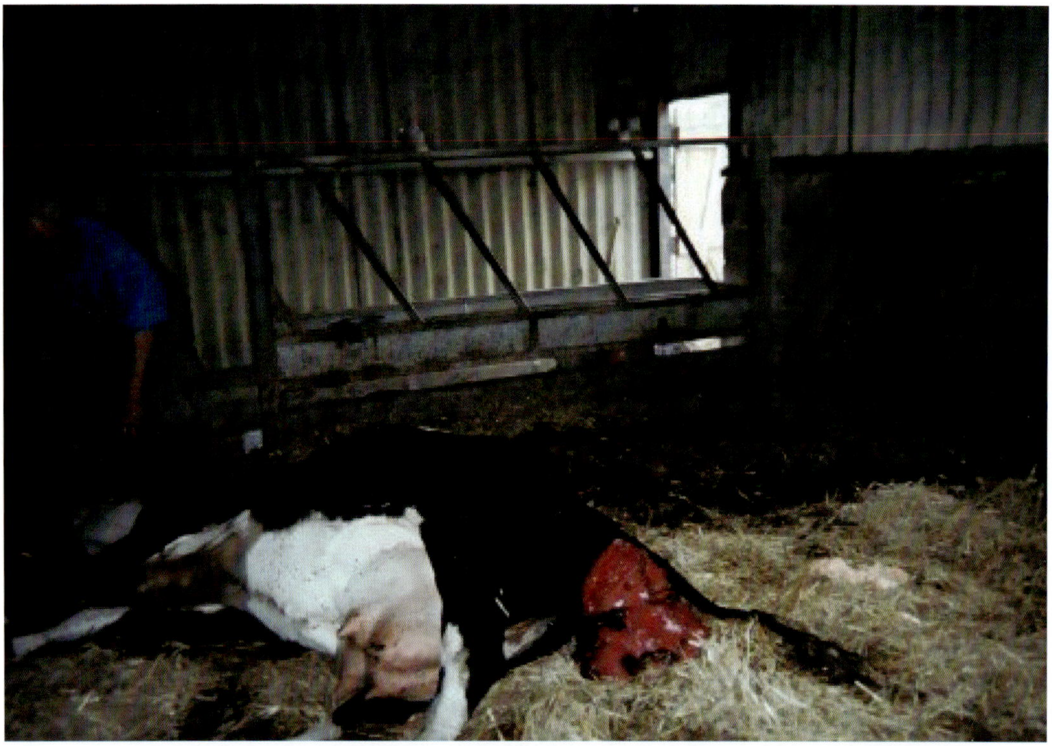

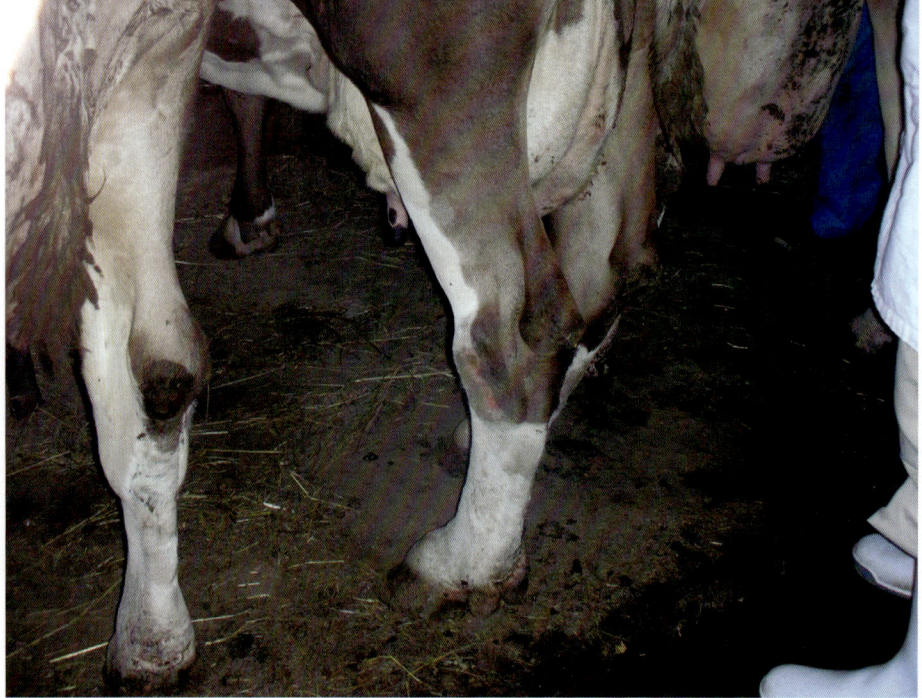

8

Plate 7. Prolapsed uterus in a cow.
Plate 8. Hock bursitis in a cow.

9

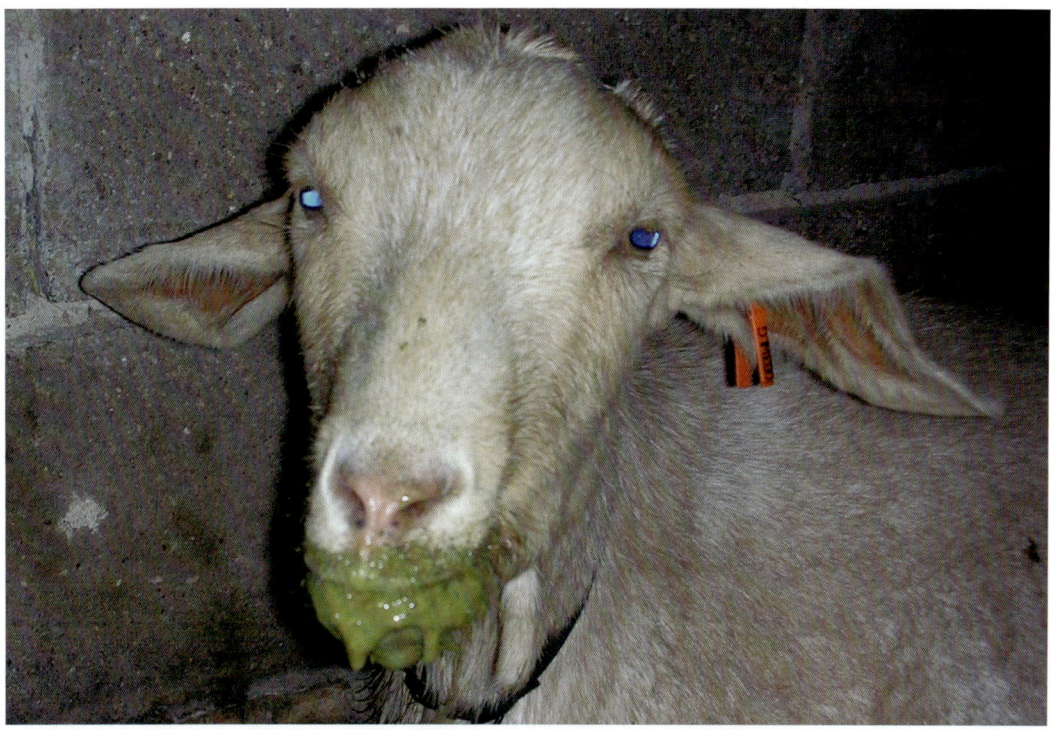

10

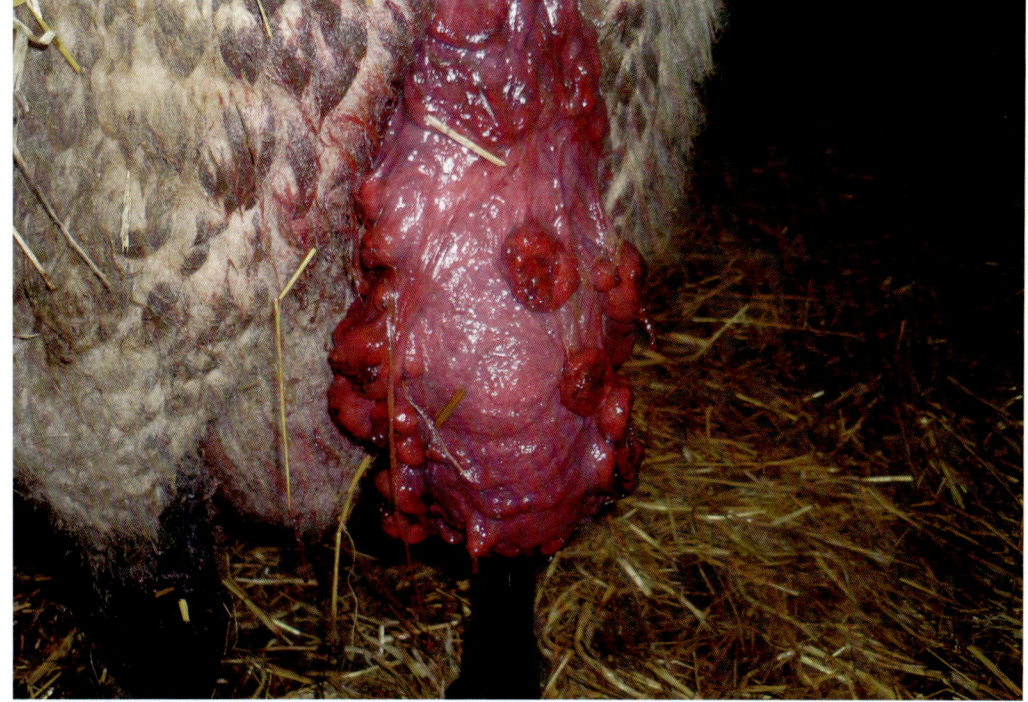

Plate 9. Goat with rhododendron poisoning.
Plate 10. Uterine prolapse in a sheep.

11

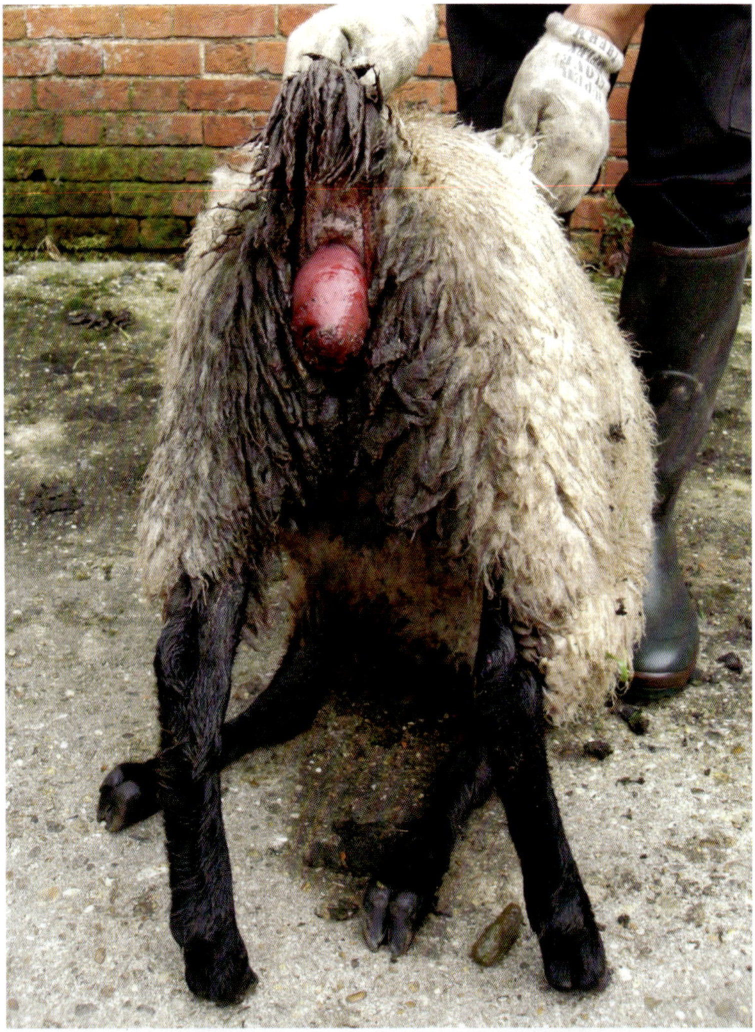

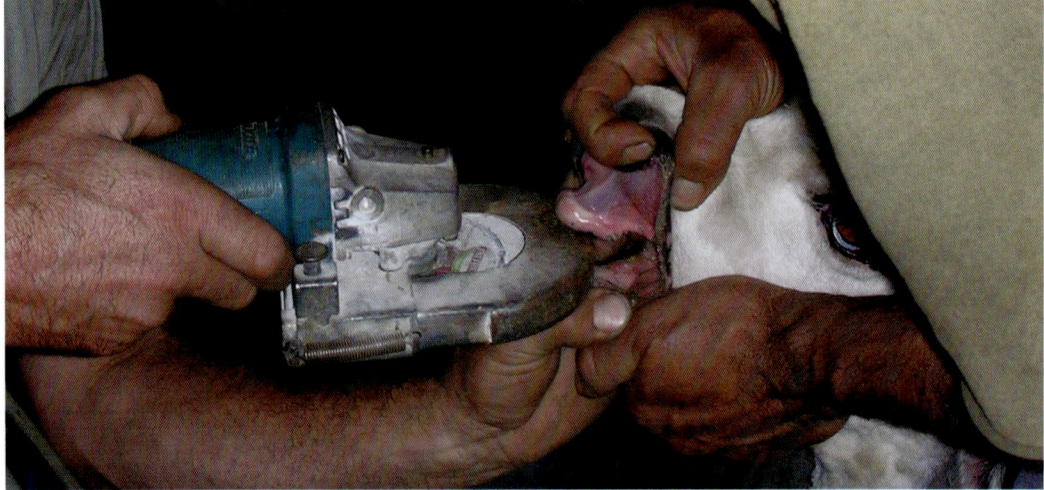

12

Plate 11. Vaginal prolapse in a sheep.
Plate 12. Grinding of the incisors in South American camelids is inhumane.

13

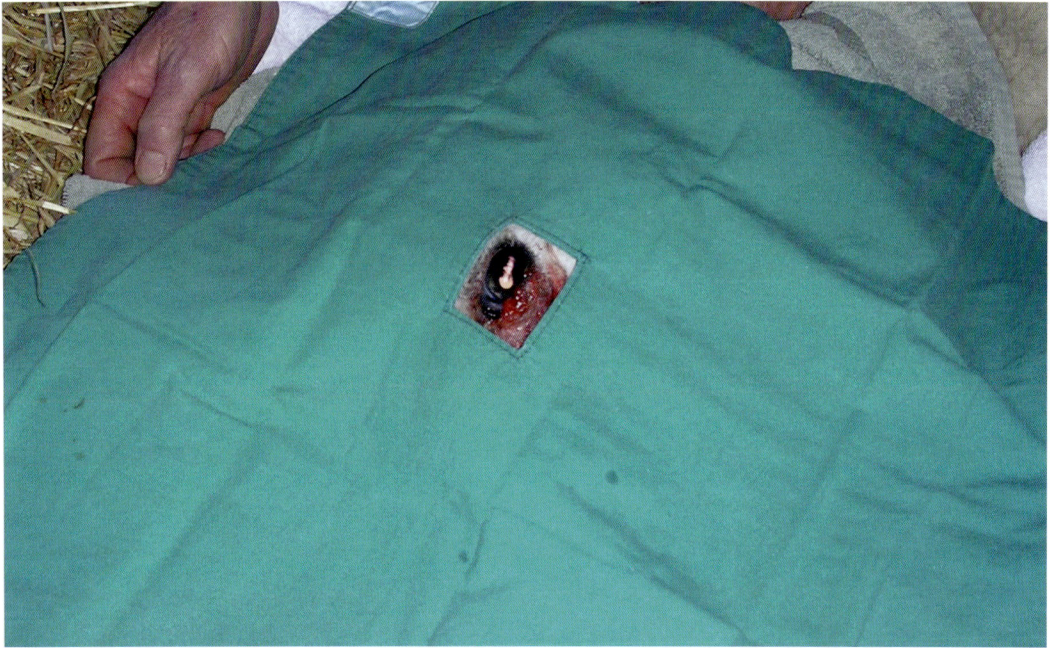

14

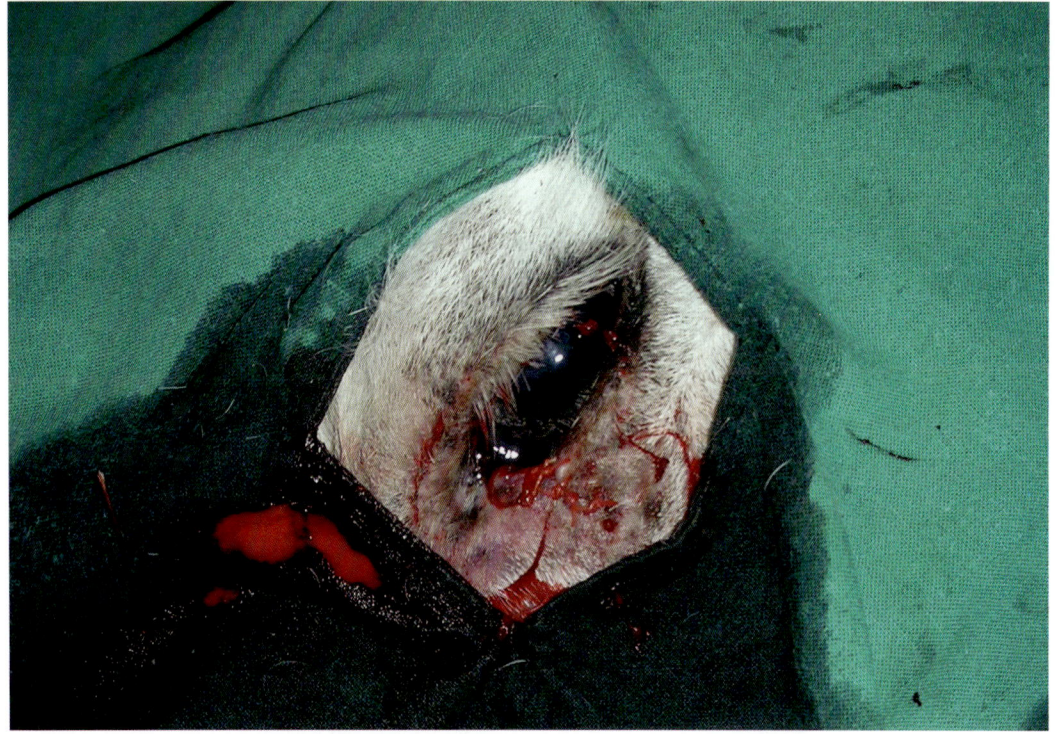

Plate 13. Removal of an eyelid tumour in South American camelids. Surgery to section the third eyelid is straightforward.

Plate 14. Removal of an eyelid tumour in South American camelids. After surgery to section the third eyelid, haemorrhage is minimal.

15

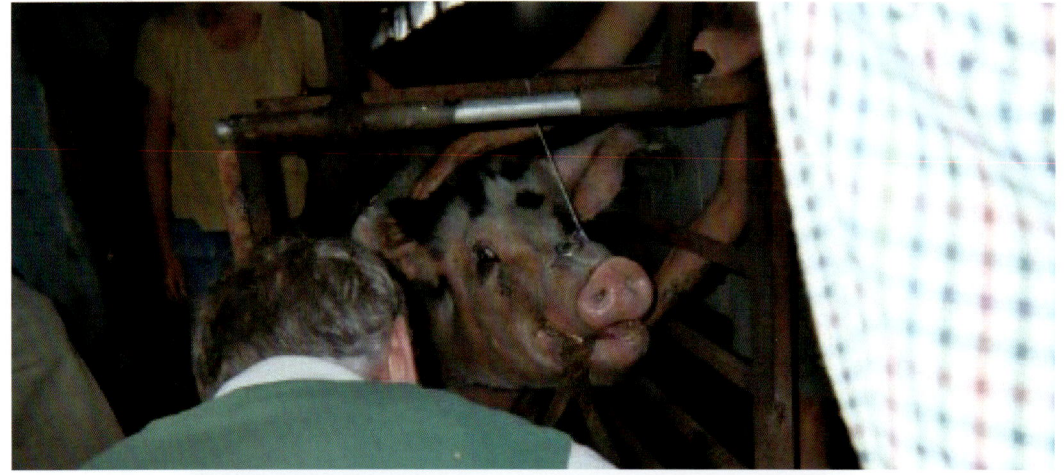

16

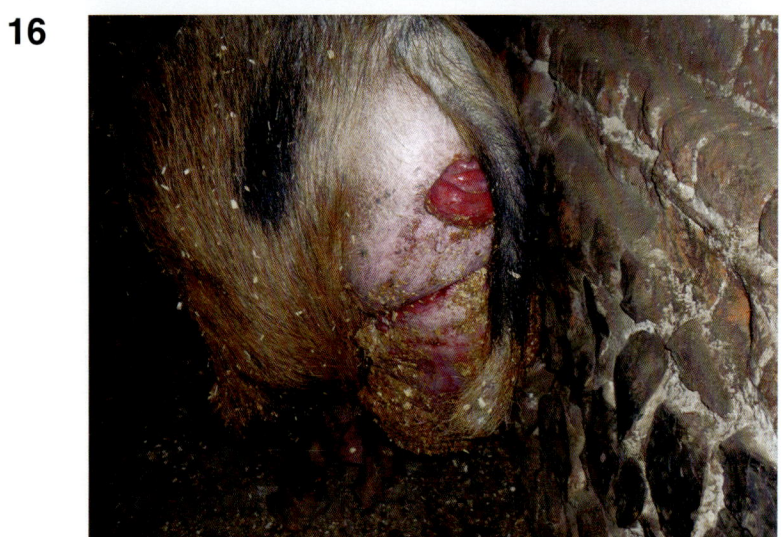

17

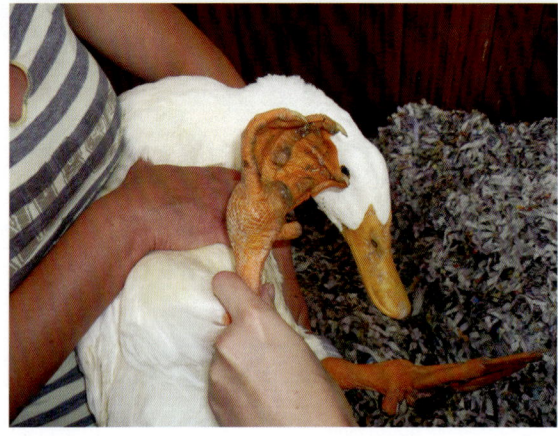

Plate 15. Detusking a boar.
Plate 16. Uterine prolapse in a sow.
Plate 17. Bumblefoot in a goose.

should be pointed out that there are two different dosages: the dosage for cattle is 2 ml and that for sheep is 1 ml for sheep. SACs should receive the sheep dose.

Struck is caused by *Cl. perfringens* type C. As the name suggests, it causes sudden death.

Tetanus is caused by *Cl. tetani*. Vaccination is advisable. Animals will appear stiff and reluctant to feed. They often appear slightly blown and movement in C3 will be absent. The neck will be straight out and there may well be saliva coming from the mouth. Initial treatment should be large doses of tetanus antitoxin (TAT) and also large doses of penicillin. Animals may recover if they are given adequate nursing. Acetylpromazine given twice daily by im injection at 0.1 mg/kg may help to control the tetanic spasms.

Escherichia coli (E.coli) O157

E. coli O157 is not a pathogen in SACs but it is carried by them and therefore they are a danger to man. Precautions must be taken by owners, particularly those with farms open to the general public. In the UK, the organism is found by routine testing to be present in approximately 3% of samples of alpaca faeces.

Escherichia coli

Pathogenic strains are rare in crias. *E. coli* infection is largely about poor management rather than virulent pathogens. *E coli* with the K99 antigen is only found in 2% of herds. With this disease, there is nearly always a septicaemia. The condition may be peracute so that death may occur before the cria is seen to scour. Amoxicillin with clavulanic acid is likely to be the antibiotic of choice, both orally and by injection.

Johne's disease

Alpacas and llamas with Johne's disease, or paratuberculosis (caused by *Mycobacterium paratuberculosis – M. avium* subsp. *paratuberculosis*) do not suffer from scour but from ill thrift. In all animals, once clinical signs develop the disease is always fatal. Euthanasia

is the only option. The normal method of transmission is from dam to offspring soon after birth through colostrum, milk and faeces. Trans-placental infection can also occur, particularly in animals showing advanced signs of ill thrift.

The disease can be diagnosed by an ELISA blood test, which is fairly sensitive once the animal shows signs of the disease, although it is too insensitive to be used as a screening test in clinically normal animals. Faecal smears stained with Zeihl-Neelson (ZN) have a high specificity but a sensitivity of only 30%, as the shedding of the organism is very intermittent in SACs. The strains found in alpacas and llamas are very difficult to grow on culture. Three months is required as a minimum for a negative result, which may then not be that sensitive. Control of Johne's disease in SACs is possible using the Weybridge vaccine. Crias should be given half the cattle dose into the brisket at less than 4 weeks of age. Owners should be warned of the unsightly lumps which may occur at the site of injection.

Enteric diseases caused by protozoa and their treatment

Coccidiosis

This is one of the most frequently diagnosed diseases of British SACs, with affected animals usually showing clinical signs of weight loss and diarrhoea (Twomey *et al.*, 2010). There are five species involved: *Eimeria alpacae*, *E. lamae*, *E. macusaniensis*, *E. ivitaensis* and *E. punoensis*. The most pathogenic are the two larger species, *E. macusaniensis* and *E. ivitaensis*. The average life cycle takes approximately 3 weeks and starts in the small intestine.

Symptoms consist of weight loss and hypoproteinaemia with little diarrhoea until the infection spreads to involve the spiral colon and large intestine. Thus, there may be extensive damage to the small intestine before it is possible to diagnose the infection via faecal samples. Although immunity does develop with age, it is *Eimeria* species specific, so such individuals remain susceptible to new species and any immunity will wane in geriatric animals. Even immune animals may continue to shed, leading to huge environmental contamination which can be exacerbated by overcrowding. Animals can maintain infectivity for many years. Pastures can also maintain infectivity for several months when not grazed.

Diagnosis is straightforward in chronically infected animals by flotation techniques on faeces samples. It is very important that laboratories give the practitioner an estimate of the numbers of the large and the small species found in the faeces. The problem diagnosis is within the prepatent period when the animals can be very sick and yet are not shedding oocysts.

There are old-fashioned treatments using amprolium as a drench at 10 mg/kg for 3 weeks, or sulfonamides (160 mg/kg sulfamethoxine twice daily for 5 days followed by 80 mg/kg for 10 days as a drench), or decoquinate at 0.5 mg/kg for 28 days mixed in the feed. Sulfonamides have been proven to be effective in crias but they are poorly absorbed from the gastrointestinal (GI) tract in adults and therefore this treatment is not recommended for adults. Also, oral sulfonamides upset the flora in C1 of adults. On the whole, clinicians are likely to advise modern treatments licensed for sheep and cattle: diclazuril at 1 mg/kg as a drench repeated in 3 weeks, or toltrazuril at 5 mg/kg also as a drench. Both these treatments effect all intracellular stages, and hence will not only cure the infection but also reduce oocyst shedding.

Cryptosporidiosis

This is caused by *Cryptosporidium parvum*, which will cause diarrhoea in crias and will also affect humans. *C. parvum* has a direct life cycle with infection occurring by the faecal–oral route. The highest mortality rates occur in crias under 21 days of age. The oocysts are fully sporulated and infective when they are excreted in the faeces. Very large numbers are excreted during the prepatent period, resulting in heavy environmental contamination. Transmission can occur directly from cria to cria, or indirectly via a fomite, which may be a human. For bottle-fed llamas or

alpacas, infection can be via contaminated milk. For suckling crias, infection can occur from dirty contaminated teats.

In clinical cases in crias, the faeces tend to be pale and liquid. Fresh blood may be seen but tenesmus is not a feature. In severe cases, the animal will be depressed and dehydrated. Abdominal pain is common. The condition is easy to diagnose as large numbers of oocysts will be seen in the infected faeces. Control of the condition requires attention to detail in all aspects of hygiene to lessen cross-contamination and auto-infection. Halofuginone lactate can be used for prophylaxis and treatment and is available as an oral solution containing 0.5 mg/ml halofuginone lactate. The dose is 2 ml/kg daily for 7 days. Cryptosporidiosis does not seem to be a problem in adult SACs, only in young animals.

Giardia

This is a zoonotic pathogen which is transmitted by the faecal–oral route. Only young animals are affected with diarrhoea. The pathogen does not affect adults. It has a long maturation period of 2 or more weeks so it is not found in crias younger than 4 weeks of age. Treatment should be either with fenbendazole at 10 mg/kg orally for 3 days or metronidizole at 25 mg/kg given either orally or as an enema for 3 days.

Enteric diseases caused by parasites and their treatment

Intestinal cestodes

Adult tapeworms do occur in SACs. *Moniezia expansa* occurs in the UK and worldwide. *M. benedeni* and *Thysaniesia giardi* are found in Peru. The secondary host is an oribatid mite found on the pasture. The prepatent period is 40 days. Some authorities suggest that these cestodes are of no clinical significance, but in large numbers they may cause ill thrift and intussusceptions. They are well controlled with albendazole. *Thysanosoma actinioides* lives in the bile ducts and the pancreatic ducts and is found in the Rocky Mountains in North America. The clinical signs vary from mild to violent diarrhoea and liver failure. Liver enzymes will be raised in serum samples. Control is not easy; weekly dosing with double-strength albendazole for three treatments is recommended.

Intestinal nematodes

These are a problem in SACs as they can become infected by species found in ruminants, e.g. *Haemonchus contortus*, but they can also be infected by species specific to SACs, e.g. *Lamanema chavezi*, which is a problem in South America but not in the UK. Diagnosis is not straightforward as clinical disease may occur before high faecal egg counts (FECs) are seen. Diarrhoea is not a constant sign. Assessing the pallor of the mucous membranes is helpful. Raised serum pepsinogen levels will indicate encysted *Ostertagia* spp.

As resistance to anthelmintics is widespread, the aim of the practitioner and the owner must be to minimize the use of anthelmintic treatment. Anthelmintics should *only* be used when it is necessary to prevent clinical disease. There are no licensed products for SACs. General advice would be to use twice the sheep dose with benzamidazoles and avermectins, which have a wide safety margin. Levamisole does not have a wide safety margin and so the dose can be increased to one and a half times the sheep dose but no higher than this.

Trematodes

Fasciola hepatica is becoming a massive problem in the UK. The distribution is dependent on the presence of the snail intermediate host, *Lymnaea truncatula*. This aquatic snail is now fairly ubiquitous. The eggs hatch in water in the warmer months (>10°C), releasing motile miracidia. These infect the snails in which the development continues through sporocyst and redia stages to the release of cercariae. In wetter summers, there is a massive shedding of cercariae on the pasture during August to October.

The cercariae encyst into metacercariae on the herbage and are ingested by the SAC. The immature flukes migrate through the liver to the bile ducts. This migration will cause severe disease in SACs, with massive damage to the liver resulting in death from acute fascioliasis. In the UK, deaths will occur from September to December. More chronic infections are seen in llamas and alpacas with adult flukes in the bile ducts, and these will occur in February and March. Mild winters increase the numbers of hibernating snails, which shed more cercariae in the following spring.

Llamas and alpacas with chronic fascioliasis will be weak, anaemic and show weight loss. The classic sign is oedema in the mandibular space, known as 'bottle jaw'. Some animals will show pain and recumbency. Diarrhoea is not a feature. Fluke eggs may be seen in the faeces by using a sedimentation test. The bovine PCR test has not been validated in SACs. Eggs will only be present in the chronic cases after the long prepatent period. Treatment is with oral triclabendazole 10 mg/kg.

Conditions of the stomachs and intestines

Anatomy of the gastrointestinal (GI) tract

SACs have a long oesophagus which leads to their stomachs. Examination of the viscera in the abdomen of a camelid from the left-hand side reveals instead of a reticulum, rumen, omasum and abomasum as in a ruminant, three compartments – called compartments 1, 2 and 3 (C1, C2 and C3). There are no papillae but there is glandular tissue in all three compartments.

C1 occupies the entire left-hand side of the abdomen except for the triangular spleen which lies caudally; it has cranial and caudal sacs which are separated by a horizontal pillar. The oesophagus enters C1 midline from a cranio-dorsal aspect. There is only a single lipped oesophageal grove. Looking from the right-hand side directly behind the diaphragm, a small part of C2 and C3 can be seen but the rest will be hidden behind the liver which lies entirely on the right and has a fimbriated caudal border. Camelids do not have a gall bladder. Behind the liver will be seen part of C1. Both C1 and C2 have glandular saccules which contain mucus-producing glands.

C2 lies on the cranio-dorsal aspect of C1 with C3 lying as a long slipper-like organ on the cranio-mesial aspect of C2. Only the final fifth of C3 contains true gastric glands and is the true acid-forming stomach. C3 has five longitudinal ridges of mucosa-like pleats. The lesser omentum has no sling. The greater omentum is attached along the greater and lesser curvature of C2 and C3 and along the right surface of C1.

The duodenum is dorsal to the right-hand side of C1 running into the jejunum which is folded around the root of the mesentery in the right caudal abdomen. The jejunum joins with the ileum which begins ventrally and courses medially and dorsally to enter the large intestine at the caeco-colic junction. The caecum lies midline and runs towards the pelvis. The colon is roughly similar to that of ruminants in that it runs cranially and ventrally before entering a spiral loop. There are five coils in the spiral colon, contrasting with three in the sheep. The colon narrows from a diameter of 5 cm to 2 cm in the spiral colon but widens again as it becomes the transverse colon, which runs caudally to the rectum.

Diagnosis

RADIOGRAPHIC IMAGING OF THE ABDOMEN This is best performed with the animal standing. However, this may not be possible in severe colics and therefore radiographs in these cases should be taken in lateral recumbency. If there is distension of C1, there will be cranial distension of the diaphragm and compression of the thorax. There may be displacement of the intestine into the pelvis. Small gas pockets or fluid lines in C1 are abnormal. Gas-filled intestines indicate intestinal obstruction. Bezoars (concretions) may be seen.

TRANS-ABDOMINAL ULTRASONOGRAPHY OF THE GI TRACT This is useful to aid in the diagnosis of sick SACs. Starting on the right flank, the liver will be seen ventral to the diaphragmatic lobe of the right lung. C2, C3, the intestines and the right kidney can be seen. If time is taken to watch compartmental contractions fluid movement will be seen. On the left side, C1 can be seen. With careful observation

the sacculated and non-sacculated regions can be seen together with their motility patterns. The left kidney is superficial to C1 and immediately caudal to the spleen. Ventral to the kidney will be seen small intestine and the spiral colon. The larger diameter loops of the colon will contain more echo-dense fluid than the small intestine. Visceral oedema will possibly be seen ventrally between C1 and C3 in the right para-lumbar fossa. Visceral oedema may also be seen in the left para-lumbar fossa near the left kidney, spleen and C1.

Differentiation between surgical and medical cases

In camelids, differentiating between surgical and medical cases of gastroenteric disease is difficult even for experienced clinicians. Restlessness is a key sign. Constant shifting indicates pain, and trembling more severe pain. If clinicians are in any doubt, a laparotomy must be performed even if the case turns out not to be a surgical case.

Colic

This is extremely rare, but it does pose a diagnostic challenge to the practitioner. Cases need to be differentiated as whether surgical or medical. Recognition of colic in camelids has two major difficulties as many clinicians expect it to be an active violent process as in equine practice; equally, inexperienced owners may mislead clinicians by over-interpreting non-specific signs such as sternal recumbency, anorexia and lack of faeces, so many animals which do not have colic will be included.

At first, animals will appear bright and alert when handled, but they will lie down when left alone. They may appear restless and will be constantly getting up and down. Then they may go from sternal to lateral recumbency. They may keep stretching out their legs. Signs may become more violent or may lessen if shock sets in. The mucous membranes will be helpful in diagnosis, as will be the tightness of the skin. The heart rate will be high and continue to rise. The respiratory rate will be raised in severe cases. Mouth breathing will occur in animals which are just on the edge of *in extremis*. The rectal temperature will be raised with peritonitis, pancreatitis, nephritis or hepatitis, but otherwise will be subnormal in most cases of colic where shock is setting in. Gastric atony will occur. A tense painful abdomen is a more serious sign.

Most GI colic is due to ischaemia, inflammation or a fluid-distended gut tugging on the mesentery. Large-diameter gastric compartments, full of fibrous material, empty into the small intestine which is not only narrow but tortuous. Intra-luminal obstruction can occur in the duodenum or the first two-thirds of the jejunum. The last third of the jejunum to the transverse colon and the spiral colon has long mesenteric attachments, and these pendulous parts of the bowel are very susceptible to torsion, entrapment or strangulation, i.e. these are surgical cases.

Abdominal distension due to the accumulation of fluid within the gastric compartments is commonly seen with phyto/trichobezoars (plant fibre/hair balls) or other obstructions between the pylorus and the cranial jejunum. Only mild colic signs will be seen with cranial intra-luminal obstruction. Faeces distal to the obstruction will continue to be passed for 24 h. With enteritis or pancreatitis, diarrhoea as well as colic signs will be seen. Small amounts of raspberry jam faeces will occur in cases of intussusceptions.

Tenesmus without diarrhoea is often seen with faecoliths (a hardened mass of faecal matter), other obstructions or impactions in the large intestine. Tenesmus will also be seen in colitis, peritonitis and peri-rectal abscesses. Tenesmus with diarrhoea may also be indicative of internal parasites. The diameter of the spiral colon decreases rapidly. It has short mesenteric attachments between loops. In the lumen, the faeces are dehydrated. Whether the cause is due to impaired motility, too rapid dehydration of faeces or abnormal material in the faeces is unknown and probably varies from case to case, but this part of the gut is very susceptible to impaction or faecolith obstruction. These are normally medical cases in adults, but will require surgery in crias (see 'Spiral colon impaction' below).

Torsion of the spiral colon may well be linked with coccidiosis as nearly all cases have a significant coccidian burden.

Intussusceptions are extremely rare in the jejunum but are not that uncommon at either the ileo-caecal junction or at the caeco-colonic junction. In theory, visualization should be possible with ultrasound, but this is not easy. All that can be seen is an excess of fluid. As these cases are likely to be surgical, the clinician has little choice but to perform an exploratory laparotomy.

Gastric ulceration

This is a common problem. It is important to treat the acidosis before gastric ulcers develop as they are a very serious sequel, which may cause the death of the animal if an ulcer should perforate. Treatment for acidosis if ulcers are not suspected should be prompt and aim to correct dehydration and systemic acidosis. Fluids administered iv and containing magnesium bicarbonate or magnesium hydroxide are ideal. If iv fluids are not practical then oral fluids containing magnesium oxide should be given.

Antibiotics such as penicillin or ceftiofur should be given by injection together with B vitamins to prevent secondary complications. Cover with NSAIDs by injection is useful, together with activated charcoal by mouth. Most affected animals will survive with immediate diagnosis and this treatment. A few, however, may become chronic poor doers with intermittent fever, depression, hypoproteinaemia and weight loss. These animals will be likely to have gastric ulcers. Ulcers are often seen in the mouths of these cases. These are secondary to uraemia due to renal failure from acute nephritis which is seen in the end stages of these cases. *Cl. perfringens* and other *Clostridium* spp. are known to cause disease in camelids. It is possible that these organisms – which cause haemorrhage in the bowel wall – might cause ulceration. Gastric ulcers are generally chronic in nature and only cause acute disease on perforation.

Treatment of ulcers is difficult as there are no licensed medicines in the UK. On being faced with a possible acute ulcer liable to perforate, a human drug, sodium pantoprazole (marketed as PROTIUM i.v.™ by Nycomed GmbH, Konstanz, Germany) should be injected iv after dissolving the 40 mg powder in the vial in water for injection. Injections should be repeated daily either iv at 1 mg/kg or sub cut at 2 mg/kg. Pain can be controlled with NSAIDs but these should be discontinued as soon as appetite is re-established.

Gastroliths

Adult SACs suffer from gastroliths, which are formed as follows. The non-keratinized epithelium of the gastric saccules is protected from the abrasive action of ingested fibre by muscular sphincters coated with keratinized squamous epithelium. If large particles, e.g. large grains, pass this sphincter, they are trapped in the saccular lumen. Once in the lumen, minerals are laid down around them forming stones. These stones, which are very common in adult SACs, can be seen on radiography, although the animals will rarely show clinical signs.

Grain overload

Camelids are very susceptible to grain overload. They are discriminate feeders and thus not prone to engorgement, but high-density confinement increases competition between animals and alters feeding behaviour. Camelids with access to highly fermentable feedstuffs will certainly gorge themselves. The signs will include acute depression, gastric atony and subnormal temperature, as well as neurological signs, including pain. Confirmation of a diagnosis of acidosis can be made by taking a sample from C1 with a long 16G needle through the flank. This avoids salivary contamination. The normal pH of the contents of C1 is 6.4–6.8. Camelids suffering from acute acidosis will have ph values lower than 4.5, but in reality anything under pH 6 is suspicious.

Spiral colon impaction

This is a relatively common condition in crias under 4 months of age. There are known trigger factors, e.g. recent diet change, recent diarrhoea, parasitism, pneumonia and hospitalization. The animals do not normally show colic but have a reduced appetite with reduced GI sounds and faecal output.

Ultrasonographic examination is useful. The small intestine will appear to have a thinner wall with an increase in fluid showing as black rather than grey loops. The blood picture will show a raised total protein and an increase in polymorphs. Diagnosis is straightforward on laparotomy. Enterotomy should be avoided as such surgery lowers survival rates. The obstruction should be milked through, giving a possible survival rate of 33.3%.

The liver

In the SAC, the liver is very different in gross appearance from that of a ruminant. It is multi-lobulated with a fringed pattern, and no gall bladder (as already noted). Abscesses are commonly caused by *E. coli*. Clinically, the animals will be ill with pyrexia. Jaundice may be a feature. A diagnosis may be made from raised liver enzymes. Aggressive antibiotic treatment is indicated. Fascioliasis is the most important liver disease in SACs, although hyperlipaemia is also an important condition.

Diseases of the Neurological System

Congenital conditions

Atlanto-occipital malalignment

This may be iatrogenic from rough correction of a neck deflection at parturition, and it is important that at this time practitioners place the head rope behind the ears and through the mouth like a bit rather than around the neck. Animals can also have atlanto-occipital malalignment without any interference at parturition. The prognosis is extremely guarded.

Hydrocephalus

This is rare and is thought to have a hereditary element. The skull is rarely large enough to cause parturition difficulties.

Kyphosis

This is mainly seen in premature fetuses. It could be an inherited condition, but this is unlikely.

Infectious diseases caused by various agents

Equine herpesvirus (EHV)

This is exceptionally rare. It has been reported in SACs running with zebras, when EHV 1 was the virus type isolated (Rebhun *et al.*, 1988).

Listeriosis

This is caused by *Listeria monocytogenes* and has an acute onset with a marked fever and severe neurological signs, including seizures. Diagnosis can be confirmed with a cerebrospinal fluid (CSF) tap. This will show a raised protein, raised creatine kinase (CK) and a large number of monocytes. Tetracycline or florfenicol is the antibiotic of choice for treatment. These should be coupled with NSAIDs and careful nursing.

Louping ill

This viral disease, which is caused by a *Flavivirus*, is manifest as ataxia, seizures, opisthotonos and sudden death. Diagnosis can be confirmed by virus isolation. There is a PCR test available.

Meningeal worms

These are contracted in North America from the white-tailed deer, *Odocoileus virginianus*. It is the migrating larvae of the causative nematode, *Parelaphostrongylus tenuis*, which causes the problems. These are ingested by SACs when eating infected snails which, in their turn, have eaten the worm eggs. Signs take over a month to develop. The infection causes an inference with the gait, starting with the hind legs. This sign may lead to ataxia and recumbency. Recumbent animals have a poor prognosis. The specific therapy is fenbendazole 50 mg/kg for 5 days. The definitive diagnosis is made by a CSF tap, which will show eosinophilia and raised protein.

Otitis media

This very painful condition is rare in SACs. Foreign bodies, e.g. barley awns, may cause problems, as can functional narrowing of the ear canal. The tympanic membrane is very difficult to visualize in SACs, but there may be a head tilt and facial nerve deficits, e.g. flaccidity of ear and lip with a deviation of the muzzle. Treatment should include parenteral antibiotics and NSAIDs, which will need to be given long term.

Protozoal meningitis

This condition is caused by a *Cryptococcus* sp. and has been found in a CSF tap in an 8 year old alpaca which died showing neurological signs in Australia (Goodchild *et al.*, 1996). It is likely that this is not a primary pathogen.

Rabies

This notifiable disease, which is caused by a rhabdovirus, will only be seen in endemic areas. It will be caused by a bite from a carnivore.

Septic bacterial meningitis

This is seen mainly in crias below a year of age. The invading organism is usually *E. coli*. The antibiotic of choice is a combination of penicillin and gentamicin. Other authorities suggest florfenicol.

West Nile fever

This is caused by *West Nile virus* (WNV), a *Flavivirus* which is spread by mosquitoes. No live virus has been found in the UK, but it is widespread in the USA. The clinical signs are ataxia, general weakness and general torpor. Treatment can only be supportive. Control is through vaccination which is very effective in horses and may well be very effective in SACs.

Miscellaneous conditions

Facial paralysis

This is normally seen immediately after trauma. Antibiotics and NSAIDs should be given as the condition may not be permanent.

Heat stroke

This is confirmed by a high rectal temperature. The animals will show tachypnoea and tachycardia. Recumbency carries a poor prognosis. The animals need to be immersed in ice-cold water until the rectal temperature returns to normal. This should be carried out immediately. No time should be lost while a drip is set up. Corticosteroids iv are helpful.

Hypothermia

This is seen in young crias born in the winter or very early spring and left in exposed conditions. If it does occur in crias over 24 h old it is vital that they receive a glucose enema before they are warmed up, otherwise the central nervous system (CNS) will die through lack of glucose. If the cria is under 24 h old, it should be tubed with colostrum. Obviously the crias need to be warmed up. The use of hot-air blowers should be avoided as initially they cause a drop in core temperature as a result of the latent heat of vaporization.

Polioencephalomalacia

This is similar to cerebrocortical necrosis (CCN) in sheep. It responds to treatment with thiamine (vitamin B_1) injections, ideally 15 mg/kg iv at 6 h intervals, but these can also be given sub cut. The prognosis is good provided the SAC is not recumbent. It is mainly seen in year-old or young adult animals following a change of diet or overfeeding of concentrates. Animals are blind and wander away from others. They are depressed but will eat if the food is in front of them. Their rectal temperature, heart rate and respiratory rate are normal.

Tumours of the brain and spinal cord

These are extremely rare.

Musculoskeletal conditions

Peripheral nerve damage

This can occur to any nerve. The most important condition is radial paralysis, which will give the impression of forelimb fracture.

However, if the leg is placed for the animal it can bear weight without pain. It is miraculous how in 6–10 weeks the animals will learn to flick the foreleg forward and appear normal.

Toxic conditions

Botulism

This is very rare. Animals will drool and may become recumbent. The pathognomic sign is the flaccid anus on taking the temperature. These animals may recover with good nursing. Penicillin and NSAIDs should be given.

Ionophore toxicosis

This type of poisoning occurs if animals gain access to food destined for chicken feed that contains common anti-coccidial and antibacterial additives (ionophores). Animals will be recumbent and then show convulsions. Euthanasia is advised.

Ryegrass staggers

This is caused by an endophyte which grows on ryegrass, particularly in dry weather. The main signs are ataxia and a head tilt. Normally, animals recover if moved to a new unaffected pasture.

Tetanus

This condition is always a potential threat (see above under 'Diseases of the Gastroenteric System', 'Enteric diseases caused by bacteria and their treatment', 'Clostridial diseases').

Traumatic conditions

Cerebral hypoxia

This occurs with a delayed parturition. Crias will not lift up their heads and certainly will not make any effort to get up. Euthanasia is indicated.

Fractured vertebrae in the neck

These are commonly reported. Vertebral body subluxation requires prompt treatment with realignment under general anaesthetic (GA). Vertebral body fractures may survive with good neck support, but usually they are fatal or require immediate euthanasia.

Eye disorders

Eye disorders and visual defects in neonatal crias

CATARACTS These are usually congenital and may be inherited. There is no treatment. If the cria has some vision, it is reasonable to wait to see how it will adapt. However, if it is totally blind euthanasia should be performed.

NON-PIGMENTED IRIS This does not cause problems.

Eye disorders and visual defects in older crias and adults

VITAMIN A DEFICIENCY This is irreversible. The animals have fixed dilated pupils. In advanced cases, they will be ataxic and may show head pressing.

Metabolic Diseases

Hepatic encephalopathy

This will occur in advanced liver disease. The animal will show acute neurological signs indicating pain, i.e. head pressing. Liver enzymes will be raised. Treatment is with concentrated vitamin B injections and dexamethazone (assuming that the animal is not pregnant).

Hypocalcaemia

This is a metabolic condition of the lactating female 3–6 weeks after parturition. The animal will be off food with atony of C1. Treatment is with calcium borogluconate daily.

Hypoglycaemia

This is a condition of the newborn cria and is often linked with hypothermia (see above

under 'Diseases of the Neurological System', 'Miscellaneous problems'). If the cria is less than 24 h old it should be given warm colostrum. If it is older than 24 h it should be given plasma (see below under 'Diseases of the Reproductive System', 'Diseases of the mammary gland', 'Failure of passive transfer (FPT)'). If this is not possible, then warmed glucose should be given *per rectum* (20 ml of a 40% solution).

Hypomagnesaemia

This is extremely rare. Animals will be showing neurological signs, generally convulsions. Treatment is 60 ml of a 25% solution of magnesium sulfate sub cut.

Uraemic encephalopathy

This is the terminal condition of several other syndromes, e.g. intestinal volvulus or ruptured gastric ulcers. There will be ulcers in the mouth and there will be a strong smell of urea on the breath. There is renal shut down and the prognosis is normally hopeless.

Diseases of the Respiratory System

Non-infectious conditions of the upper respiratory tract

Hyperplasia of the soft palate

This is a rare condition of unknown aetiology. The main clinical sign is a rattling noise on inspiration. The animals do not appear to be ill or to suffer from respiratory distress. Neither antibiotics nor anti-inflammatories seem to alleviate the signs.

Rhinitis

This is extremely rare and is thought to be an allergic rhinitis. The main sign is an intermittent clear nasal discharge from both nostrils. Sneezing is not seen but there is an eosinophilia on blood testing. Antibiotics and NSAIDs do not seem to be helpful, nor do antihistamines. In the UK, the condition seems to get better in the autumn. Owners think that nasal nets are helpful but the author is not convinced.

Infectious conditions of the upper respiratory tract

Nasal myiasis

This is caused by the sheep nasal botfly, *Oestrus ovis*, in SACs in the UK and Europe, but it is extremely rare. The adult fly deposits larvae around the nostrils, and these invade the nasal cavity and develop into second-stage instars which then invade the sinuses in the head. The mature larvae are sneezed out up to a year later. The signs of sneezing can be controlled by eliminating the larvae with ivermectin treatment (0.2 mg/kg sub cut).

Non-infectious conditions of the lower respiratory tract

Aspiration pneumonia

This often called 'inhalation pneumonia' and is a real danger in SACs undergoing a GA, particularly if a gaseous anaesthetic is used. The occurrence can be lessened by careful monitoring of the animal on recovery. Aspiration pneumonia can also occur after using a faulty drenching technique in adults. This is particularly common in SACs which have not been handled regularly. It is also seen in lactating females which have hypocalcaemia and have been treated *per os* by the owner.

Diaphragmatic paralysis

This occurs in young SACs between the ages of 2 months and 3 years. It tends to occur in the winter in the northern hemisphere. The cause is unknown but might be traumatic damage to the phrenic nerve, which comes from the lower cervical region and supplies motor nerves to the diaphragm. The main clinical signs are tachypnoea and dyspnoea. There is an abdominal effort and paradoxic breathing, i.e. the chest goes out as the flank goes in. Often the animal will adopt a dog-sitting posture. Diagnosis is on clinical signs after ruling out upper airway obstruction. Diaphragmatic hernia and pneumothorax can be ruled out by radiography. Diaphragmatic paralysis is better seen on fluoroscopy. Treatment is non-specific and supportive. Survival rates are 75%.

Drowning

SACs can swim well. However, in winter in the UK they become exhausted if they are not able to get out of the water on account of their heavy fleeces. If artificial respiration is attempted, expiration may be aided by pressing the ribs firmly behind the shoulder with the animal in lateral recumbency. Blowing into the nostrils does not seem to inflate the lungs and so inspiration can be aided by lifting the ribcage behind the last rib. This same procedure can be used very carefully in newborn crias.

Pleural effusion

This will occur with infectious pneumonia and with tuberculosis (TB). It will occur idiopathically. The animal will be in respiratory distress and will be mouth breathing. There will be dullness on percussion of the ventral thorax and a fluid line may be seen on ultrasound. Clear straw-coloured fluid may be drawn off by aspiration below this line. This will bring about some clinical improvement, but if this is not sustainable then euthanasia is warranted.

Trauma

The most important cause in adults is road traffic accidents causing rib fracture. These will be seen on radiography. Trauma can also occur when there is fighting between males resulting in thoracic penetration by bite wounds. Aggressive antibiotic treatment is required. NSAIDs are useful in both incidences. Trauma of the ribcage can occur in crias from problems at parturition. Owners should be urged to take care when assisting birth and when trying to revive crias.

Infectious conditions of the lower respiratory tract

Infectious pneumonia

This is extremely rare and is a very serious condition if not treated promptly with broad-spectrum antibiotics and NSAIDs. Bovine respiratory viruses could affect SACs if cattle and SACs are housed closely together. Equally, SACs can develop pasteurellosis if they are housed closely with sheep and goats. The disease is particularly prevalent in 1–2 year old animals which have been stressed by travelling or have been in the same airspace as infected lambs or calves. Diagnosis can be confirmed by culture of nasal swabs or paired serum samples. Clinicians should note that the 'Pasteurella vaccines' prepared for cattle or sheep do not seem to provide immunity in SACs. Other organisms causing pneumonia in SACs include *Equine herpesvirus* which has been isolated from SACs in close proximity to infected zebras and *Rhodococcus equi* which has been found in SACs in close contact with infected foals.

Lungworms

In the main, these are of no real significance. There is one exception: when there is mixed grazing with cattle *Dictyocaulus filaria* can cause real problems in younger animals, i.e. first-season crias. This lungworm has a direct life cycle in SACs so that cattle are not required to continue an infection. While still out at grass in late summer, the infected animals will have a rasping cough. Although ivermectins by injection will eliminate the adults in the lungs, supportive therapy with antibiotics and NSAIDs is useful. A second dose of ivermectin should be given after an interval of 3 weeks. The pasture will be contaminated in the following year so it is advisable for it to be used as a hay or silage field until later in the season.

Streptococcus equi

SACs can become infected by *Streptococcus equi* but this is rare in the UK, although it is relatively common in Peru, where it causes 'alpaca fever'. This is a very serious disease in crias and young adults, causing a high fever and pneumonia. Animals should be treated with high doses of penicillin.

Tuberculosis (TB)

TB is increasing rapidly in prevalence in SACs in the UK which is a worrying phenomenon and in some way mirrors the increase in bovine TB. As the disease is particularly difficult to diagnose in live SACs, because the skin test is unreliable, the industry and the government regulatory body in the UK (Defra, Department for Environment, Food and Rural Affairs) is left in a difficult position. There is a blood test for TB, the Chembio Rapid Blood test, but this is hardly any better than the insensitive skin test. The main pathogen is *Mycobacterium bovis*, but *M. microti* and *M. avium* also occur.

The clinical signs of TB are very confusing as individuals vary enormously. There may be ill thrift and loss of weight. Coughing may be a feature, but it does not occur in all lung cases and certainly does not occur if another organ, e.g. the liver, is infected. Occasionally, a peripheral lymph node will be swollen. Cutaneous lesions are often linked with a discharging superficial lymph node. *M. bovis* has been isolated from a mammary gland in an alpaca (Richey *et al.*, 2011). Practitioners should be aware that there can be severe side effects following the skin test which appear to be linked to actual infection.

Diseases of the Circulatory System

Diseases of the cardiovascular system

Iliac arterial thrombosis

The main sign is hind limb lameness. The condition can be confirmed by rectal ultrasound examination. Treatment should be antibiotics and NSAIDs for 10 days. The lameness should make a steady improvement.

Vegetative endocarditis

There are a variety of bacteria which can cause the condition but a common cause is *Erysipelas rhusiopathiae*. Animals should be treated for at least 2 weeks with antibiotics.

Ventricular septal defects

These are relatively common in crias.

Viral myocarditis

This is associated with FMD and results in sudden death.

White muscle disease

This will affect crias in their first few months. Cases may be found dead or very ill. Vitamin E and selenium injections are rarely successful.

Diseases affecting the haemopoietic and lymphatic systems

Anaplasmosis

This is a tick-borne disease caused by an obligate intracellular bacterium, *Anaplasma phagocytophilum*. The predominant vector in the UK is *Ixodes ricinus*. The clinical signs are very variable but include fever, lethargy and anorexia. Some animals may show neurological signs, mainly ataxia, which are thought to be caused by focal CNS lesions secondary to localized vasculitis. Cytoplasmic inclusions are commonly seen in the neutrophils and are diagnostic. The diagnosis can be confirmed by a PCR test on anticoagulant-treated blood. Treatment is 20 mg/kg tetracycline on alternate days for a minimum of 10 days.

Babesiosis

This is a tick-transmitted disease caused by protozoal parasites of the red blood cells. In the UK, SACs can be infected with *Babesia motasi* caught from sheep and *B. capreoli* caught from red deer. Diagnosis can be confirmed by identification of the parasite in Giemsa-stained red blood smears. Treatment

is with imidocarb which is supplied in a multi-dose vial as a 12% solution; 1 ml/100 kg should be given im. Abscess formation is possible so owners should be warned.

Mycoplasma haemolamae

Animals infected by *M. haemolamae* are not necessarily anaemic but normally will show an acute onset of weakness, fever, depression and recumbency. They will have pale mucous membranes and are often anorexic. They often show respiratory distress. The disease can affect all ages. The organism can be seen in thin blood smears stained with Giemsa and examined under the oil immersion power of a microscope. The blood film should be examined immediately after collection to avoid missing the organism, which can also be positively diagnosed by a PCR test on a blood sample collected in EDTA. Large doses of tetracycline i.e. 20 mg/kg every other day for 10 days should be used for treatment.

Diseases of the Urinary system

Congenital and hereditary conditions of the urinary system

Renal agenesis

This may be hereditary. It is normally seen as a terminal condition and so euthanasia is advised. It is often linked to gonadal agenesis. If the condition is unilateral both renal agenesis and gonadal agenesis may well go unnoticed in females. In males, there may be a misdiagnosis which considers the SACs to be rigs.

Medical conditions of the urinary tract

Nephritis

The presenting sign will be general malaise and low-grade abdominal pain. The most common bacterium isolated is *E. coli*. Yeasts, namely *Candida albicans*, have been isolated on rare occasions.

Prostatitis

This is seen in young males when stressed at weaning. Signs will look like those of cystitis or bladder stones. Indeed, struvite crystals will often be seen in the urine which is usually alkaline with a pH of 9. The presence of struvite crystals is difficult to interpret as they are seen in normal urine that is allowed to stand. Long-term antibiotic treatment with penicillin and NSAIDs should be given. Glycosaminoglycans might be used in treatment following the model of idiopathic cystitis in other animals.

Diseases of the Reproductive System

Abortion and its causes

- Allergies
- Anaphylaxis
- Deficiencies of vitamins A or E, copper, iodine or selenium
- High dietary levels of toxic chemicals e.g. nitrates, selenium and arsenic
- Physiological stress
- Thermal stress
- Vaccination against clostridial disease
- Various poisonous plants

The most notable poisonous plant is the ponderosa pine (*Pinus ponderosa*) whose needles, whether fresh or dry, have definitely been indicated as a cause of abortion. The problem with vaccination against clostridial disease is handling stress rather than the vaccine itself.

A list of infectious causes of abortion might well include:

- *Campylobacter fetus* subsp. *fetus*. This organism will cause abortions, stillbirths and weak crias. Placentitis is easily seen.
- Chlamydophilosis. *Chlamydophila* is rare in SACs but it will cause abortions in late pregnancy. Female SACs that are in contact with *Chlamydophila* could be given a long-acting dose of oxytetracycline to try to limit the number of abortions and reduce the excretion of organisms.

- *E. coli*. This organism has been isolated in pure culture from aborted fetuses.
- Leptospirosis. *Leptospira* serovar Hardjo of cattle origin has been isolated from aborted fetuses.
- Q fever. This has been diagnosed in SACs in the UK and elsewhere in the world but not in New Zealand. The causal rickettsia, *Coxiella burnetii*, is shed intermittently in the milk, faeces, vagina and placenta. The latter has a gritty feel. Abortions normally occur within 6 weeks of the expected parturition date. There are also stillbirths and weak crias. The organism can stay in the environment for a considerable length of time. Problems are mainly seen in the first pregnancy. Prophylactic antibiotics do not seem to be helpful. The best diagnostic tools are PCR and ELISA tests. The complement fixation test (CFT) is unreliable.
- Toxoplasmosis. This condition (causal organism *Toxoplasma gondii*) is extremely rare in SACs. However there is a fairly long window during pregnancy when the SAC dam can become infected. Infection is acquired from cat faeces on the food. Up to 2 months of pregnancy the SAC will appear to have absorbed the fetus and be barren, but from then on until the 10th month of pregnancy the dam will either abort or have a stillborn full-term cria.

The following organisms are likely to cause abortions but, as yet, there have been no published isolates in the UK:

- *Bluetongue virus*.
- Bovine viral diarrhoea (BVD). This has been widely reported as causing abortion in the USA. The virus can be readily found in the saliva and in the salivary glands. Antibody-positive animals are readily found in infected herds with occasional PI crias being seen. These are defined as virus positive but antibody negative despite repeated tests. Such crias may be slightly underweight and woolly looking but are impossible to definitely detect clinically. Some PCR-positive animals have become positive only at 15 weeks of age. This implies that it is possible that not all animals identified as PI animals are in fact

persistently infected, but instead are slowly developing an antibody response and combating the disease. True PIs may show a reduced growth rate and be prone to infections or sudden death. In the USA, the virus in SACs is related to diarrhoea but in the UK respiratory signs are more common.

- *Brucella* spp.
- *Equine herpesvirus* 1 (EHV 1). This has only been isolated when the SACs are in very close proximity to equines.
- Infectious bovine rhinotracheitis (IBR, caused by *Bovine herpesvirus 1*).
- *Listeria monocytogenes*.
- *Salmonella* spp.

Embryonic death

Causes are largely unknown but some of those considered to be likely reasons for embryonic deaths are listed below:

- age (or more likely, parity)
- endocrine imbalance (may be an oestrogen/progesterone imbalance)
- gamete ageing
- genetic incompatibility
- immunological incompatibility
- infection (no recognized bacteria, but streptococci, staphylococci, coliforms, clostridia, *Actinobacillus pyogenes*, peptostreptococci and *Bacteriodes* spp. have been isolated)
- physiological stress
- polyspermia
- poor nutrition (unlikely but mouldy feedstuffs or feedstuffs with high oestrogenic activity may be responsible)
- stress of lactation (may be because of too early post-partum breeding)
- thermal stress
- uterine crowding (twins are extremely rare in SACs)

Diseases of the mammary gland

Mastitis

This is a very rare condition in SACs. It is often brought on by trauma, e.g. dog bites or animals jumping out of pens soon after parturition. A variety of organisms can be involved. Treatment with parenteral antibiotics and NSAIDs is required (intramammary preparations should *not* be used). SACs will develop peracute mastitis immediately after parturition if there is failure of sucking. The causal organism is either *E. coli* or *Klebsiella pneumoniae*. The condition is more likely with human interference, e.g. hand stripping. Owners should be urged to be hygienic. The condition has a poor prognosis and if the animal is severely shocked and toxic with a low rectal temperature, euthanasia should be carried out. If clinicians feel that there is a chance of recovery, treatment should be aggressive, i.e. hospitalization, warmth, iv fluids, NSAIDs and appropriate antibiotic treatment for Gram-negative organisms. *Mycobacterium bovis* has been found to cause mastitis in an alpaca (Richey *et al.*, 2011).

Failure of passive transfer (FPT)

This is common. The aim is for crias to receive 12% of their body weight of colostrum in the first 12 h of life. FPT occurs with weak crias or ineffective nursing from blocked teats, mastitis, poor milk production and poor maternal instincts. It can be monitored by measuring the birth weight and reweighing at 8 h. The treatment for FPT is to give plasma collected from a healthy animal in the same environment. The argument against ip transfusion versus iv transfusion is that it is not so effective and might cause peritonitis; however, ip transfusion is much less stressful for the cria and is much quicker as administration can be done in 10 min after careful aseptic preparation. Collection of plasma ideally needs to be done in advance and then the plasma is stored in a deep freeze on the client's holding.

Cross matching of plasma is not required as SACs have only one blood group with one factor. Before use, the plasma needs to be defrosted very slowly in a water bath at 37°C over a period of 20 min. A microwave should not be used as there is a danger that some of the proteins will be damaged. The plasma can then be given iv or ip.

Acquired infertility in females

This is common as there is often a very short length of time between parturition and subsequent mating. Vaginal infections as a result of trauma at parturition will require aggressive antibiotic treatment of penicillin given parenterally and 20 IU oxytocin injected im. Sexual rest should be advised with small doses of prostaglandin (125 mcg cloprostenol) given by im injection. Cystic ovaries are very rarely seen on ultrasonography. If present, they should be treated with injections of gonadotrophin-releasing hormone (GnRH) as 0.004 mg buserelin im not only before mating but after service. Manual popping of cysts should be avoided on account of the danger of trauma to the rectum and possible haemorrhage from the ovary. The latter can be life threatening or can lead to adhesions which would render that ovary unable to deliver eggs.

Male infertility

The majority of infertility cases in male SACs are actually immaturity rather than infertility. No SAC should be said to be infertile or even sub-fertile until it is over 3 years of age. Sperms need to mature in the male so that although there is adequate libido and intromission takes place, pregnancy does not necessarily follow. Given a few more months, such males will become fertile. Heat stress and diseases causing pyrexia will cause transitory infertility for some weeks but fertility normally returns after 3 months.

There are certain physical congenital problems which will cause infertility in unproven males:

- persistent frenulum
- corkscrew penis
- preputial stricture
- hypospadia
- hypoplastic testicles
- cystic testicles

There are other physical problems which will cause infertility in previously fertile males:

- preputial tears
- scarring strictures

- haematomas
- adhesions

Diseases of the Integument

Viral skin diseases

Bluetongue disease

This systemic viral disease causes hyperaemia of the oral mucosa with excoriations of the tongue, lips and gums that become ulcerative and necrotic. There is also a coronitis with hyperaemia and swelling around the coronet which leads to obvious lameness. See also above under 'Diseases of the Gastroenteric System', 'Enteric diseases caused by viruses and their treatment', for more information.

Contagious pustular dermatitis

This is primarily a disease of sheep but it can affect SACs as well. The initial lesion consists of a number of red papules within which vesicles develop, rupture and form a thick scab. Proliferative changes may then occur, resulting in papillomatous lesions. Secondary bacterial infection is common with all lesions, and in females with mastitis deaths may occur. Difficulty in sucking may cause weight restriction in crias and lesions on the coronary band may result in lameness. The disease will spread rapidly. Although the causative agent is a virus, a blanket dose of a penicillin/streptomycin injection is very helpful. Really bad lesions should be treated with oily creams.

Foot-and-mouth disease (FMD)

This notifiable viral disease will cause vesicles on the oral mucosa and the coronary band. See above under 'Diseases of the Gastroenteric System', 'Enteric diseases caused by viruses and their treatment', for more information.

Malignant Catarrhal Fever (MCF)

MCF is caused by a systemic virus which will produce severe generalized alopecia with granulomatous mural folliculitis. A definitive diagnosis may be made by a PCR test. The condition is normally fatal. There is no treatment and so euthanasia is recommended if a definitive diagnosis has been made. See above under 'Diseases of the Gastroenteric System', 'Enteric diseases caused by viruses and their treatment'.

Bacterial skin diseases

Actinobacillosis

This condition (causal organism *Actinobacillus*) is characterized by thickening of the skin with multiple granulomatous swellings often associated with the lymphatics. These swellings are unrewarding to lance as the pus is only in small pockets. Treatment with prolonged daily dosing with streptomycin is usually effective. A minimum of 10 mg/kg for 10 days is suggested.

Actinomycosis

This condition (causal organism *Actinomyces bovis*) occurs in the soft tissues of the mouth. Treatment with streptomycin at a minimum of 10 mg/kg for 10 days is suggested.

Caseous lymphadenitis (CLA)

This is caused by *Corynebacterium pseudotuberculosis*. Abscesses develop in the lymph nodes under the skin. It is a contagious condition and can be spread by the shearer. If incised the abscesses take on an onion-like appearance with concentric rings of fibrous tissue and inspissated pus. There is no effective treatment.

Clostridial cellulitis

This is called malignant oedema. It is most common in males as a result of fighting wounds. The causal organism is *Cl. septicum*. It is a very serious condition. The area of swelling, which is initially hot and painful with crepitus, then turns cold and gangrenous. Treatment may be attempted if the disease is caught in the febrile stage. High doses of crystalline penicillin should be given iv together with NSAIDs.

Dermatophilosis

This is caused by the bacterium *Dermatophilus congolensis*. It is also called 'fibre rot'. The disease is manifest as an exudative dermatitis affecting the back and flanks, and is progressive. It starts with an exudation which then crusts and scabs. The initial penetration by *D. congolensis* is facilitated by prolonged wetting of the fleece during periods of protracted wet weather. Diagnosis may be made on clinical grounds and confirmed by Giemsa staining of the scabs. Treatment in severe cases is parenteral antibiotics and antibiotic cream on the raw areas. Most mild cases will heal spontaneously.

Necrotic dermatitis

This is caused by *Pseudomonas aeruginosa*. It is a very serious condition as it is very difficult to treat. Large areas may be involved and the local lymph nodes become swollen. The diagnosis can be confirmed on culture. Treatment is parenteral broad-spectrum antibiotics together with local creams containing miconazole nitrate, prednisolone acetate and polymyxin B sulfate.

Periorbital eczema

This is usually caused by a *Staphylococcus* sp. The condition characteristically affects trough-fed SACs. The early lesion is seen as a small inflamed and scabbed area on one or other of the bony prominences of the face or, less commonly, on the nose. This extends, usually around the eye, hence the name, to give an alarming scabbed, discharging sore. Severe cases may require aggressive antibiotic treatment. The author recommends daily injections for 3 days with amoxicillin with clavulanic acid and local treatment with the same antibiotic (which is available as an intra-mammary preparation for cows).

Staphylococcal folliculitis

This is a benign condition which affects young crias. It is caused by *S. hyicus*. The condition will generally resolve without treatment in a few days.

Fungal skin diseases

Ringworm

This is caused by *Trichophyton verrucosum* which is normally contracted from cattle, but it can also be caused by *Microsporum canis* contracted from dogs and by *T. mentagrophytes* contracted from goats. The clinical picture of round crusting lesions is the same with all three species of fungi. Pruritis is more marked with *T. verrucosum* infection. Only debilitated animals will develop a bad infection. In normal animals, the infection is self-limiting in a few months. If treatment is required for special animals, e.g. showing animals, there are topical fungicides such as natamycin and oral antibiotics such as griseofulvin.

Parasitic skin diseases

Blowfly strike

This is caused by secondary strikers (*Lucilia sericata*). The condition, if advanced, can be life threatening and so treatment needs to be aggressive. The animal should receive antibiotics and NSAIDs immediately. The area around the strike is trimmed of fibre and cleaned. *All* the maggots are removed with warm salty water, but if this is difficult a hair drier can be used (author's practice). Cypermethrin in a 1.25% w/v non-aqueous liquid is applied to all the affected parts at the rate of 2.5 ml/100–150 sq. cm (roughly the size of a hand). The whole wet area is dressed with oily cream, usually a mixture of acriflavin and benzene hexachloride (BHC).

Lice

Bovicola breviceps is the only louse confirmed in the UK (Foster, 2008). It causes pruritis. The safest treatment is fipronil applied as a spray or cypermethrin diluted and applied as a spray. All louse treatments require a repeat treatment in 10 days to control the unhatched eggs.

Mites

CHORIOPTES MITES These are the most common mites found in SACs in the UK. They cause mild pruritis, alopecia and scaling. Lesions are commonly found on the head, ears, feet and perineum but can also extend to the limbs and ventral abdomen. A high prevalence has been reported (D'Alterio *et al.*, 2005) in the south-west of England. Over 20% of alpacas were affected and mites were identified in 40% of these cases; 55% of animals which actually had no skin lesions were found to be harbouring mites. The most likely area to find mites was in the interdigital space. The most effective treatment is topical application of either eprinexin diluted with dimethyl sulfoxide (DMSO) to affected areas weekly for 3 months or fipronil spray applied weekly for a similar length of time.

PSOROPTES MITES These are also found on SACs. They are indistinguishable from the mites causing sheep scab (*P. ovis*) and so it is to be expected that SACs become infected from this source. Treatment with injectable avermectins three times at weekly intervals is normally successful.

SARCOPTES MITES These may well be more common in SACs than was previously thought. They cause more intense pruritis than *Chorioptes* spp. Mites can be found all over the body, and there will be hyperaemia, papules and pustules with crusting. As the mite seems to burrow deeper than *Chorioptes* treatment with regular avermectins by injection seems to be effective.

Vitamin and mineral related skin diseases

Cobalt deficiency

This results in rough brittle hair coat or wool. Other deficiency signs, e.g. weight loss, may be severe.

Copper deficiency

This causes important systemic disease. Black SACs will also show a lack of pigment. Fibre animals will show a lack of crimp.

Iodism

Alopecia and scaling occurs in SACs if they are fed foods very rich in iodine, e.g. seaweed, over long periods of time.

Sulfur deficiency

This deficiency causes fleece biting and alopecia. Diagnosis can be made from serum or liver samples.

Vitamin A deficiency

This is extremely rare. The coat will show a generalized seborrhoea. The main sign is an irreversible retinal atrophy causing blindness.

Vitamin C deficiency

This is seen as a non-pruritic alopecia with some scaling. It may not be a true deficiency but rather a vitamin C-responsive alopecia.

Vitamin E deficiency

This deficiency is not a real deficiency but rather a vitamin E/selenium-responsive dermatosis. The animals appear healthy and are non-pruritic but lose their hair.

Zinc deficiency

This is really a zinc-responsive condition. There is marked scaling and crusting. Clinicians should remember that any blood samples for zinc levels must be taken into bottles without rubber stoppers or erroneous results will be obtained.

Physical causes of skin disease

Frostbite

This is seen when animals are outside in extreme weather conditions. It is usually the ears which are affected. The skin will slough. The animals should be given antibiotics to prevent secondary bacterial infection and NSAIDs to lessen the pain.

Photosensitization

This occurs on the non-pigmented areas of the animals that are free from fibre. Diagnosis may be made on clinical grounds with confirmation by demonstrating raised serum levels of phylloerythrin and, in the case of hepatogenous disease, raised levels of serum liver enzymes. Animals should be housed and any severely affected areas treated with oily creams.

Sunburn

This is caused by the harmful effects of ultraviolet radiation from direct sunlight in newly shorn alpacas, and should not be forgotten as a potential cause of skin damage, particularly in areas where there is no shade. Encrustment of the non-pigmented skin, with ultimate necrosis of the epidermis, upper dermis and superficial sebaceous glands, may occur. Animals should be housed and oily creams applied to the affected areas. Antibiotics and NSAIDs may be required in severe cases.

Trauma

This is the most common physical cause of skin disease. Airgun pellets will cause abscesses, normally on the flank. These may be found when the abscesses are lanced or confirmed quite simply with a rectal linear ultrasound scanner. Tethered animals will develop tether galls or bell strap galls. Working llamas may get saddle sores. Animals may also be attacked by magpies. Shearing wounds are common. Burn cases will often result in keloids and crusty nodules.

Neoplastic conditions

Malignant tumours

These may occur in the skin anywhere on the body. They include histiocytomas, lymphosarcomas, malignant melanomas and squamous cell carcinomas. The latter occur in the conjunctiva, on the third eyelid, on the penis and on the vulva. Melanomas are not restricted to white animals.

Skin diseases of uncertain aetiology

Pemphigus foliaceus

This is an autoimmune-mediated disease. Bacteria, fungi and even parasites may well be found as secondary invaders. If the skin condition persists after treatment for these last three infections, the practitioner should suspect pemphigus, which can be confirmed by a biopsy. The main presenting signs include a generalized severe pustular eruption involving most of the body. Treatment is difficult as all the secondary bacteria, fungi and parasites have to be removed before regular steroid treatment is carried out. Dexamethazone should be given orally at 2 mg/kg every other morning.

Common Causes for SACs to be Found Dead

Iatrogenic causes of sudden death

Sudden death is a misnomer. In reality it means that death has occurred since the animal was last seen. The owner will very rarely see an animal die. It is even rarer for the clinician to see death. Sadly, when such deaths do occur it is usually at the time of veterinary treatment. The likely causes of iatrogenic deaths in SACs are shown in Table 7.1.

Reasons for animals to be found dead

True sudden deaths are very rare. Possible causes of such deaths in SACs are shown in Table 7.2.

Table 7.1. A list of possible iatrogenic causes of sudden death in South American camelids.

Anaphylaxis from administration of medicines
General anaesthesia
Intra-arterial injection
Intravenous (iv) injection
Lumbar/sacral collection of cerebrospinal fluid (CSF)
Massive haemorrhage (this could occur at parturition where there is no human involvement)
Sedation

Table 7.2. A list of the causes of sudden death in South American camelids.

Anthrax
Cast on the back
Chemical poisons
Clostridial disease
Drowning (this may occur at dipping or in deep water)
Electrocution
Hypomagnesaemia
Lightning strike
Poisonous plants
Ruptured aneurysm
Ruptured uterine artery
Snake bite
Trauma (mainly road traffic accidents or fighting in males)

8

South American Camelid (SAC) Surgery

Introduction

The chapter starts with a discussion of general points for all surgery on SACs, and is followed accounts of basic procedures in general and regional anaesthesia. This is followed by an account of surgical conditions and procedures which is organized by system. The first three systems covered are the gastroenteric system, the neurological system and the urinary system. The reproductive system is then discussed in two separate sections: the first is devoted to the female reproductive system, and includes accounts of reproductive ultrasonography, parturition, dystocia and associated conditions and surgical procedures; the second looks at the male reproductive system. The locomotory system is covered next. Lastly, there is a brief section on euthanasia.

General Points for All Surgery

Tetanus cover

SACs are very prone to tetanus. Full vaccination involves a double dose of vaccine separated by 4 weeks. The boosters should be given at 6 monthly intervals. If the animal has had an initial course to two doses of vaccine some time ago a single booster dose will be sufficient. If this has not been done, it is suggested that the patient should receive its primary dose of tetanus vaccine and 3000 IU of tetanus antitoxin (TAT). This could be reduced to 1500 IU in very young animals.

Antibiotic cover

In elective procedures, antibiotic cover should ideally start 24 h before surgery. Penicillin is the antibiotic of choice.

Analgesia

The analgesic drug of choice with both sedation and anaesthesia is butorphanol. This can be given post-operatively as well as pre-operatively at 0.1 mg/kg every 6 h either im, sub cut or iv. Nonsteroidal anti-inflammatory drugs (NSAIDs) can be given at the same time except it should be remembered that they are nephrotoxic and so should be avoided if there is likely to be any kidney damage.

Sedation

Xylazine

Xylazine is very effective, and 1 ml of a 2% solution given im will certainly sedate a llama, which may well then 'kush'. For a large male alpaca, 0.75 ml of 2% solution is quite sufficient.

Acepromazine

Acepromazine is not a very useful sedative in SACs as it really only gives mild tranquillization at standard doses of 0.03 mg/kg iv or 0.05 mg/kg im. However, it is useful in maiden females who are reluctant to allow crias to suckle. A single injection of 5 ml acepromazine (5% solution) and 2.5 ml oxytocin (10 IU/ml) given im as soon as the problem is realized is helpful.

Diazepam

Diazepam is a useful sedative for use in small crias. It can be given either iv or im at 0.1 mg/kg, and at this dosage, it will give safe profound sedation. It is not nearly so effective in older and larger animals.

General Anaesthesia (GA)

Gaseous anaesthesia

This is hazardous as there is a considerable danger of regurgitation, which is described as either passive or active. Passive regurgitation occurs under deep anaesthesia and is manifest as a continual flow of stomach contents through the mouth. Active regurgitation occurs during light anaesthesia and is projectile, as it is in fact antiperistalsis. It is extremely dangerous and can lead to inhalation pneumonia, particularly if it occurs during intubation. Adult SACs should be fasted for 12 h before surgery, and water should be withheld for 8 h. Premedication with atropine 0.04 mg/kg im is worthwhile; premedication with xylazine 6 mg/10 kg im will give deep sedation. Ketamine is the induction agent of choice given at 2.2 mg/kg iv.

This will allow intubation and gaseous anaesthesia with isoflurane. An adult alpaca will require an 8 mm endotracheal tube and an adult llama will require a 10 mm endotracheal tube. A laryngoscope with a 20 cm blade will be required. With the animal in sternal recumbency, the neck should be stretched vertically. The top and bottom jaws should be held open by an assistant with two loops of bandage. The tube can then be inserted into the trachea with the laryngoscope. This will be aided by an aluminum rod inside the tube to add rigidity.

Recovery from gaseous anaesthesia

SACs are obligate nasal breathers and gas exchange must be confirmed immediately after the endotracheal tube has been removed as the airway may be compromised during the transition from endotracheal tube breathing to nasal breathing. SACS tend to relax after the endotracheal tube is removed as the stimulus is also removed. The tube should be left in place until the patient is able to swallow, chew and cough, and is actively trying to expel the tube. The tube is then liable to damage but at least the animal is not put at risk. If regurgitation has occurred, the tube should be withdrawn with the cuff inflated until the cuff reaches the larynx. Any ingesta must be removed from the pharynx or buccal cavity. The animal's head should be kept elevated. Human assistance must always be present until a SAC is fully recovered.

Injectable anaesthesia

This is the method preferred by the author and involves an im injection of an anaesthetic cocktail into the quadriceps muscle. The dose for a typical 18 month old llama weighing 80 kg (a common time for castration) is 5 ml ketamine (10% solution), 2.5 ml xylazine (2% solution) and 0.5 ml butorphanol (1% solution). All these three medicines should be given in the same syringe. This will give 20 min of anaesthesia after an induction period of 5–10 min. Larger or smaller animals can be anaesthetized with different dosages on a pro rata basis.

Another method which is also recommended is a combination of ketamine and diazepam following xylazine sedation. For a 50 kg animal, sedation involves 0.75 ml 2% xylazine (20 mg/ml) im. The animal is then catheterized (a bleb of local anaesthetic should be given under the skin); 1 ml 10% (100 mg/ml) ketamine is injected iv followed by 1 ml 0.5% (5 mg/ml) diazepam iv and 2 ml atropine sulfate 600 mcg/ml iv. Anaesthesia can be maintained by giving 0.5 ml 2% xylazine, 0.5 ml 10% ketamine and 0.5 ml 0.5% diazepam every 30 min.

Regional Anaesthesia

Epidural anaesthesia

The normal site used by practitioners is the sacrococcygeal space. A 4 cm 20 G needle should be used perpendicularly to the spine. The dose is 2 ml of 2% lignocaine for an adult llama; 0.25 ml of 2% xylazine can be added to this to give a longer action and some slight sedation. The dose of both lignocaine and xylazine should be reduced by 25% in alpacas.

Regional anaesthesia of the lower limb

A tourniquet should be applied immediately above the carpal or tarsal joint. Two small rolls of bandage should be inserted either side of the Achilles tendon when applying the tourniquet to the hind leg. The mid area of the metacarpus or metatarsus should be clipped and surgically cleaned. A suitable superficial vein should be selected. Location is not easy. A bleb of local anaesthetic should be put under the skin using a 25 G needle. Next, using a 2 cm 23 G needle, 2.5–10 ml (depending on the size of the animal) 2% lignocaine should be injected extremely slowly into the vein. Full regional anaesthesia will be achieved within 5 min, and will last for over an hour. Anaesthesia will cease as soon as the tourniquet is removed.

Surgical Conditions of the Gastroenteric System

Choanal atresia

Non-patency of the choanae can be bilateral or unilateral. The former will result in the cria having to mouth breathe and has a hopeless prognosis, so euthanasia is advised. Unilateral cases can survive, but as the condition is very likely to be inherited animals should not be bred from. The condition can be differentiated from a cleft palate by visually looking into the mouth. It can also be differentiated because milk comes down the nose when a cria with a cleft palate sucks, and this does not happen in choanal atresia.

Congenital and hereditary conditions

Atresia ani

This will present in neonates as a swelling below the tail and an absence of an anus. A small bleb of local anaesthetic (1 ml) should be injected over the swelling where there should be an anus. A small stab incision is made with a very small scalpel blade into the swelling and faeces will be extruded. Sutures are not required and normally the anus will remain open if the owner cleans the area for a couple of days.

For other congenital and hereditary conditions see Chapter 7.

Fracture of the mandible

Radiographs should be taken under heavy sedation. The wound should be cleaned and debrided as necessary. The mandible should be stabilized with wire using the incisors, canines and rostral cheek teeth. Any loose teeth should be left *in situ* as they will often re-anchor. Any fractured teeth should be removed as fractured enamel cannot repair. The soft tissue should be sutured. The animal should be given antibiotics, NSAIDs and TAT. It should be fed on a sloppy diet or lush grass. The wire should be removed in 3 weeks.

Problems with teeth

Problems with cheek teeth

Normally, a tooth problem is manifest as a slowly progressive hard swelling which fistulates and is related to the mandible or, less commonly, to the maxilla. Extremely rarely, there will be a malodorous unilateral nasal discharge or a tooth root abscess will drain into the mouth. Long-term antibiotics may be tried but the result is rarely satisfactory. At least a month of daily injections of penicillin or ceftiofur have been tried. A ten-shot series of florfenicol at the higher dose given every 4th day is claimed to have a success rate of 50%. The fistula may appear to close but will re-open when the antibiotic cover ceases.

Tooth removal is the only option. The author's preference is removal *per os* with the SAC held in the 'kush' position under very light sedation with xylazine at 0.05 mg/kg (0.125 ml of a 2% solution per 50 kg) im. Radiographs should be taken to accurately pinpoint the diseased tooth. A second holder, using both hands, should keep the gag open and in the correct plane. The tooth to be removed should be examined with a head torch and then the gingival mucosa should be elevated on both the lateral and medial aspects of the tooth using a very small equine dental pick. The dental pick should be forced between the tooth and the alveolar socket. A pair of small molar separators should be placed rostral and caudal to the tooth to try to obtain some tooth movement. The tooth should then be grasped with a pair of small right-angled molar extraction forceps. A careful, persistent medial/lateral rocking motion should be commenced. When the tooth is loose it should be elevated using a long pair of artery forceps as a fulcrum.

Antibiotic cover and pain relief should be maintained for several days. The alveolar socket does not require packing but flushing through the fistula daily is helpful. The socket rapidly granulates.

Problems with fighting teeth

These are very vicious weapons and can inflict severe wounds on other animals, particularly other mature uncastrated males. The general opinion of eminent veterinarians in the UK and elsewhere is that the erupted crown of these teeth should be removed at the age of 2–3 years. This procedure will have to be repeated at regular intervals of roughly 2 years. It needs to be carried out in a human manner under a short-acting anaesthetic using embryotomy wire which is continuously bathed in cold water to prevent excess heat.

Problems with incisor teeth

These are common. There are inherited problems of overextension of the mandible (prognathia) and of under-extension (brachygnathia). Animals with these conditions do not suffer from any degree of 'dysprehension' and therefore suffer no problems with loss of weight. Routine grinding of these incisors should not be carried out as it is inhumane and is being used to mask an inherited conformation fault (see Plate 12).

Prolapsed rectum

The causes of this very rare condition are obscure. It has been suggested that homosexual behaviour might be a cause, and it does appear to be more prevalent in males. With the SAC either in the standing position or in the 'kush' position, an epidural regional anaesthetic should be given. The perineal area should be cleaned before a purse-string suture is put in place. It is important that this is placed before replacement of the rectum, otherwise the rectum will re-prolapse while the suture is being placed. After replacement of the rectum, and using plenty of obstetrical lubricant, the purse-string should be drawn tight to only allow one finger in the orifice. The animal should be kept on a laxative diet and regularly checked. The suture should be removed in 10 days. In the majority of cases, it will remain *in situ*. If the rectum re-prolapses, euthanasia is indicated unless the rectal mucosa can be carefully resected. This surgery is beyond the experience of the author.

Umbilical hernia

Umbilical hernias are extremely rare in SACs, but they have a high heritability and so repair should not be carried out in males unless the animals are castrated. It is reasonable to repair an umbilical hernia in a female which is being kept for breeding on the understanding that her progeny will not be kept for breeding. Repair of umbilical hernias should be delayed until the cria is at least 4 months of age. Often, with increasing age there is little reason to repair the hernia as the abdominal opening is relatively small.

If no more than three fingers can be inserted into the abdominal opening, the hernia can be closed with an elastrator ring. The cria is placed in dorsal recumbency and the hernia sack raised to ensure there are no bowel contents. A rubber ring is then placed as near to the abdominal wall as possible.

If the abdominal opening is larger than three fingers wide, a full surgical operation will need to be carried out under GA. The cria should be anaesthetized as above, and the area should clipped and surgically prepared. An elliptical skin incision is made around the hernia sack. The skin is removed with blunt dissection. With great care, and again with blunt dissection, the hernia sac is undermined from the abdominal wall without entering the abdomen so that there is a rim of 1 cm around the orifice. Sterile nylon mesh is then sutured to an abdominal ring over the orifice with monofilament nylon continuous stitches. After closing the dead space with a continuous layer of subcuticular sutures of absorbable material, the skin is closed with single horizontal mattress sutures of monofilament nylon. The cria should be confined for a minimum of 10 days before the sutures are removed.

Surgical Conditions of the Neurological System

Enucleation of the eye

In all cases where there is no chance of any eye condition recovering, enucleation should be considered on welfare grounds. This can be carried out under heavy sedation, normally with xylazine. Local anaesthetic should be instilled all around the orbit, not only under the skin but also into the deeper tissues with a single very deep injection of 5 ml behind the eye to block the optic nerve. The eyelids should then be sutured together and the whole area clipped and prepared aseptically. A careful incision is then made through the skin parallel to the upper eyelid margin, but not entering the conjunctival sac. Using blunt dissection, the eye muscles are sectioned around that half of the eye. The same procedure is then carried out on the lower half. Eventually, a pair of curved scissors can be used to section the optic nerve and the eye can be removed. The remaining socket can then be obliterated with subcuticular suturing with absorbable material and the remaining eyelids sutured with nonabsorbable material. The animal should receive antibiotics and NSAIDs for a minimum of 5 days. The sutures should be removed in 10 days.

Eye disorders

Eye disorders and visual defects in neonatal crias

ENTROPION   This is extremely rare. It should be corrected surgically by carrying out a 'cake slice op'.

EYELID HYPOGENESIS   This is extremely rare. Surgery may be possible.

Eye disorders and visual defects in older crias and adults

TUMOURS OF THE EYELIDS   These are common, particularly squamous cell carcinomas of the third eyelid. They have a good prognosis if they can be removed before the tumour has invaded the conjunctiva. Surgery is straightforward as the eyelid can be removed with a pair of scissors under anaesthesia (see Plate 13). Haemorrhage is minimal and suturing is not required (see Plate 14).

See Chapter 7 for other eye disorders.

Surgical Conditions of the Urinary System

Persistent patent urachus

This is usually a congenital condition as the urachus fails to close at birth. If it occurs a few days after birth it is likely to be as a result of a septic omphalophlebitis. If the urachus remains patent at birth, it can be ligated immediately together with the vessels lying beside it, without need for anaesthesia. Prolonged antibiotic cover is vital as if sepsis develops further difficult surgery will be required.

In the event of the urachus not closing with this treatment, or if it has become patent some days after birth as a result of infection, more aggressive surgery needs to be carried out. The cria should be anaesthetized by masking down with halothane or isoflurane and surgically prepared. The practitioner should perform a laparotomy so that the urachus can be traced back to the bladder. It should be sectioned and the bladder closed with a double layer of continuous Lembert sutures of an absorbable material. The umbilical vessels should be ligated proximally to any infected and diseased tissue. This tissue should then be totally removed. Once the diseased tissue has been removed the urachus and the vessels will need to be ligated inside the abdomen. Drainage will have to be established so that the healing can occur from within. Further broad-spectrum antibiotic cover will be required as well as wound flushing with dilute povidone iodine.

The abdomen should be closed with interrupted sutures of monofilament nylon. These all should be laid individually before any are tightened in a 'vest over pants' configuration. When the practitioner is satisfied that there are enough sutures to close the abdomen and that no small intestine is trapped the sutures can be tightened. It is very important that no extra sutures are added after this on account of the danger of perforation of the small intestine. A subcuticular layer of continuous sutures of an absorbable material should be laid before the skin is closed with interrupted horizontal mattress sutures of monofilament nylon.

It is also important that the animal receives aggressive antibiotic treatment until 10 days later when the sutures, if clean and dry, can be removed. If there is any doubt, they should be left in place and further antibiotic treatment should be given.

Ruptured bladder

This condition does not seem to occur at birth in male alpacas or llamas as it does in horses. It can though occur in both males and females which are subjected to violent trauma from road traffic accidents (RTAs) or falls from high places. It has also been reported that a bladder has been ruptured during rectal examination. The more common cause is rupture as a result of urethral obstruction. In case of the incidence of trauma, the repair needs to be carried out as soon as possible and does not carry any welfare or ethical considerations. Diagnosis of bladder rupture is not easy, and if it is suspected, the delay in waiting for confirmation of raised blood urea will not be helpful. A peritoneal tap is required. Normal peritoneal fluid has a potassium concentration of below 5 mEq/l; urine has a potassium level of ten times that figure.

Repair should be carried out under GA with the animal in dorsal recumbency. In the male, an incision will have to made paramedian to get as much access to the bladder as possible. The bladder should be closed using a double layer of continuous inverting sutures. The abdomen should be flushed after closure of the bladder before closing with two layers of continuous sutures. The skin should be closed with single layer of interrupted sutures of monofilament nylon.

The welfare and ethical dilemma arises when the bladder has ruptured because the urethra of a male has become blocked with calculi. If these calculi can be flushed out, the bladder can be repaired as described above, but if the urethra cannot be cleared the clinician has a dilemma. Several surgical approaches have been described. These include ischial urethrostomy, urethrotomy and marsupialization. The problem is that invariably there is urine scalding. At best, there is continual pyoderma, and at worst there will be continual acute skin inflammation with fly strike in the summer. The author's opinion is that euthanasia is required (based on his own poor surgical results in other species, though in other surgical hands the outcome may well be more favourable).

Urethral obstruction

This is seen typically in young males fed on dry concentrate diets. Surgery as described for a ruptured bladder is possible but carries severe welfare implications.

Surgical Conditions of the Reproductive System

Surgical conditions of females

Parturition

NORMAL DELIVERY   This occurs from the standing position between dawn and noon. Before parturition, the dam makes no effort to leave the herd. After the delivery, she tends to show little in the way of mothering behaviour while being watched, but can be surprisingly aggressive if she thinks the cria is being threatened. Supervision should not be too intense or the mother will become distracted. It is important that the cria suckles as soon as possible, as it needs to consume 10% of its body weight of colostrum within the first 24 h. Most crias will get up and be steady on their legs within 2 h.

The placenta is usually shed in 2 h; 10 IU oxytocin may be given at this time sub cut. Normally, a placenta is said to be retained if it has not been shed within 6 hours (see below). The navel of the cria should be dressed only after 2 h if the parturition has been unassisted, using iodine or tetracycline spray. If the cria has not been seen to suck after 2 h the mammary gland should be checked for mastitis. The wax plugs that are present are *normal* and should be left *in situ*. They will act as an indicator that each individual teat has been sucked. The cria should pass the meconium in 36 h. If not, it should be given an enema; there are several

suitable human preparations freely available. SACs have a very small milk cistern for each teat so that frequent sucking is required. This is normal and does not necessarily mean that a female does not have enough milk. It is also normal for the cria to keep moving between teats. Exogenous oxytocin can be given in small doses, i.e. 10 IU to aid milk let-down.

Induction of parturition

This intervention should not be encouraged as service dates are often unreliable. If owners insist, it is best achieved with a prostaglandin injection (187.5 mcg cloprostenol, which is equivalent to 0.75 ml standard solution) im. This should be followed by 125 mcg cloprostenol (equivalent to 0.5 ml standard solution) injected 24 h later. Fluprostenol 40 mg im can also be used to induce parturition in SACs within 10 days of their due date. Parturition will occur on average 21 h later (Bravo *et al.*, 1996). Neonatal survival is not affected. Neither dexamethasone nor oxytocin are suitable for inducing parturition in SACs.

Dystocia

Dystocia in SACs is relatively uncommon with less than 5% of animals requiring any assistance. Dystocia may be defined as failure of transition from stage 1 to stage 2 of labour, or when little or no progress is made for 30 min or more after the start of stage 2 of labour. Stage 1 of labour for a veteran female will not last more than 4–6 h but may last for up to 24 h in a maiden.

The most common cause of dystocia is fetal malpositioning. Relative fetal oversize is an extremely rare occurrence. Poor cervical dilation, similar to ring womb in sheep, is also extremely rare. Other reasons for dystocia include uterine torsion and pelvic problems, e.g. fractures, tumours and abscesses.

Guidelines for when a Caesarean section should be carried out include the following:

- The cervix is inadequately dilated or the pelvis is of an inadequate size to extract the fetus.
- The pelvis is too small to allow a hand to be introduced to manipulate the fetus.

- The uterus has insufficient room to grasp and manipulate the fetus.
- There is insufficient room for a fetotomy to be performed on a dead fetus.

CAESAREAN SECTION A recovery area heated to 90°F (32°C) should be prepared for the cria. Caesarean section can be performed with a ventral midline laparotomy. The thin, tense abdominal musculature and friable linea alba present problems. GA allows a midline approach and leads to good relaxation and repair but decreases the chances of the survival of the cria. Not only is the cria depressed by the drugs used, but it then receives no immediate attention from the dam as she needs time to recover.

The author favours a left para-lumbar fossa approach. Sedation, if there are good handlers, is rarely required. If needed, 0.1 mg/kg xylazine and 0.1 mg/kg butorphanol can be given in the same syringe im in the quadriceps. Lignocaine without adrenaline is then infiltrated at the proposed incision site. This should be kept to the minimum as an overdose can be toxic. No more than 4 mg/kg should be given; this is 15 ml of a 2% solution of lignocaine for a 75 kg alpaca. Systemic antibiotics and NSAIDs should be given and the tetanus status checked.

An oblique (30° from vertical) skin incision and then a muscle incision should be made, following a line between the tuber coxae and the angulation of the ribs. This follows the aponeurosis of the internal abdominal oblique muscle and also mimics the line of the uterus (thus making the uterus easier to exteriorize). The incision does not need to be long; only a hand's width is sufficient. If possible, the uterus should then be exteriorized to lessen contamination. This is usually possible, as 95% of pregnancies are in the left horn. After removal of the cria, the placenta needs to be peeled away from the uterus.

The uterus should then be closed with a single inverting layer of Lembert sutures using synthetic absorbable suture material. If the uterus is oedematous and friable, a second layer of sutures should be put in. Obviously, clinicians should be mindful of subsequent pregnancies. The uterus is more vascular than the ruminant but there is no need to place an inner blanket layer as in the horse; 20 IU of oxytocin should be injected im after replacement of the uterus. Intra-abdominal antibiotics should be instilled before abdominal closure with two layers of continuous sutures of synthetic absorbable suture material. The deepest layer must include the peritoneum. The skin should be closed with single interrupted mattress sutures of monofilament nylon. Antibiotics should be continued for 5 days and NSAIDs for 3 days.

EMBRYOTOMY AND 'HUNG CRIA' In cases where the cria is putrid and rotten, the vagina will be dry and swollen. The cria will be emphysematous and cannot be delivered *per vagina*. Caesarean section carries a very poor prognosis and therefore unless a decision is likely to be made to destroy the animal on welfare grounds, a simple embryotomy can be performed.

The animal should be given antibiotics and NSAIDs. If the cria is in anterior presentation, a rope should be put around one carpus with the aid of a large amount of obstetric lubricant or 'J lube', and the leg should be drawn out as far as possible. An incision should be made with a scalpel on the medial side of the leg to allow the insertion of a disposable embryotomy knife. The knife should be put up the leg as far as possible to cut the skin up into the axilla and, if possible, over the shoulder joint up to the top of the scapular. All of the attachments of the shoulder blade to the chest wall should be broken down with an outstretched hand while pulling the leg constantly. The whole front leg can then be removed after cutting the remaining skin. This process should be repeated on the opposite side. A loop of a lambing rope is then placed on the head over the ears and in the mouth. The whole of the rest of the cria can then be removed.

In the case of a 'hung cria', i.e. when the head is out and the legs cannot be felt, it is vital to make 100% certain that the cria is dead. If this has been definitely ascertained, the head can be cut off as near to the body as possible to allow the forelegs to be located and extended. The cria can then be drawn out. If the cria is alive, it is generally possible to repel the head, after putting a rope over the poll and into the mouth, and locate the legs. It is best if both legs are extended before drawing the cria.

However, if one leg is in extension and the other is totally back against the body, it is usually still possible to draw the cria. If the cria is in a posterior presentation it can also usually be drawn. If it is dead and emphysematous an embryotomy may be required. In that case, the hocks should be brought caudally and the legs sectioned with embryotomy wire just distal to the hocks. The ropes can then be attached to the hock joint and the cria can be drawn using a large amount of lubricant.

RETAINED PLACENTA   Removal should be attempted within 6 h of parturition, stimulated by 30 IU oxytocin given im. Antibiotics and NSAIDs should also be given. If the placenta is still *in situ* in a further 6 h more oxytocin should be given. This should be repeated in a further 6 h if necessary. Gentle traction will then normally accomplish removal.

UTERINE TORSION   This condition, which is actually torsion of the anterior vagina does occur in SACs at parturition. It should be corrected by rolling. At least three people will be required. The animal should be rolled in the direction of the twist and allowed to get up immediately. If the twist has been corrected but the cervix is only partially dilated the practitioner should not delay but apply traction after making sure the fetus is in the correct position. This traction will naturally dilate the cervix, but if the practitioner delays, the cervix will become indurated and fail to dilate and Caesarean section will have to be performed.

Uterine torsion can also occur in the last third of pregnancy and not at parturition, as in the mare. This is a true torsion of the body of the uterus and not of the anterior vagina. Diagnosis is difficult as it is inadvisable to perform a rectal examination. The presenting sign will be colic. As most SACs are very stoical this will not be very violent. In any cases of colic in pregnant animals well on in their pregnancy, uterine torsion should be suspected. Rolling could be tried in an ad hoc manner. The most likely direction is clockwise, so this should be tried first. The animal should then be allowed to stand for 10 min to access any improvement in pulse rate and pain. If there is no improvement, rolling in the opposite direction should be tried. Still failing any improvement a left-flank laparotomy should be carried out to make a diagnosis of the problem. If there is torsion of the spiral colon this will not be affected by rolling but it will be discovered promptly. Obviously, if there is a uterine torsion it should be corrected, leaving the *in situ* fetus to come to full term.

Fusion of the vulval lips

This is quite a common finding. If it is total it will be observed within 48 h of birth as a fluid-filled swelling below the anus. A small bleb of local anaesthetic should be inserted over the position where the vulva should be. An incision should then be made with a scalpel and urine will pour out. The incision may have to be enlarged slightly with a pair of straight scissors. Suturing is not required. Often the labial fusion is not complete so that urine will be seen to come out of a small hole in a thin stream. Occasionally, the condition will not be observed until the first mating. The correction at that time is similar to that carried out in neonates.

Persistent hymen and vaginal aplasia

If this condition is really a persistent hymen it is relatively easily rectified. It also does not hold any ethical problems, unlike the similar but rarer condition of vaginal aplasia. This latter condition is genetic and so surgery should not be attempted. The sign shown by the affected animals by both of these conditions will be that of the male failing to fully penetrate the female. Normally the hymen, which contains uterine mucoid secretions, can be perforated with a finger. The secretions are voided and the animal can be bred from in the normal manner. There is no need for further treatment. If this cannot be achieved, the animal should be examined carefully with a small duck-billed speculum. If there is a persistent hymen it will be seen bulging towards the operator and should be pieced with a stab incision with a small scalpel and widened with a finger. If there is aplasia of the vagina, the animal should be left as a fibre producer and not be considered for breeding.

Prolapsed uterus

This will occur immediately after parturition and should be treated as a real emergency. Generally, the animal will be in the 'kush' position. She should be allowed to remain in that position. It is important that no attempt is made to stretch out her hind legs as is advocated in cows because this is very painful for SACs. The uterus should be protected with a clean sheet underneath it. The afterbirth should be removed and the organ should be cleaned with warm very dilute chlorhexidine solution. An epidural anaesthetic should be given together with antibiotics and NSAIDs. The organ should be replaced into position. This is usually relatively easy to accomplish. It is vital though that the uterus is totally returned to its normal state. Oxytocin (30 IU) should be given im. The author favours using a single 'Buhner' suture of uterine tape to suture the lips of the vagina. A long Seaton needle is inserted into the skin at the ventral end of the vulva. It is pushed carefully in a dorsal direction subcutaneously and slightly laterally to emerge ventral to the anus. The tape is threaded and withdrawn. This is repeated for the other side of the vulva. The two ends are tied with a bow so that only two fingers can be inserted into the vulva. In theory though, if the uterus has been correctly replaced, this suturing should not be necessary. Antibiotics, NSAIDs and 10 IU oxytocin should be continued for 5 days. There is no evidence available to enable advice to be given on the likelihood of a recurrence at a subsequent pregnancy. However, prudence suggests further pregnancies would be unwise.

Prolapsed vagina

IN THE PREGNANT ANIMAL   With the animal in the 'kush' position, a sacrococcygeal epidural anaesthetic should be administered. In the pregnant animal, after replacing the vagina and cervix, the lips of the vulva should be sutured with a single Buhner suture of uterine tape in which the two ends are tied with a bow so that only two fingers can be inserted into the vulva (see above under 'Prolapsed uterus').

The owner is advised to untie the bow but not remove the suture if the animal is thought to be parturient. If this is the case, the cria can be drawn and the suture removed as the condition should not recur in the non-pregnant animal. If the cervix is closed and the animal is not parturient the suture should be retied as the condition will recur until parturition has occurred. The animal should not be bred from as the condition will also recur at a subsequent pregnancy.

IN THE NON-PREGNANT ANIMAL   The prognosis is guarded. Under epidural anaesthesia, the vagina should be cleaned and replaced and then a 'Caslick's' operation should be performed as in the mare. A strip of mucosa should be removed from both sides of the vulva, including the dorsal end. The lips should then be sutured with single interrupted sutures of monofilament nylon. A small orifice should be left at the ventral end of the vulva to allow for urination. The animal should be given antibiotic cover and pain relief with NSAIDs for 10 days, when the sutures can be removed.

Reproductive ultrasonography

EARLY PREGNANCY EVENTS   The corpus luteum is first visible trans-rectally at 6 days post breeding, i.e. 4 days post ovulation. The initial diameter is 8–10 mm, and this will increase to 13–14 mm 20 days post ovulation. The conceptus may be visible as early as 10 days post ovulation. Uterine contractibility and embryo motility can be observed up to 35 days.

PREGNANCY DIAGNOSIS   There are dangers in carrying out a rectal diagnosis of pregnancy using a rigid guide for the rectal probe, but this can be carried out at 30 days post service. In the UK, the Veterinary Defence Society (VDS) do not advise the practice, having lost a test case in the courts. It is safer to delay pregnancy diagnosis until 60 days post service when it can be performed trans-abdominally using a 3 MHz probe (Fig. 8.1). After 90 days, a 5 MHz probe is more useful. Lubricant can be used, but most operatives prefer isopropyl alcohol (surgical spirit should not be used as this will damage the probe). The probe should

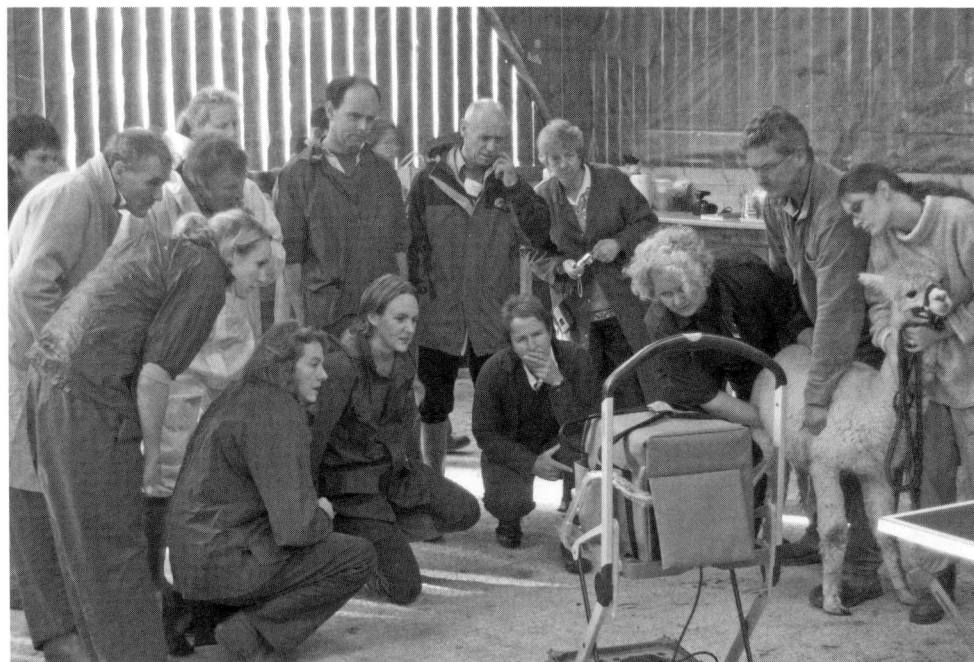

Fig. 8.1. Trans-abdominal ultrasonography of a camelid.

be pressed firmly high up in the inguinal region. The left or right side may be used at this stage. After locating the bladder the uterine bifurcation should be visualized.

The skull of the fetus can be seen in a pregnant animal but the vertebrae will not be seen until 67 days post service. By 83 days, the skull can be measured and the ribcage can be seen. Twins are extremely rare. However, they can reach maturity and be viable. If trans-rectal ultrasonography is used, the normal non-pregnant uterus will appear as mid-'echogenic' dense tissue with no fluid and an indistinct lumen. In a case of 'mucometra', usually caused by a persistent hymen, the uterus will be fluid filled without membrane folds or a fetus, and will have a 'snowy' appearance. In contrast, a 'pyometra' will have a thick uterine wall without membrane folds or a fetus, and will have a 'cloudy' appearance. A heart beat should be visible from day 25. The cross-sectional horn diameter will be 8–10 cm at 60 days.

Fetal loss is high in SACs. Although fertilization rates are high, with 85% of ovulating females having an egg fertilized, only 50% of embryos survive after 30 days. About 10% of confirmed pregnancies are lost up to day 45. The 'normal' abortion rate is around 5%.

As well as confirmation by reproductive ultrasonography, pregnancy can also be confirmed with a progesterone assay. Ideally, blood should be collected 20 days after breeding and again 30 days after breeding. Any progesterone value over 1 ng/ml on both occasions is likely to indicate a positive result.

INFERTILITY INVESTIGATION   This has to be carried out per rectum. It is prudent for practitioners to require owners to sign a disclaimer. The probe, with a rigid guide, should be inserted into the rectum using plenty of lubricant. Unless the animal has just urinated, the bladder should be easily located as a fluid-filled ball. On moving slightly more cranially, the body of the uterus should be visualized. Rotation of the probe will reveal the horns. In maidens, the uterus is just above the bladder. In older animals, it will be more cranial. The normal diameter of the uterine horn of a maiden SAC is 25–30 mm. A diameter of 20 mm would indicate immaturity and would not necessarily indicate hypoplasia unless the animal was over 3 years old. The normal ovaries should be round. Ovarian hypoplasia is very difficult to evaluate on a scan. It is easier to take a blood sample 5 days post mating to measure progesterone levels. This can be repeated in another 5 days for further confirmation. In maidens, the most common abnormality is either a persistent hymen or vaginal aplasia (see above). Both of these conditions will be seen on ultrasound as a mucometra.

Uterine cysts are much more common than uterine tumours, but differentiation is difficult. Animals are able to get pregnant with a uterine cyst in the wall of the uterus. Ovarian cysts are also much more common than ovarian abscesses, but again, differentiation on scan is difficult. Size is the only differential between a follicle and a cyst. A female with a follicle in excess of 4 mm in diameter is worth mating. A follicle up to 13 mm across might be normal. Mating should be carried out with an injection of gonadotrophin-releasing hormone (GnRH) as 0.0084 mg buserelin given 30 h after service. If the follicle or cyst is still present after 10 days it is likely to be a cyst. In this case, mating should be carried out again with 1500 IU of chorionic gonadotrophin given iv on the day of service. Practitioners should be aware that in rare cases pregnancy will be achieved with a cyst on one ovary. Rarely, females will accept the male when pregnant.

Conditions of males

Castration

There is a myth, strongly held by owners of SACs, that castration should be delayed until puberty, i.e. 18 months old. They feel that if animals are castrated before sexual maturity they will get weak long legs. It is difficult to disprove this opinion as owners are reluctant to allow a clinical audit.

CLOSED CASTRATION   The animal should be given a GA and placed in dorsal recumbency with the area around the penis and the scrotum surgically prepared. One testicle is pushed cranially into a pre-scrotal position, and a careful incision is made over it. It is then drawn out within its tunics. Two pairs of artery forceps are then clamped above the testicle. The pair nearest to the testicle is removed and a tight ligature of absorbable material is placed in the groove that has been made. The testicle is then removed distal to the second pair of artery forceps. These forceps are then removed carefully, allowing the stump to return to its normal position in the scrotum. This process is repeated with the second testicle through the same incision. The skin is then closed with a single continuous sub-cuticular suture of absorbable suture material. The area is covered with antibiotic spray. With skill and forethought, there is time to perform this surgical procedure under im anaesthesia without a top-up, provided the surgeon is assisted by a competent theatre nurse who can prepare the patient and the instruments while the surgeon is scrubbing up.

OPEN CASTRATION   Ideally, the animal is well restrained behind a solid gate, e.g. in the front of a cattle trailer with an inner partition. Access can be provided from behind, e.g. via the 'jockey' door. The use of a trailer spares the surgeon from having to kneel down. Of course, if there is no trailer the animal can be made to 'kush' or be 'chukkered' on the ground. It is useful to lay a towel under the hind quarters to keep the surgery site as clean as possible. Local anaesthetic (5 ml in total) is injected under the skin into the scrotum and up into the cord on each side. The area is thoroughly cleaned. A testicle is squeezed into the scrotum. An incision is made over the testicle and through the tunics. The testicle is then drawn from the scrotum and from the abdomen by pulling and twisting. Any scrotal fat should be removed. This procedure should be repeated for the second testicle. The wound should be covered with antibiotic spray. If castration is carried out in the summer in the UK, some sort of fly control should be considered.

CASTRATION OF ANIMALS WITH A RETAINED TESTICLE (RIGS)   Retained testicles are very rare in SACs, but there is every reason to suspect that retained testicles are more likely to become cancerous. Therefore, these animals will need to be castrated. Such an operation should not be undertaken lightly as some retained testicles may be up near to the kidney. In these instances, the best method is to carry out the removal laparoscopically.

In most cases, the testicle will lie just inside the inner inguinal ring. Under these circumstances, a straightforward surgical procedure can be carried out under GA. The scrotum and the surrounding area should be clipped and surgically cleaned. An incision should be made over the external inguinal ring. The tunics covering the retained testicle will be found by blunt dissection over the inguinal ring. These should be grasped by a large pair of artery forceps and the small soft testicle should be drawn, slowly and carefully, to the exterior. A transfixing ligature of absorbable suture material should be placed around the tunics dorsally to a second pair of artery forceps. The testicle should then be removed and the subcuticular tissues should be closed with a continuous row of sutures of absorbable material. The skin should then be closed with single horizontal mattress sutures of monofilament nylon.

Before deciding that an animal is a rig, clinicians should examine the groin very carefully, not only to see previous scars but also because often testicles have descended and do not lie in the scrotum but cranial to the scrotum lateral to the penis.

Inguinal hernia

Inguinal hernias are extremely rare in male SACs and are not seen in female animals. They are the result of a genetic recessive disorder and therefore they should only be repaired after castration. The left side is more commonly affected. If there is a strangulation of the intestine within the hernia, the animal will show colic-type pain. Because of the stoical nature of SACs, these affected animals are often found dead before diagnosis.

The animal should be given a GA and placed in dorsal recumbency. The area is surgically cleansed in the normal manner. A careful scrotal incision is made over the testicle, taking care not to incise the tunics. The testicle

is drawn through the skin incision, milking any abdominal contents back into the abdomen. When the surgeon is 100% certain that this has been accomplished, two large pairs of artery forceps (haemostats) are placed over the cord. The proximal pair is removed and a transfixing ligature is tied in the groove left by the artery forceps. The testicle is then removed distal to the remaining pair of haemostats. When the testicle has been removed the skin should be sutured with horizontal mattress sutures. Similar surgery should be carried out on the other side even if there is no inguinal herniation.

Vasectomy

This operation is not required under normal circumstances though it may be required for reproduction studies. The scrotum is not pendulous and so the operation is best performed under GA in dorsal recumbency. The scrotal area, and the area cranial to it, are prepared for surgery. A 5 cm incision is made cranial to the scrotum over the spermatic cord but slightly medial to the cord. The spermatic cord is then exteriorized by blunt dissection. A pair of artery forceps is positioned between the skin and the cord. The shiny vas deferens will be seen on the medial aspect of the spermatic cord. This can be grasped with a pair of rat-toothed dressing forceps. A 2 cm length is removed after ligaturing both ends with absorbable suture material. The skin is closed with two horizontal mattress sutures of similar absorbable material. The process is repeated on the other side.

Surgical Conditions of the Locomotory System

Angular limb deformity

This type of deformity will be observed soon after birth. Such deformities should be monitored but no immediate action should be taken and the cria allowed to mature for 6 weeks (Fig. 8.2). Radiographs should then be taken of the carpus and metacarpus, or in the case of the extremely rare hind limb

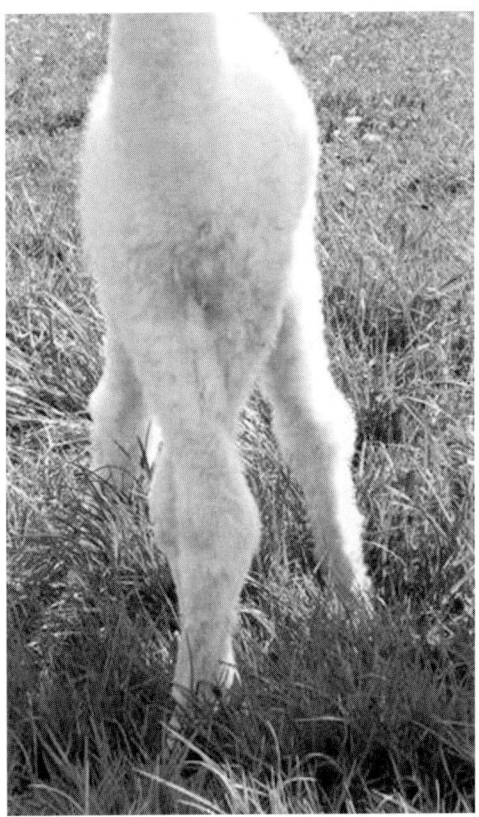

Fig. 8.2. Angular limb deformity in a cria. No immediate action should be taken.

deformity, of the tarsus and the metatarsus. If the carpus or the tarsus is deformed, euthanasia should be advised.

Only if the metacarpus or metatarsus is bent should surgery be attempted. The author advises a periosteal strip, as no specialized instruments, screws, etc. are required and neither is a second operation. The cria should be masked down with halothane or isoflurane and the limbs prepared for surgery. Depending on whether the deformity is varus or valgus, a 1 inch long vertical incision should be made on the lateral or medial aspect of the metacarpus. The periosteum should be scratched off the metacarpus for a length of 1 cm and width of 0.5 cm. The skin should be closed with small interrupted skin sutures or staples, to be removed in 10 days. The wound should be covered by a protective bandage.

Bilateral luxating patellae

This condition is probably present at birth but is only noticed by the owner as the cria grows and becomes more mobile. Diagnosis is not difficult. Surgical repair is extremely difficult and likely to be unsuccessful. As the condition is inherited, euthanasia is a more humane option.

Digital amputation

This procedure should be considered if there is chronic septic arthritis in one intraphalangeal joint. It is best to carry out the surgery under light sedation and a regional block. A tourniquet is required for both the regional block and for the operation. The whole leg below the middle of the metacarpus or metatarsus is clipped and surgically prepared. A length of embryotomy wire is positioned between the cleats. With an assistant holding the affected cleat with a pair of vulsellum forceps the cleat is sawn off with the wire at a 45° upward angle. This cut will be made in the middle of the second phalange.

The stump is then dressed with a suitable antibiotic cream and covered with a suitable dressing. The whole foot and leg to mid carpus/tarsus is bandaged with thin cotton wool and standard bandages. The bandaged area is then covered by gaffer tape, taking care that the tape does not actually touch the skin. The animal is kept under antibiotic and NSAID cover for a minimum of 10 days. The dressing should be changed twice in this period. If a good healthy bed of granulation tissue has been formed a lighter protective bandage can then be applied.

Dropped pasterns

This is hyperextension of the metacarpalphalangeal joint and is primarily a condition of old llamas. Most affected llamas can live normal lives but there are concerns over the wisdom of pregnancy. There is no treatment.

Flying scapula

This is seen after weaning but before maturity. The muscles securing the scapula to the ribcage become weak and rupture to some extent so that the ribcage drops. The spine is then lower in the thoracic area than in the lumbar–sacral area. The animal is still mobile. The condition is irreversible.

Fractures

These occur particularly in crias on account of the length of their long bones. Certain old SACs may suffer from osteoporosis and will often develop multiple fractures. See also 'Spondylosis' below.

Scapulo-humeral joint luxation

This has been reported in alpacas by a group of authors in the USA (Rousseau *et al.*, 2010).

Sequestrations

These can form in the bones of young growing animals from 1 week old onwards. The common presentation is peracute lameness. Radiography will not reveal a fracture at this stage and there are no other radiological signs, but these will develop later. Clinicians should radiograph the affected limbs in a further 2 weeks. Dead bone fragments will then be seen. There is no known definite aetiology of this condition. Surgery appears to be the only worthwhile treatment. Surgeons should cut down on the sequestrum and remove it. There is no need to splint or bandage the leg.

Spondylosis

This is a slow-onset condition of geriatric animals. The pathology is the formation of excess sponge-like bone in the lumbar area of the spine. The excess bone pinches on the nerves as they emerge from the spine. The most common chronic manifestation is that the animal will drag the toes of its hind legs. The condition does not seem painful but is progressive. NSAIDs are often given but they rarely appear to be beneficial. In certain cases, the extra bone, the spondyle, may fracture. This will cause acute lameness with pain and even crepitus over the area. The animals can recover though because as this is a small fracture it can repair. See also 'Fractures' above.

Tendon contraction

If the limb or limbs can be extended but the crias chooses not to, the author gives the cria an injection of 500 mg oxytetracycline. There is considerable doubt as to the effectiveness of this treatment, but its virtue is that it gives 48 h for further evaluation. It is not prudent to immediately splint or cast the limbs in cases of tendon contraction as many cases will self-cure. Splinting or casting is very hazardous as pressure sores are likely to be created with life-threatening results.

If after 48 h the limbs can be extended, then the owner should be instructed to house the cria and its mother. Then, as many times as possible every day, the limbs should be forcibly extended. In the author's experience, this will have a 50% success rate. Should this fail, or if the tendons are so contracted that the limb cannot be extended, then surgery should be attempted under GA.

The cria should be masked down with halothane or isoflurane and the limbs prepared for surgery. A 1 inch long incision is made centrally in the palmer aspect of the metacarpus in the direction of the limb. The median artery and nerve will lie medially and the ulna nerve will lie laterally. These should be reflected medially and laterally so that the two branches of the superficial digital flexor tendon can be severed. The skin should be sutured with small interrupted skin sutures or staples. The wound should be covered with a padded support bandage. The weight of the cria will hopefully stretch the deep digital flexor tendon.

Total spasticity of the limbs

This is seen in neonates. The outcome is hopeless if the animal is quadriplegic. However, if the animal can use its front legs normally but it is only paralysed behind, time and good nursing may bring about a recovery.

Euthanasia

Chemical euthanasia

This is the normal method of euthanasia for SACs. For skilled veterinarians who are used to giving iv injections in these animals, there are few problems in injecting either a large volume (approximately 100 ml of triple-strength barbiturate solution) or 25 ml of a solution containing 400 mg/ml quinalbarbitone and 25 mg/ml cinchocaine hydrochloride.

Normally, the skin of SACs is too thick to allow the jugular vein to be visualized so inexperienced veterinarians will find this difficult, particularly if the SAC is large and poorly handled (Fig. 8.3). In these instances the SAC can be heavily sedated with 2% xylazine given im (5 ml for a large male llama) or actually anaesthetized by a cocktail of agents given im. The triple-strength barbiturate or

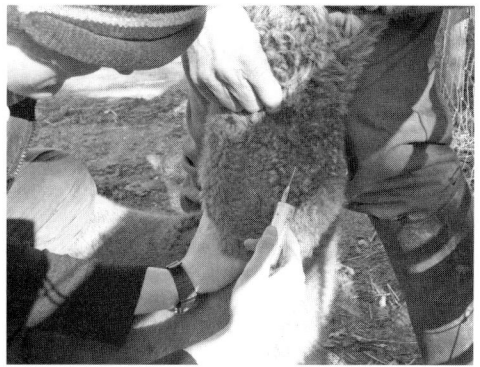

Fig. 8.3. The skin of South American camelids is too thick for the jugular vein to be visualized for use in euthanasia.

the solution containing quinalbarbitone and cinchocaine hydrochloride can then be given iv when the animal is in lateral recumbency.

Small crias can be destroyed by injecting 15 ml of triple-strength barbiturate into the jugular vein. In the author's experience, this may be difficult in a totally collapsed moribund cria. In these cases, it is humane to inject the triple-strength barbiturate straight into the heart. To do this, the cria should be held by the assistant either in lateral recumbency or with both arms across the assistant's chest.

9

Pig Medicine

_____

Introduction

The chapter covers commercial and pet pig medicine. It starts with a brief section on clinical examination of and history taking in pigs. The rest of the chapter is organized by system, with sections on diseases of the gastroenteric tract, diseases of the neurological system, metabolic diseases (which can also be viewed as a category of neurological diseases), diseases of the respiratory system, diseases of the urinary system, diseases of the reproductive system and diseases of the integument. The last section briefly covers common reasons for pigs to be found dead.

Clinical Examination, Including History Taking

Medical conditions pose a particular challenge to the practitioner when carrying out a clinical examination of pigs. Basically, they are not easy to examine with a stethoscope because of the thick layer of fat under the skin and because of their loud squealing. The normal pulse rate for an adult pig is 70–80 beats/min. The respiratory rate can also be observed; the normal for adults is 10–20 breaths/min, but this rises to 20–30 in growers and 40–50 in newborn piglets. The rectal temperature is a useful sign too; the normal range is 38.4–40°C. In white pigs, the skin reveals some helpful signs as well. The age of the pig is very important, so practitioners are advised to concentrate on systems and age groups. Diseases that affect multiple systems add problems. A history of the animal/s should include any changes or movement of pigs together with any changes in diet.

Practitioners should record:

- number of pigs on the holding
- number of pigs in the affected group
- number of pigs affected
- number dead
- age and sex of affected pigs
- predominant signs shown

Diseases of the Gastroenteric System

The predominant signs

- Diarrhoea
- Anorexia
- Pyrexia
- Vomiting
- Dysentery
- Tenesmus

Diagnosis

Apart from observing the clinical signs and knowing the age of the pigs, a faeces sample (rectal swabs are not normally sufficient) will probably be required to make a diagnosis. As stated earlier, any change in diet is significant.

Mode of infection

Pet pigs are likely to become infected by faeces on visitors' boots, and commercial pigmen, however well meaning, should be kept away from backyard pigs. Commercial pigs are particularly vulnerable to incoming stock and transport lorries.

Prevention

- Avoid bringing live pigs on to the farm.
- All outgoing pigs to be taken and loaded outside the perimeter.
- All dead pigs to be either incinerated on farm or taken outside the perimeter for collection.
- All visitors to have been pig free for 3 days before entry.
- All visitors to wear boots and overalls provided by the farm at the gates. Veterinarians particularly should remember to up hold strict biosecurity. This should involve using overalls and boots provided by the farm and leaving their own vehicles outside the farm gates.

Causes of enteric disease

- Viruses
- Bacteria
- Protozoa
- Endoparasites
- Poisoning
- Change of nutrition (as a rule of thumb epidemic enteric disease is seen less in backyard pigs than in commercial pigs, but problems with nutrition are more common in backyard pigs)

Enteric diseases caused by viruses and their treatment

Epidemic diarrhoea

This is caused by a coronavirus and is similar to transmissible gastroenteritis (TGE, see below) but less common. There is a specific monoclonal antibody test available to differentiate the two diseases. Epidemic diarrhoea may cause vomiting, but the mortality is less than with TGE. There is no treatment or vaccine available.

Foot-and-mouth disease (FMD)

FMD, swine vesicular disease (SVD, see below under 'Diseases of the Neurological System', 'Neurological diseases caused by viruses') and vesicular stomatitis (VS, see Chapters 3 and 12) are termed 'vesicular diseases' and are best grouped together. SVD and VS are not important as such, except that they initially look like FMD and may delay its diagnosis. An FMD-infected pig excretes 3000 times as much virus in its exhaled breath as an infected bovine animal. It is therefore vital that the disease is diagnosed immediately.

No household scraps should be fed to pigs. However, this rule may be disobeyed by pet pig owners and therefore a pet pig might easily be the focus of an outbreak of FMD.

It is necessary to clean the feet of pigs being examined to determine whether vesicular lesions are present. It is important to use only clean water, as detergents and disinfectants will kill the FMD virus and make confirmation difficult. Vesicles are more common on the feet than on the tongue, lips or snout. *FMD should always be suspected if vesicular lesions are present, particularly if there is a high mortality in baby pigs.* In older pigs, morbidity is high but mortality is low.

The most common finding in FMD is the sudden onset of severe lameness. There is a high fever – up to 41°C – and the affected animals will have arched backs and be reluctant to move. If goaded, they will squeal pitifully. They are depressed and anorexic. The incubation period may be as short as 2 days.

Other than SVD and VS, there are additional conditions that may cause confusion with FMD and these should be included in a list of differential diagnoses, as follows:

- Chemical burns: these are seen on the side of the face at the same time as on the feet. They have definite crust appearance.
- Contact dermatitis: the lesions in this condition are seen all over the lower part of the leg and are not confined to the coronary band.
- Swinepox: this disease is characterized by papular lesions, which occur all over the body and are not confined to the feet (see below under 'Diseases of the Integument', 'Skin diseases caused by viruses'.
- Traumatic lesions: traumatic lesions on the feet may look like old vesicular lesions, particularly if the diet is deficient in biotin. However, close examination should reveal the absence of fresh vesicular lesions. The snout and the tongue should also be examined, as lesions at this site are unlikely to be traumatic.

FMD is also listed as a cause of abortion in pigs (see below under 'Diseases of the Reproductive System', 'Abortions, stillbirths, and weak and mummified piglets').

Rotavirus

Rotavirus is a killer of very young pigs but older pigs are more resistant. Diagnosis is by a fluorescent antibody test (FAT) on a faeces sample. Post-mortem shows a typical milk-filled intestine. Supportive antibiotics and fluids help to reduce the mortality. The virus spreads relatively slowly through a litter.

Transmissible gastroenteritis (TGE)

This is a highly contagious disease caused by a coronavirus which causes 100% mortality in baby pigs but no symptoms in adults. Diagnosis is by FAT on a faeces sample. There is an ELISA test and a specific monoclonal antibody test available. There is no treatment, but immunity is rapidly established in a herd. It is suggested that dung from infected piglets is given to in-pig sows to establish an immunity which can then be passed on as a passive immunity to the piglets. Such procedures are not without hazard and so should be given very careful consideration. TGE is only likely to attack the small pig herd which is buying in gilts.

Vomiting wasting disease

This disease is caused by a coronavirus which affects piglets of 5–20 days old. As the name suggests, they vomit, slowly lose weight and die. They also appear to become hairy. There is a FAT for the faeces available. There is no treatment and euthanasia is indicated. Passive colostral immunity will protect the piglets from disease.

Enteric diseases caused by bacteria and their treatment

Campylobacter *enteritis*

This normally affects young piglets from 3 days to 3 weeks of age. The most noticeable feature is the mucoid quality of the diarrhoea. The main organism responsible is *C. coli* but other *Campylobacter* spp. may also be involved. There is a sharp loss of condition but death is rare. Neomycin or tetracyclines are the preferred antibiotics given by the oral route.

Clostridial diarrhoea

This is quite common in outdoor pigs. It can be caused by *Clostridium perfringens* type A or C. Type A causes less severe diarrhoea than type C, which causes 100% mortality in piglets less than a week old. The faeces are claret coloured. Older pigs may survive but will be stunted. At that stage, euthanasia should be strongly advised. Susceptible pigs can be given hyperimmune antiserum at birth. Sows can be vaccinated with the correct clostridial vaccine 2 weeks before farrowing.

Escherichia coli *diarrhoea*

This normally starts with diarrhoea but quickly progresses to septicaemia and death if there is no treatment. It is a disease of the neonatal piglet, the suckling pig and the weaned pig. Certain specific strains of *E. coli* are involved, particularly those with the O and K antigens. Laboratory confirmation is important for the strain, so that the appropriate vaccine can be given to the sow and the appropriate antibiotic to the piglets. *E. coli* may be seen as oedema disease (bowel oedema) in very rapidly growing newly weaned pigs. The eyelids will be oedematous and the squeak will be higher pitched than normal. This may be seen as a neurological condition. Antibiotics will help, as will the giving of a less nutritious diet.

Helicobacter pylori

This organism, which might give rise to human isolates, has been found in the pig. Its significance is unknown but it might cause gastritis.

Proliferative enteropathy

This is an infectious bacterial condition of the mucosa of the small and large bowel. It underlies necrotic enteritis, regional ileitis and proliferative haemorrhagic enteropathy. It is a stress-related syndrome. The causal bacterium, *Lawsonia intracellularis* is, as the name suggests, intracellular. Affected pigs lose weight and appear pale. They may die suddenly with clotted blood in the small bowel. Tylosin is the antibiotic of choice although some authorities favour tiamulin.

Salmonellosis

This is a real problem in pigs, particularly in the UK. The specific pig bacterium is *Salmonella choleraesuis* (more recently designated *Salmonella* serovar Choleraesuis), which normally affects bigger growing pigs in the 10–16 week old range. It causes a high morbidity and mortality. There is a high fever, sometimes with pneumonic signs as well as diarrhoea. There may also be nervous signs and severe skin discoloration. Other *Salmonella* species are likely to be significant as well, e.g. *S. typhimurium*. Laboratory confirmation is important in this zoonotic disease which may cause disease in all ages of pig, although it should be remembered that pigs in many herds do not show disease signs. Hygiene

precautions are very important. See also below under 'Diseases of the Reproductive System', 'Abortions, stillbirths, and weak and mummified piglets', '*Salmonella* spp.'.

Swine dysentery

This is a condition of larger growing pigs and adults, and is caused by *Brachyspira* (formerly *Sepulina* or *Treponema*) *hyodysenteriae*. As the name suggests, dysentery is a feature. The pigs will show a high fever and quickly die without treatment. Tylosin used to be the drug of choice but now most isolates are resistant to this and tiamulin (by injection) would now be the drug of choice. Confirmation of the diagnosis is not easy, as the organism really needs to be seen in wet smears examined on farm, and even then there may be confusion as there is another similar condition called spirochaetal diarrhoea. This is a syndrome of younger pigs, mainly newly weaned pigs and is caused by spirochaetes other than *B. hyodysenteriae*. In this disease, dysentery is nothing like so marked, there is often no fever and deaths are rare. Treatment is the same as for swine dysentery.

Yersinia

Yersinia can cause human disease but is very rare in pigs. The two main causal organisms are *Y. enterocolitica and Y. pseudotuberculosis*. These have been associated with mild diarrhoea in pigs. Supportive treatment is rarely required.

Enteric diseases caused by protozoa

Coccidiosis

This occurs in baby pigs. There are eight *Eimeria* and one *Isospora* species affecting pigs but only *I. suis* is considered to be of clinical importance. This has a prepatent period of less than 1 week, and causes profuse diarrhoea in 7–10 day old unweaned piglets. There are two licensed products available for treatment: toltrazuril, which can be given as a one-off oral dose of 20 mg/kg at 3–5 days old and sulfadiazine/trimethropin which can be given as a single im injection of 25 mg/2 kg sulfadiazine and 5 mg/2 kg trimethropin. Improving the hygiene of the farrowing accommodation will help to reduce the incidence of the condition but treating the sows is not helpful.

Cryptosporidiosis

This is caused by *Cryptosporidium parvum*. The organism is present in healthy pigs but the organisms have been found in large numbers in piglets with diarrhoea. The hygiene of farrowing accommodation is important. There are no licensed medicines in the UK, but halofuginone lactate can be given orally under the cascade principle at 1 mg/10 kg. It should be remembered that this is a zoonotic disease.

Enteric diseases caused by endoparasites

Ascaris suum

This is the large roundworm, which actually only rarely causes ill thrift in growing pigs but does cause liver condemnation at slaughter. It also very rarely causes small intestinal obstruction. Ascarid eggs are extremely resistant and can survive on fields for many years. High faecal egg counts (FECs) will be seen and there is an ELISA test available.

Hyostrongylus rubidus

This is the red stomach worm, which mainly affects adults. The worms are 1 cm in length and may cause gastric ulceration and ill thrift. Sows will show high FECs.

Oesophagostomum dentatum and O. quadrispinulatum

These are the nodular worms which mainly live in the colon and caecum of adult pigs. They are about 1.5 cm in length and may cause ill thrift and even torsion of the colon. Sows will show high FECs.

Trichuris suis

This is the pig whipworm, which is about 1.5 cm long and lives in the caecum. It only causes problems in young growing pigs if there are heavy infestations. Ulceration and high FECs will be seen.

Control and resistance to anthelmintics

So far, resistance of helminths to anthelmintics has not been found to be a problem in pigs. Treatment should be carried out in adults on a 6 monthly basis, with outdoor pigs being moved to clean pasture and indoor pigs having their accommodation steam cleaned. Growing pigs should be treated at 8 weeks of age and then every 2 months until maturity. It is important to remember to reduce the risk of resistance by treating animals up to weight. Only licensed medicines for pigs should be used. Control of helminths in pigs can be easily accomplished in commercial herds by in-feed ivermectin or fenbendazole given at 6 monthly intervals. Individual treatments can be given by im injection of doramectin at 3 mg/10 kg or by sub cut injection of ivermectin at 300 mcg/kg. Small group treatment may be carried out by in-water medication of flubendazole at 1 mg/kg for 5 days or fenbendazole oral pellets at 5 mg/kg as a single dose. As with all medication, meat withdrawal periods must be followed.

Enteric diseases caused by poisons

Aflatoxin B1

This poisoning occurs from feeding badly stored feed. There is fatty degeneration of the liver. Pigs will scour and may show terminal signs of jaundice and convulsions. There is no specific treatment other than removing the contaminated feed and treating symptomatically.

Enteric diseases of unknown aetiology

Intestinal haemorrhagic syndrome

This is a condition which is normally associated with the feeding of whey, and is seen rarely in pigs fed on other regimes. It is a peracute disease of fattening pigs, which are often found dead. Treatment has been recommended with oxytetracycline at 20 mg/kg given im.

Diseases of the Neurological System

The predominant signs

These are best observed before handling. They are:

- stupor
- head tilt
- facial paralysis
- ocular discharge
- nystagmus
- aural discharge
- circling
- abnormalities of gait
- high stepping gait
- lack of pedal withdrawal
- loss of balance
- abnormal posture
- hyperaesthesia
- mania
- tremor
- flaccid tail
- unable to stand
- paddling
- opisthotonos
- convulsions

Diagnosis

For making a diagnosis, an accurate history with careful observation is required. The age and rectal temperature are very relevant.

Causes of neurological disease

- Viruses
- Bacteria
- Protozoa
- Poisoning
- Miscellaneous

Neurological diseases caused by viruses

African swine fever (ASF)

This is notifiable in the UK. The peracute nature of this disease may give rise to nervous signs but they are not a consistent feature.

See also below under 'Diseases of the Reproductive System', 'Abortion, stillbirths, and weak and mummified piglets'.

Aujeszky's disease

This is notifiable in the UK. Nervous signs are more prominent in baby pigs. See also below under Diseases of the Reproductive System', 'Abortion, stillbirths, and weak and mummified piglets'.

Classical swine fever (CSF)

This disease is notifiable in the UK. As with ASF, the peracute nature of this viral disease may give rise to nervous signs, particularly in baby piglets. See also below under 'Diseases of the Reproductive System', 'Abortion, stillbirths, and weak and mummified piglets'.

Rabies

This is a notifiable disease which is not likely to be seen in the UK. It is extremely rare in pigs even where rabies is endemic. Pigs do excrete the virus in their saliva, so practitioners should take care. The dumb form of rabies with excessive salivation is the most common in pigs but the 'rage' form is also seen.

Swine vesicular disease (SVD)

Encephalitis is seen in pigs with SVD. Young pigs will scream when they move. The problem is that the lesions cannot be differentiated from those of foot-and-mouth disease (FMD; see 'Diseases of the Gastroenteric System', 'Enteric diseases caused by viruses and their treatment'). Both diseases are notifiable in the UK.

Talfan disease

This is a notifiable disease which has been very rarely recorded in the UK. It is thought to be a mild form of Teschen disease and is mainly seen in piglets rather than older pigs. There is an ELISA test is available.

Teschen disease

This is a notifiable disease which has nervous signs but has never been recorded in the UK.

It is seen in central Europe. Marked pyrexia and severe neurological signs are seen. There is an ELISA test is available.

Neurological diseases caused by bacteria and their treatment

Abscesses

If abscesses occur in the brain or spinal cord they are normally as a result of tail biting. Large doses of antibiotics together with non-steroidal anti-inflammatory drugs (NSAIDs) can be tried but are rarely successful.

Actinobacillosis

This disease is caused by two organisms, *Actinobacillus suis* and *A. equuli*. It is not really known as a disease of the nervous system but there may be neurological signs in the pera-cute form in piglets up to 6 weeks of age. There is septicaemia, arthritis and endocardi-tis. In older pigs, the disease is less acute with skin lesions and a necrotizing focal pneumo-nia. Adults may die with an endocarditis. Antibiotics given as a treatment are rarely successful but can be used to reduce the inci-dence of the disease. See also below under 'Diseases of the Respiratory System', 'Respiratory diseases caused by bacteria'.

Bowel oedema

This is really an enteric disease, but the asso-ciated acute septicaemia can cause oedema of the central nervous system (CNS) and so give nervous signs. Oedema of the eyelids will also be seen and will aid in diagnosis. Pigs should have their rations reduced and be given antibiotics in the water.

Haemophilus parasuis *meningitis*

This is part of the Glasser's disease syndrome. All serous surfaces are affected, including the meninges, so neurological signs can be a fea-ture of this disease as well as respiratory signs. The disease is sporadic. Antibiotics are rarely useful for treatment. See below under 'Diseases of the Respiratory System',

'Respiratory diseases caused by bacteria' for more information.

Leptospirosis

Certain *Leptospira* spp. cause liver toxicity, which results in jaundice. Affected animals may show neurological signs. The antibiotic of choice for treatment is streptomycin. Practitioners should remember the zoonotic implications.

Listeriosis

This zoonotic disease is caused by *Listeria monocytogenes*. The organism has been found in normal pigs at slaughter. Deaths in neona-tal pigs showing neurological signs have been recorded. It is an extremely rare disease in pigs. Treatment and prevention can be attempted with oxytetracyclines.

Middle ear infection

The main sign will be shaking of the head. Aural haematomas may be seen in adult lop-eared breeds. The infection is likely to follow mange. Treatment must involve treating the sarcoptic mange as well as the secondary infection (see below under 'Diseases of the Integument', 'Diseases caused by parasites'). Obvious aural haematomas may be treated as in dogs under a general anaesthetic (GA) in a variety of surgical ways. However, in view of the dangers of anaesthetics in adult pigs, this procedure cannot be recommended. Equally, practitioners should *not* be tempted to release the swelling by cutting the aural skin. The resulting haemorrhage will be very signifi-cant and not appreciated by the pig owner. If the mites and the bacteria can be controlled, the head shaking will stop and the ear will heal as a cauliflower.

Salmonellosis

This zoonotic disease causes a high fever which may give nervous signs in young pigs. It is normally considered as an enteric dis-ease. See above under 'Diseases of the Gastroenteric System', 'Enteric diseases caused by bacteria and their treatment' for more information.

Streptococcal meningitis

This is one of the most common neurological diseases to affect pigs. The most usual condition occurs in the 8–12 week old age group. Pigs may be found dead, but the condition is more commonly seen as pigs that are unable to sit up and are paddling. Antibiotics, normally penicillin, are very helpful. A small dose of dexamethasone will cut down the inflammation in the CNS. Survival will also be aided by supplying fluids by mouth. Care must be taken not to choke the pig. An old teapot is useful to pour a stream of water for the affected pig to lick. There is a much less common streptococcal condition shown in fat pigs which is called 'type 2 meningitis' in which pigs are normally found dead.

Tetanus

This disease is very rarely found in pigs as they are very resistant to the tetanus toxin so routine antitoxin injections need not be given in this species. The pig will appear rigid with the tail sticking out. Penicillin may be given but the clostridial bacteria are likely to be dead long before the symptoms appear. Recovery is normally complete over a 10 day period.

Neurological diseases caused by protozoa

Coccidiosis

This disease may cause severe enteric signs in baby pigs. The dehydration may result in neurological signs.

Neurological diseases caused by poisoning

Arsenic poisoning

This should be a condition of the past, as arsanilic acid is no longer used in the treatment of swine dysentery. Progressive paralysis and blindness follow tremor. Pigs will recover if kept warm and given ad lib fluids by mouth. If they have not considerably improved in 3 days, euthanasia should be advised.

Congenital tremor

This is a condition of the newborn piglet. Historically it was associated with CSF affecting the sow in late pregnancy. It may be seen after any acute disease in the pregnant sow and even after organophosphorus poisoning. It is an alarming condition. Often the piglets will survive if they do not shake so much that they cannot hold the teat.

Iron toxicity

This can occur from overdosing injectable iron in piglets. Death is usually within 6 h of the injection.

Metaldehyde

This is the active ingredient in molluscicides used in the control of snails and slugs. Excess salivation and nervous signs are seen and death is rapid. There is no specific antidote but anaesthetizing the pigs ip with barbiturates might be helpful. When they recover from the anaesthetic the pigs may have stopped fitting and can make a recovery.

Nitrite/nitrate poisoning

This is a condition recorded in whey fed pigs kept in very poorly ventilated conditions. The lack of fever will help diagnosis in pigs found in such conditions. Pigs will show respiratory signs as well as neurological signs.

Salt poisoning

This is really water deprivation and is one of the most common causes of neurological signs in growing pigs. It occurs if the water supply is turned off or frozen up. A growing pig weighing 15 kg requires 2 l water a day, and a 100 kg finishing pig requires 12 l daily. Pigs do not like to queue so adequate sources of water should be available. Nervous signs are more prominent in growing pigs. The renewal of the water should be controlled. Dexamethasone injections may help with recovery.

Selenium poisoning

This is extremely rare. The author has seen the condition in pigs which were given a large amount of an equine supplement. The pigs remained mentally alert but were reluctant to rise. They recovered with careful nursing.

Neurological diseases caused by miscellaneous causes

Heat stroke

This will cause neurological signs which are very similar to those caused by water deprivation (salt poisoning). Overfat pot-bellied pigs are very susceptible. Sunburn may complicate the condition in white pigs. The pigs should be cooled rapidly with buckets of cold water or a hose. If they are *in extremis* dexamethazone iv will be helpful. If the pigs have sunburn they will require antibiotics, NSAIDs and topical oily creams.

Metabolic Diseases

Copper deficiency myelopathy

This is extremely rare. It may be associated with iron deficiency in commercial indoor pigs.

Hypoglycaemia

This is seen in neonatal pigs which have not received adequate energy, e.g. in very cold conditions when a sow has farrowed outside in winter. Convulsions will be seen in piglets. Hypoglycaemia can also be brought on by various low-level infections in piglets. The farrowing fever complex syndrome (see Chapter 10), which will decrease milk output, will put piglets at risk. Treatment is with proprietary energy fluids by mouth.

Osteomalacia

This condition will only be seen in very badly fed adult or very aged backyard pigs.

Calcium has to be virtually absent from the diet. The bones are very brittle. The pig may have multiple long bone fractures and be unable to rise. Prompt euthanasia is the only course of action.

Vitamin A deficiency

This will cause blindness and so the pigs will appear to show nervous signs. The condition is certainly a possibility in badly fed backyard pigs. Once there is blindness, recovery is impossible even with vitamin A injections. Single or pairs of affected pigs might be thought to have a reasonable quality of life but euthanasia should be seriously considered.

Vitamin B deficiency

This may occur in backyard pigs fed either a very fat diet or fed solely on bread. Normally pigs go off their hind legs, and this is followed by a progressive paralysis. They may recover with good nursing and a proper diet.

Diseases of the Respiratory System

Predominant signs

- Dyspnoea
- Tachycardia
- Pyrexia
- Coughing
- Snout deviation

Diagnosis

For an accurate diagnosis, a post-mortem with viral and bacterial examination will be required. In commercial units, regular lung examination at the abattoir is well worthwhile.

Mode of infection

- Mixing pigs
- Incoming pigs
- Pigs going to shows

Prevention

Prevention is much better than treatment and so keeping a closed herd is well worthwhile. There are some very useful vaccines available. Good ventilation for indoor pigs is vital.

Causes of respiratory disease

- Viruses
- Bacteria
- Endoparasites

Respiratory diseases caused by viruses

Inclusion body rhinitis

This is a very rare viral disease which is lethal to young piglets, but signs, except for transitory sneezing, are rarely seen in adults.

Porcine reproductive and respiratory syndrome (PRRS)

This syndrome will cause reproductive problems in sows. It is caused by an *Arterivirus*. Fattening pigs will show respiratory signs. The adult pigs do not normally show a fever but laboured breathing and inappetence. Skin changes occur more commonly in growing pigs which show the classic blue ear appearance. Baby pigs often show oedema of the eyelids and conjunctivitis. Mortality may not be high in well looked after piglets. Treatment with oral paracetamol or aspirin in the early stages is worthwhile. There is a commercial vaccine available. See also below under 'Diseases of the Reproductive System', 'Abortions, stillbirths, and weak and mummified piglets'.

Post-weaning multi-systemic wasting syndrome (PMWS)

PMWS is extremely important in commercial pigs and is clinically similar to PRRS. It is caused by a *Circovirus*, and is obviously important in backyard pet pigs obtained from commercial stock. There is a vaccine available. Ideally, backyard fattening pigs should be vaccinated before movement. Naturally, good hygiene practices should be paramount, as well as avoiding stress. Once the pigs are showing signs of the syndrome antibiotic treatment is rarely worthwhile and so euthanasia should be carried out.

Swine influenza

The virus that causes swine influenza is specific to pigs and causes coughing and dyspnoea. Fever is very severe for the first 24 h. The pigs will be prostrate. With warmth, recovery is quite rapid without treatment, but may be accelerated by oral aspirin. Adult pigs as well as growing pigs are affected. See also below under 'Diseases of the Reproductive System', 'Abortions, stillbirths, and weak and mummified piglets'.

Respiratory diseases caused by bacteria

Actinobacillosis

This is a highly contagious respiratory disease caused by *Actinobacillus pleuropneumoniae*. There is a fibrinous pleurisy, which may be heard on auscultation. The disease is often fatal, particularly if other respiratory pathogens are involved. Antibiotic treatment is rarely effective, as the antibiotics do not reach the affected areas. There is a commercially available vaccine. See also above under 'Diseases of the Neurological System', 'Neurological diseases caused by bacteria and their treatment'.

Atrophic rhinitis

This shows as sneezing in young piglets. It is rarely fatal, but causes atrophy of the turbinate bones with distortion of the nasal septum, resulting in shortening and twisting of the upper jaw. It is caused by a combination of *Pasteurella multocida* and *Bordetella bronchiseptica*. Deaths occur if there is an additional *Mycoplasma* infection.

Enzootic pneumonia

This is caused by *Mycoplasma hyopneumoniae*. It is not only a highly contagious pulmonary disease but also affects the joints. It is likely to be seen in pigs soon after arrival on a new holding. They will show mild lameness and/or coughing. Temperatures will be raised initially. Treatment with oxytetracycline or tylosin by injection is the recommended treatment. This should be followed with water medication. NSAIDs are helpful. The disease is unlikely to be fatal but may be very persistent. There are several commercially available vaccines.

Glasser's disease

This is an infectious disease caused by *Haemophilus parasuis*, which is often fatal in growing pigs. There is a polyserositis, a polyarthritis and sometimes meningitis. Bronchitis may occur in adults. The classic scenario is the stressed pig arriving in a contaminated environment.

There is a sudden onset high fever. Lung sounds and pericardial rubbing will be heard on auscultation. Very soon, the arthritic signs will be seen. If the pig survives, the disease will be manifest in the joints as a chronic arthritis. Meningitis can occur at this stage. Euthanasia is then the correct procedure and would also be appropriate if there is bowel obstruction from intestinal adhesions. There is a commercially available vaccine either on its own or linked with enzootic pneumonia vaccine.

Pasteurellosis

This is an infectious disease seen in the older growing pig and caused by *P. multocida*. It is often secondary to infection by *H. parasuis*, *A. pleuropneumoniae* and *M. hyopneumoniae*. There is fever and a nasal discharge. Lung sounds are loud and breathing laboured with mouth breathing. Aggressive antibiotic treatment should be tried but is unlikely to be effective.

Respiratory diseases caused by endoparasites

Ascaris

Ascaris spp. are not respiratory endoparasites but their migration phase through the lungs can cause respiratory distress and is very important in backyard pigs. The signs are similar to asthma in man, to heaves in horses and to fog fever in cattle, but the pathological lesions are different. Prevention by good helminth control is important and affected pigs should be treated.

Metastrongylus

This lungworm is found in outdoor pigs. It rarely causes any respiratory signs.

Miscellaneous causes of respiratory disease

Warfarin poisoning

Warfarin, when used as a rat poison, can cause poisoning in pigs. Pallor and haemorrhages are seen, together with vomiting and the coughing of blood. Treatment is large doses of vitamin K (20 mg vitamin K_1 im per piglet).

Diseases of the Urinary System

The predominant sign is haematuria.

Diagnosis

Urine can be collected for examination for blood, crystals and bacteria. The rectal temperature is an important diagnostic sign.

Mode of infection

This is normally at parturition or after service.

Urinary diseases caused by bacteria

Cystitis/Pyelonephritis

This clinical entity is normally caused by *Actinobaculum suis*, *E. coli* or *Klebsiella* spp. These organisms are widespread in the prepuce of boars. It is not known why in certain cases the infection is not killed by the sow's immune mechanisms. It becomes an ascending infection through the bladder, ureter and on to the kidney. The temperature is rarely raised. Blood or pus maybe seen in the urine. Prolonged treatment with antibiotics will be helpful provided that both kidneys are not affected.

Porcine dermatitis and nephropathy syndrome (PDNS)

This is a syndrome which is covered in the section on 'Skin diseases caused by bacteria' under 'Diseases of the Integument' above. It is a serious condition which tends to occur in large fattening pigs. The rectal temperature will be raised.

Miscellaneous urinary diseases

Urolithiasis

This caused by calcium carbonate and is seen in sows and neonatal pigs. It is rare in finishing pigs. It can be prevented by providing a good diet.

Diseases of the Reproductive System

Abortions, stillbirths, and weak and mummified piglets

With all infectious or toxic causes, the time in the pregnancy will affect the outcome for the sow and subsequent breeding. Thus, if the agent affects the sow in the first 5 weeks of pregnancy, there is likely to be a vulval discharge, with a subsequent return to service. If the agent affects the sow between the 6th and 8th week of pregnancy, some or all of the piglets are likely to be mummified at term. If the agent affects the sow after the 8th week of pregnancy, there is likely to be abortion, or stillbirths or weak piglets at term. It should be remembered that any disease causing a fever might cause an abortion. So-called 'barker' piglets are thought to be just a manifestation of prematurity.

The common causes are as follows.

Aujeszky's disease

This disease used to be called pseudorabies and is caused by *Suid herpesvirus 1* (SuHV-1), a *Varicellovirus*. It is a notifiable disease in the UK and is likely to cause 100% mortality in newly born piglets and 60% mortality in older piglets, with nervous signs. There may be few signs in adult sows except abortion and small herpes cold sore-type lesions on the snout.

Blue eye paramyxovirus

This virus causes abortions in parts of Mexico.

Brucellosis

Brucella suis does not occur in the UK or Eire, but it is found on mainland Europe and in the USA. Ensuing abortions may not be widespread but there will be signs of orchitis in boars and a severe endometritis in sows. Both sexes will suffer severe painful septic arthritis. Euthanasia is indicated.

Carbon monoxide

This poisonous gas can cause abortion. Fetal tissue will be cherry red. Pigs should not be kept in garages.

Erysipelas

This condition may cause abortions on account of the high fever shown by some animals. There is a good vaccine available. See below under 'Diseases of the Integument', 'Skin diseases caused by bacteria' for more information.

Foot-and-mouth disease (FMD)

This highly contagious viral disease is notifiable in the UK and will cause abortions in pigs in other parts of the world. See above under 'Diseases of the Gastroenteric System', 'Enteric diseases caused by viruses') for more information on FMD.

Japanese B encephalitis virus

Pigs amplify this zoonotic *Flavivirus* which is not found in the UK. There is a vaccine available.

Leptospirosis

There are many serotypes and serovars of this disease, all of which have been implicated in causing abortions. Some will cause the sow to be ill and show icterus. See also above 'Diseases of the Neurological System', 'Neurological diseases caused by bacteria and their treatment'.

Mycotoxins

There is a variety of mycotoxins. Infection will mainly come from dirty food bins or food bags stored in damp conditions. The piglets will be seen to have enlarged teats. Early embryonic death is the most common manifestation.

Porcine circovirus

Porcine circovrus-2 is ubiquitous will cause abortion. There is a vaccine available.

Porcine parvovirus

Porcine parvovirus only causes reproductive disease. There is a very effective vaccine. After an abortion the sow will be immune to further infection.

Porcine reproductive and respiratory syndrome (PRRS)

This disease is commonly called 'blue ear disease'. The acute respiratory disease is shown in growing pigs but it is very transitory in adults which will abort. There is a vaccine available. See also above under 'Diseases of the Respiratory System', 'Respiratory diseases caused by viruses'.

Salmonella *spp.*

These bacteria cause pyrexia and abortions. See also above under 'Diseases of the Gastroenteric System', 'Enteric diseases caused by bacteria', 'Salmonellosis'.

SMEDI (stillbirths, mummification, embryonic deaths and infertility)

This is caused by an *Enterovirus* and is difficult to distinguish from the disease caused by *Porcine parvovirus*.

Swine fever

Both ASF and CSF are notifiable diseases in the UK. There are highly virulent strains which will kill sows. There are less virulent strains which will cause abortion. There are good vaccines available for CSF but these are not permitted in the UK or in the USA. See also above under 'Diseases of the Neurological System', 'Neurological diseases caused by viruses'.

Swine influenza

This virus disease mainly causes respiratory signs (see above under 'Diseases of the Respiratory System', 'Respiratory diseases caused by viruses'), but also pyrexia and abortions.

Toxoplasmosis

In theory, this zoonotic disease, caused by the protozoan *Toxoplasma gondii*, which is harboured by cats, might cause abortion in pigs, although it has only been confirmed in isolated cases.

Vitamin A deficiency

This condition is only seen in backyard pigs receiving a poorly balanced diet.

Chronic mastitis

One or more mammary glands will be large, swollen and non-productive. They are rarely painful. The condition may be caused by a variety of organisms. Antibiotic treatment, even if prolonged, will not be effective. The gland should not be lanced, and if it ulcerates humane destruction should be carried out.

Diseases of the Integument

Lesions on the skin can be caused by systemic diseases, e.g. PRRS, CSF and salmonellosis, which have already been described above. Only actual skin disease will be covered in this section.

Causes of skin disease

- Viruses
- Bacteria
- Fungi
- Ectoparasites
- Poisoning
- Nutritional
- Miscellaneous

Skin diseases caused by viruses

Swinepox

This is an extremely rare condition which can be congenital. Diagnosis is difficult as it often leads to severe greasy pig disease (see below under 'Skin diseases caused by bacteria').

Skin diseases caused by bacteria

Erysipelas

This has four manifestations in pigs, which are caused by *Erysipelothrix rhusiopathiae*:

1. An acute-onset febrile disease in growing pigs in which the fever and inappetance precedes the appearance of the classical raised inflamed diamond areas on the skin.
2. A subacute form in older pigs which are hardly ill but show the skin lesions.

3. Polyarthritis in growing pigs, which may occur following either of the first two types of infection.
4. The bacteraemia and endocarditis form, which maybe fatal in adult pigs.

The organism is very sensitive to penicillin. However, once the lesions are formed on the heart valves the days of the pig are numbered. The vaccine, which can be given to growing pigs and adults, is very effective. One dose followed by a second dose in 4–6 weeks and then every 6 months is the regime advised.

Greasy pig disease

This is an infectious disease caused by *Staphylococcus hyicus*. It can occur at any age but is found mainly in young growing pigs. Parenteral antibiotics with topical Savlon washes are an effective treatment. The disease can be extremely extensive but is always non-pruritic. It can lead to necrosis of the ear tips.

Porcine dermatitis and nephropathy syndrome (PDNS)

This syndrome is a complex condition which is thought to be a hypersensitivity reaction to a severe bacteriological infection. It is invariably fatal and might be confused with swine fever (see above under 'Diseases of the Neurological System', 'Neurological diseases caused by viruses'). There is no treatment. The disease normally occurs in older growing pigs and might be confused with thrombocytopenic purpura.

Skin diseases caused by fungi

Ringworm

This is very rare in pigs. It is usually caught from rats or mice and is caused by *Trichophyton mentagrophytes*. Treatment in pigs is rarely necessary, as the disease is self-limiting. It should not be confused with pityriasis rosea (see below under 'Skin diseases due to miscellaneous causes').

Skin diseases caused by parasites

Flies

There are several species of fly which are attracted to pigs and they can cause physical bite lesions. Pig muck should be well heaped and kept well away from the pigs.

Lice

Pig lice can be seen with the naked eye as they are large sucking lice of the species *Haematopinus suis*. They cause pruritis and have been implicated in the spread of pig pox and the blood-borne bacterial parasite *Eperythrozoon suis*. Control is accomplished by treatment with ivermectin or doramectin.

Sarcoptic mange

This is caused by the mite *Sarcoptes scabiei* var. *suis*. Crusting with pruritis are the main signs. Control is accomplished by treating with iver-mectin or doramectin.

Skin diseases caused by nutritional problems

Biotin deficiency

The main signs are hair loss and hoof lesions.

Parakeratosis

This is caused a deficiency of zinc in the diet or by a conditioned deficiency resulting from high levels of phytic acid in soya. It is found in young growing pigs as scaly papules. Diagnosis can be by skin biopsy as testing for blood zinc levels is unreliable. Treatment is restoring the zinc level in the diet to 100 ppm.

Skin diseases due to miscellaneous causes

Bite wounds

These are common after pig groups have been mixed and they may be severe. They require aggressive antibiotic treatment. They should not be sutured but allowed to heal by second-ary intention.

Dermatosis vegetans

This is a rare congenital inherited condition of pigs. It affects the coronary band and is common in Landrace pigs.

Epitheliogenesis imperfecta

This is a rare congenital condition which is inherited. It is also called aplasia cutis. It is likely to be more common in inbred backyard pigs.

Frostbite

This will involve the extremities of outdoor pigs in severe weather conditions. It is a very painful condition. NSAIDs are helpful.

Pressure sores

These are commonly seen in overweight adult pigs kept on concrete. Antibiotic injections and sprays are helpful. It is vital to address the cause of the problem.

Pityriasis rosea

This is an inherited condition which appears in young suckling pigs. It is self-limiting. It has no links with any fungal condition.

Sunburn

This is possible in outdoor white pigs. It is not likely in any black pigs and has not been recorded in saddlebacks or kune kune pigs.

Thrombocytopenic purpura

This is an isoimmune condition affecting young suckling pigs. The affected pigs show large cyanotic areas.

Common Causes for Pigs to be Found Dead

Iatrogenic causes of sudden death

The term 'sudden death', as normally used, is a misnomer. In reality, sudden death usually means that death has occurred since the ani-mal was last seen. The owner will very rarely see an animal die. It is even rarer for the clinician to see death. Sadly, when such deaths do occur it is usually at the time of veterinary treatment. The likely causes of iatrogenic deaths in pigs are shown in Table 9.1.

Reasons for animals to be found dead

True sudden deaths are very rare. Possible causes of sudden deaths in pigs are shown in Table 9.2.

Table 9.1. A list of possible iatrogenic causes of sudden death in pigs.

Anaphylaxis from administration of medicines
General anaesthesia
Intravenous (iv) injection
Lumbar/sacral epidural
Massive haemorrhage (this could occur at parturition with human involvement)
Sedation

Table 9.2. A list of the causes of sudden death in pigs.

Anthrax
Bowel torsion
Clostridium novyi
Drowning (this may occur in deep water)
Electrocution can occur in faultily wired pig accommodation and it is *very important* that the electricity is turned off before there is any investigation
Endocarditis
Gassing from poorly ventilated houses
Gastric ulceration
Heat stroke
Intestinal haemorrhagic syndrome
Lightning strike
Mulberry heart disease
Porcine stress syndrome
Proliferative haemorrhagic enteropathy
Ruptured aneurysm
Ruptured uterine artery
Snake bite
Trauma (mainly from road traffic accidents or fighting in males)

10

Pig Surgery

_____

Introduction

The chapter starts with a discussion of the basic procedures used for analgesia, sedation and anaesthesia, including general anaesthesia in various age groups of pigs, and epidural anaesthesia. This is followed by an account of surgical conditions and procedures which is organized by system, with sections on the gastroenteric system, the urinary system, the reproductive system, the locomotory system and the integument. Lastly, there is a brief section on euthanasia.

Analgesia

There are four useful injectable NSAIDs licensed for pigs in the UK: flunixin, ketoprofen, meloxicam and tolfenamic acid (see Chapter 2). They all follow similar pharmokinetic pathways and therefore only a single drug needs to be carried by the ambulatory practitioner. Although these four NSAIDs are not licensed for oral use in pigs in the UK, they can be used under the cascade principle as the only licensed NSAID for oral administration is sodium salicylate, which has limited usage.

Sedation

Azaperone is the only licensed sedative for use in pigs in the UK. The dose is 2 mg/kg. It is not always very effective except when given with 1 IU/10 kg of oxytocin im to gilts that are savaging their newborn piglets.

Anaesthesia

General anaesthesia (GA)

Piglets

Anaesthesia in piglets is not well documented, although masking very young piglets is quite easy with isoflurane or halothane without premedication.

Older growing pigs

Pigs in the 15–25 kg weight range can be masked down with isoflurane or halothane after premedication with azaperone at 2 mg/kg.

Large growing pigs and adults

A combination of drugs given in the same syringe im with a hard non-disposable syringe and a 14 G needle is the author's preference.

The dose is 2 mg/kg xylazine, 10 mg/kg ket-amine and 2 mg/10 kg butorphanol. It should be acknowledged that these products are not licensed for pigs in the UK either alone or in combination.

Pentobarbital (6% solution) at 1 ml/2.5 kg can be used to anaesthetize pigs by iv injection after premedication with azaperone at 2 mg/kg im. However, this is not an easy technique.

Russian veterinary surgeons inject pentobarbital at double the normal dose directly into the testicle for castration. As soon as the pig is anaesthetized, castration is performed. Thus, the source of the anaesthetic is removed and the pig can be left to regain consciousness.

Epidural anaesthesia

This procedure is very hazardous as the epidural space entered by the injecting needle in the lumbar area contains the lower spinal cord. The procedure can be used for the replacement of uterine, vaginal and rectal prolapses, but it is not recommended.

Surgical Conditions of the Gastroenteric System

Atresia ani

This is an inherited defect which will be observed soon after birth. Careful examination should be carried out to differentiate this condition from atresia coli. These latter cases should be destroyed.

Treatment for atresia ani involves first cleaning the area before placing a small bleb of local anaesthetic where the rectum bulges out. A small stab cruciate incision should then be made to allow the passage of faeces. The animal should be re-examined in 3 days to confirm the continual passage of faeces.

Gastric torsion

This can occur in adult pigs after feeding. The pig will either be found dead or bloated *in extremis*. Splenic torsion may also occur, adding to the shock. If pigs appear bloated, forced exercise has been suggested. However, in the author's experience this has not been successful.

Gastric ulceration

This is known to occur with serious diseases such as swine fever and salmonellosis. It can also occur with transmissible gastroenteritis (TGE) in adults which show very very mild signs. There has been a link with *Helicobacter pylori* postulated, but this has never been proven. The animals will have black tarry faeces. Treatment with 4 mg omeprazole daily per rectum has been suggested. See Chapter 9 for further information on these pig diseases.

Intestinal obstruction

Intestinal obstructions are caused by:

- ingestion of foreign bodies, normally stones
- intestinal volvulus
- intestine trapped in an inguinal hernia
- intestine trapped in an umbilical hernia
- intussusception of the small intestine

There is no breed, sex or geographical predilection. Outdoor pigs are more likely to ingest stones and other debris.

Clinical signs include:

- a tacky feel as the thermometer is withdrawn after taking the rectal temperature
- anorexia
- cold ears
- lethargy
- pain and swelling in the area of the hernia
- subnormal rectal temperature

Further diagnostics include:

- Ultrasonography. This should be carried out trans-abdominally. It may need to be repeated after 12–24 h as the presence of stones needs to be assessed carefully. Stones that are present in the stomach are not likely to be significant. It is their presence in the small intestine that is important. Ultrasonography might also be helpful in the diagnosis of trapped intestines in hernias.

- Radiography. Like ultrasonography, this may have to be repeated to try to decide the significance of abdominal foreign bodies that have been identified.

Treatment of intestinal obstruction caused by a foreign body, an intussusception or a volvulus

In these cases, the animal should be given antibiotics, NSAIDs and liquid paraffin. The paraffin should be poured into the only water source available to the pig. It will float on the top and so the pig will swallow some whenever it drinks. This will often help the stone to move down the small intestine. The pig will then show some clinical improvement, but then the stone will stick again and the pig will deteriorate again. As soon as the stone enters the large intestine there will be a marked clinical improvement.

Abdominal surgery is another option. This is outside the author's experience, but it is feasible, certainly in smaller pigs. If a stone can be felt in the small intestine it can be removed or milked into the large intestine. At least with a laparotomy, the extent of any disease process can be assessed so that euthanasia can be carried out promptly if necessary.

Treatment of intestinal entrapment in an inguinal hernia

The treatment options will vary depending on the likelihood of the bowel being still viable, i.e. if there is pain in the area and the pig is not cold and shocked. Surgery in smaller pigs will be possible with local infiltration of local anaesthetic. Surgery in large boars will require a GA.

The area should be cleaned with the pig held upside down or, in the case of a large boar, with the hind quarters raised. A careful incision should be made into the swollen scrotum without penetrating the tunics. If possible, the intestine should be milked back into the abdomen. The testicle should then be

the only organ within the tunic. Two pairs of large artery forceps should be placed side by side across the cord within the tunic. The proximal pair should be removed and a transfixing ligature of absorbable suture material should be applied in the groove left by the forceps. The testicle should be removed by making a cut distal to the remaining pair of artery forceps. The skin should then be closed with interrupted horizontal mattress sutures of monofilament nylon.

If the pig is very shocked and it is likely that the bowel is no longer viable, or if the bowel is viable but cannot be milked back into the abdomen, the tunics will have to be opened carefully. This is beyond the author's experience. However, the bowel should be checked for viability. If it is viable, the inguinal ring will have to be enlarged to allow its return. If it is not viable, then bowel resection will need to be carried out. In both instances, the testicle should be removed by an open method, and an attempt will need to be made to close the inguinal ring before skin closure. Antibiotics and NSAIDs should be given in all cases.

Treatment of intestinal entrapment in an umbilical hernia

A GA will be required so that the pig can be put into dorsal recumbency. The hernia sack and the surrounding area should be surgically prepared. A careful incision should be made into the hernial sack. The bowel should be carefully examined for viability. If it is non-viable, the affected part should be resected. All of the bowel should be returned to the abdomen. Horizontal mattress sutures of monofilament nylon should be laid but not tightened across the abdominal defect, making sure that the peritoneal surfaces will be in apposition when the sutures are tightened. When the surgeon is sure that sufficient sutures have been laid, they can be tightened individually. On no account should further sutures be laid once the abdomen is closed. The sub-cuticular tissue should be closed with a continuous layer of absorbable sutures. The skin should be closed with single horizontal mattress sutures of monofilament nylon. Antibiotics and NSAIDs should be given in all cases.

Prolapsed rectum

Prolapsed rectum in fattening pigs

A prolapsed rectum is caused by continuous violent coughing due to respiratory disease and can be prevented by controlling the respiratory disease with vaccination and good husbandry. When such prolapses have occurred, treatment of the underlying respiratory disease is vital. This is usually done with suitable antibiotics and NSAIDs.

There are two methods of surgical correction:

1. The conventional method. The pig should be held upside down by its hind legs. The prolapsed rectum and surrounding area should be cleaned. Local anaesthetic should be infiltrated around the anal ring. A purse string suture of thick braided nylon should be laid around the anal ring but not tied. The prolapse should be replaced using lubricant. The suture should be tied so that only one finger can be introduced through the anal ring. The pig should be fed on a laxative diet or have liquid paraffin continuously put on its water. The suture should be removed in 14 days.
2. Another possible method, mainly for non-veterinarians, requires a 10 cm long and 2.5 cm diameter piece of ridged rubber sprayer hosepipe, together with a length of uterine tape. Using lubricant, the pipe is inserted with at least half its length into the anal ring inside the prolapse. A length of uterine tape is tied around the prolapse as close to the anal ring as possible in one of the rubber pipe grooves. The pig is given antibiotics and NSAIDs. The animal *must* be kept separately until the prolapse has rotted off and a new anal ring has been formed.

A rare sequel to a prolapsed rectum is rectal stricture, although this condition can also occur in growing pigs without there having been a prolapsed rectum. The pig will appear to be bloated. On careful examination, scarring of the rectum will be seen. Only very small ribbons of faeces may be passed. In theory, careful radical surgery would cure the condition. However, humane destruction is likely to be indicated.

Prolapsed rectum in sows

This normally occurs around parturition, and can be prevented by giving sows a laxative diet at this time. There are two methods of surgical correction which are similar to those described above for fattening pigs, but on a larger scale. The sow needs to be restrained in a crate (Fig. 10.1). The purse string suture needs to be able to accommodate three fingers. The hosepipe needs to be 6 cm in diameter and 20 cm long.

Tooth problems

Tooth problems are rare in pigs except in very old backyard pigs. They will be manifest as a pig reluctant to eat nuts and spitting out other food. There will be malodorous breath. The pig needs to be examined carefully under GA using a gag and a head torch (Fig. 10.2). Rotten cheek teeth will loose and should be removed with small equine molar extraction forceps. Antibiotics and NSAIDs should be given postoperatively. Growing backyard pigs will rarely have problems with retained deciduous incisors which will generally be shed eventually before the pig reaches 3 years of age.

Old boars will develop long extremely sharp canines (tusks) (see Fig. 10.3). These may be broken off by trauma but will not cause any problems, but they are dangerous to pig handlers and also to other pigs. They do not have a pulp cavity above the gingival margin and so can be cut off at this point without causing pain of infection. Restraint is the main problem. The tusks can be cut off while a boar is mounting a sow. Ideally, equine molar shears should be used (see Plate 15). Embryotomy wire can also be used, but this will become very hot and will continually break.

Surgical Conditions of the Urinary System

Preputial damage

The cause of this is unknown but it is likely to be related to sexual work as it tends to occur in groups of boars. The prepuce becomes very inflamed and necrotic. If caught in the early

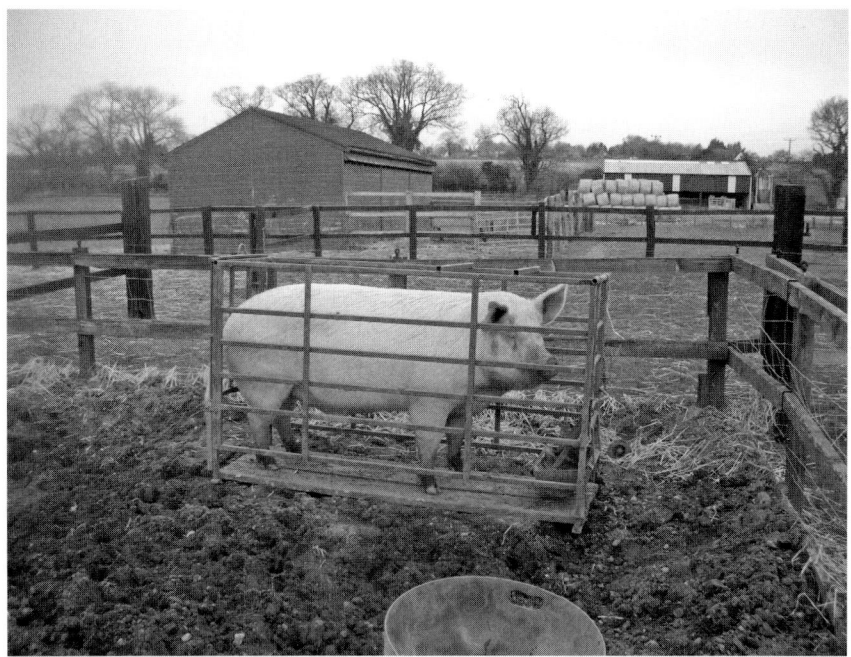

Fig. 10.1. An adult pig well secured in a crate.

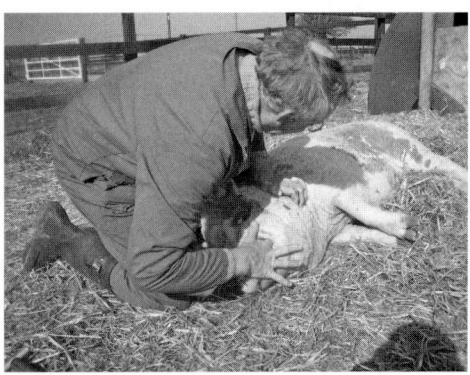

Fig. 10.2. Tooth examination of a pig under general anaesthetic.

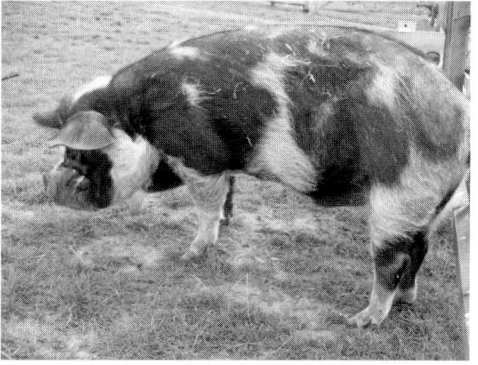

Fig. 10.3. A kune kune boar with large tusks (canines).

stages, antibiotics and NSAIDs will be curative. If the prepuce is severely damaged and the local lymph nodes enlarged, surgical debridement will have to be carried out under GA.

Retroversion of the bladder

This can occur in sows at farrowing. The inverted bladder will feel like a 15 cm ball blocking the vagina. It should be put back in place using plenty of lubricant and a horse nasogastric tube. The piglets can then be drawn. Small doses of 5 IU oxytocin should be given im at ½ hourly intervals to aid parturition, which should be supervised. Only when parturition is complete can the practitioner relax, knowing that the bladder will not retrovert again. The sow should not be bred from any more.

Surgical Conditions of the Reproductive System

Surgical conditions of females

Problems at parturition

PROLAPSED VAGINA This will occur before parturition, usually in the last few days of gestation, which is likely to be 114 days.

The treatment is to give antibiotics and NSAIDs. Local anaesthetic is injected around the vulva. A 'Buhner suture' is put in place and the vagina replaced. The suture is then tightened so that only three fingers can be placed in the vulva, and then it is tied with a bow. This is so that if the pigman thinks the sow is actually farrowing he can undo the suture without cutting it and let the sow continue to farrow. The suture can then be retied when she has finished farrowing. If the sow is not farrowing, the pigman can retie the suture immediately before the vagina re-prolapses.

FARROWING FEVER COMPLEX This is most common problem found in parturient pigs. The presenting signs are:

- a hard painful udder
- a slow parturition
- constipation
- failure to pass all the afterbirths
- inappetance
- pyrexia (a common but not invariable finding)

Examination involves taking the rectal temperature, palpating the udder and carrying out a vaginal examination. The treatment is to remove any dead piglets and remove any accessible afterbirth. Antibiotics should be given (the most likely pathogen is *E. coli*), with NSAIDs and oxytocin. If there is any likelihood of further pigs being born the oxytocin should be given as small 5 IU im doses, and vaginal examinations be repeated at 6 h intervals.

UTERINE TORSION This condition is seen in parturient pigs but it is extremely rare. There will be a total torsion of the uterus. Diagnosis is simple as the rifling of the vagina will be felt on vaginal examination.

The treatment involves giving the sow a GA and rolling it over quickly in the direction of the rifling. The sow should then be re-examined per vagina. If the twist has gone, any piglets within reach are removed, and 10 IU oxytocin im given at 30 min intervals, removing piglets until parturition is complete. Antibiotics and NSAIDs should be administered. If the twist has not gone, the procedure can be repeated once. If it is still not successful, a Caesarean section should be carried out.

Torsion of one horn of the uterus is more common. The sow will pass the pigs and afterbirth from the non-twisted horn and then parturition will cease. The torsion will be felt on a full vaginal and cervical examination. Rolling should not be attempted. A Caesarean section should be carried out.

CAESAREAN SECTION The sow is given a GA, and the upper hind leg drawn back with a rope. An area from the hind leg forward for 1 ft, and including the mammary glands and half the flank, is cleaned. As the GA is unlikely to last long enough, local infiltration should be carried out of a 9 in. incision in a para-median position just above the mammary gland. The area is then re-cleaned and antibiotics and NSAIDs given. A 20 cm incision should be made 1 cm above the mammary gland as far caudal as possible. The body of the uterus is brought up to the incision and a 12 cm incision made. An assistant should hold either side of the uterus up to the abdominal incision with two pairs of uterine forceps. All the piglets and their afterbirths are removed: very careful examination is required to make sure that *all* the piglets are removed.

The uterus is sutured with a single continuous row of Lembert sutures made with absorbable suture material, and some antibiotics placed along the suture line and into the abdomen; 30 IU oxytocin is given im. The abdominal musculature is sutured, including the peritoneum, with two rows of continuous mattress sutures made with absorbable suture material. The skin is sutured with single horizontal mattress sutures; No.1 polypropylene material on a swaged 48 mm ½ inch reverse cutting needle is very suitable for this purpose. The skin sutures need to be very close together as the piglets may try to interfere with them. The piglets should be encouraged to suckle. Antibiotics and NSAIDs should be given for a minimum of 5 days.

Problems after parturition

METRITIS   This is a common sequel to parturition and will lead to the farrowing fever syndrome described above. It may also occur after mating. The treatment is antibiotics and sexual rest.

PROLAPSED UTERUS   This is a very serious problem (see Plate 16). Practitioners must be aware of welfare issues as recovery rates are not good particularly if the prolapse is older than 3 h. Euthanasia should be carried out if hopes of recovery are poor. In commercial pigs, euthanasia is the best economic option.

In the case of pet pigs, the treatment should be as follows. The sow is given a GA and hoisted into a farrowing crate. Her hocks are tied to either side of the top of the crate. A conventional straw bale is positioned under her hind quarters so that her head and forequarters are low down at the front of the crate. The prolapsed uterus is placed on a clean polythene sack on the straw bale and checked for any damage. It is then sutured with horizontal mattress sutures of absorbable material, making sure that the peritoneal surfaces are opposed. The vulva is lubricated and one hand pushed gently into the tip of one uterine horn, which is slowly replaced into the sow. When the tip is well over the pelvic brim, a flicking motion, together with gravity, will make the uterine horn descend into the correct position. The process is repeated with the second horn and the body of the uterus. The vulva is closed with a 'Buhner' suture and 30 IU oxytocin given im. Antibiotics and NSAIDs are also given.

Surgical conditions of males

Castration

Always check for the presence of an inguinal hernia. These are particularly common in pot-bellied pigs.

NORMAL CASTRATION IN PIGLETS UNDER 2 MONTHS OF AGE   The pig is held by the hocks with its belly facing an assistant, who grips the chest of the pig between his or her knees. The scrotum is cleaned. A testicle is squeezed into the scrotum and a bold incision is made through the skin and the tunics so the testicle pops out. The testicle is pulled quickly out. The process is repeated for the other testicle and the area is sprayed with antibiotic spray.

CASTRATION IN PIGLETS UNDER 2 MONTHS OF AGE WITH AN INGUINAL HERNIA   The pig is held by the hocks with its belly facing an assistant, who grips the chest of the pig between his or her knees. The scrotum is cleaned. A testicle is squeezed into the scrotum and a careful incision is made through the skin but not through the tunics. Using blunt dissection the testicle is brought through the incision with its tunics intact and any abdominal contents are milked back into the abdomen. A pair of artery forceps is placed across the cord. A transfixing ligature of absorbable material is placed proximal to the testicle. The testicle is removed distal to the pair of artery forceps. A single horizontal mattress suture is placed in the skin. The process is repeated for the second testicle and the area is sprayed with antibiotic spray.

CASTRATION OF LARGER BOARS   This will require a GA. However the surgery is the same. There is no need to use any emasculators.

Surgical Conditions of the Locomotory System

Acute lameness

This can be caused by the following conditions.

Arthrogryposis

Welfare is paramount and so euthanasia is normally the correct course of action for this congenital condition.

Fractures

If these are low down in pet pigs, casting can be attempted but, in general, euthanasia is indicated.

Infectious mycoplasma lameness

This is caused by *Mycoplasma hyorhinitis* and *M. hyosynoviae*. It should be treated with tylosin by injection and followed by water medication.

Osteochondrosis

Osteochondrosis is a result of changes in the joint cartilage with age and should be treated with NSAIDs.

Slipped epiphysis of the femoral head

This is mainly seen in young boars. The aetiology is unknown but it may be the result of osteochondritis (damage to the cartilage experienced by the young pig). Euthanasia is recommended.

Splay leg

This is a condition of newborn piglets of unknown aetiology. If they can manage to reach a teat they will usually survive. If not, euthanasia is indicated.

Chronic lameness

This can be caused by the following conditions.

Chronic septic arthritis

Treatment is with antibiotics and NSAIDs.

Hoof abscess

Drainage should be established if possible. If not possible, then a poultice should be applied. The animal should be treated with antibiotics and NSAIDs.

Ligament damage

Treatment with NSAIDs can be tried, but if there is no response euthanasia is indicated.

Recumbency

This can be caused by the following conditions:

- A space occupying lesion in the vertebral canal, e.g. an abscess, a haematoma or a tumour. Treatment with antibiotics and NSAIDs can be tried but, if unsuccessful, euthanasia is indicated.
- Fractured vertebrae. Euthanasia is indicated.
- Trauma to the back or pelvis at mating or from fighting. NSAIDs can be tried but if not successful euthanasia is indicated.

Surgical Conditions of the Integument

Abscesses

These are a sequel to:

- bites
- burns
- cuts
- haematomas

Often, the original cause is not apparent and the abscesses may even be a sequel to haematogenous spread of bacteria to a damaged area. Treatment is first to clean the area, then to carry out a paracentesis with a 14 G needle to confirm diagnosis (but do not lance a haematoma, granuloma or a tumour). A bold incision is made large enough to allow digital palpation of the inside of the abscess after washing out any diseased contents with warm saline. Antibiotics are injected. In pigs near to slaughter weights, selection of antibiotics should be taken with care with consideration of meat withhold times.

Bites

These are caused by:

- biting of nipples by piglets
- fighting between boars (wounds will be deep and occur on the body)
- fighting between piglets (wounds occur on the face and become infected)
- fighting between sows (wounds often occur on the vulva)
- over-aggressive sexual foreplay by boars

Treatment is to inject antibiotics and NSAIDs and continue with water medication.

Topical antibiotic sprays should be applied but no sutures made.

Burns

These are caused by:

- direct burns (if heat lamps are too close)
- fires (heat lamps should always be secured with chain, not with baler twine)
- sunburn (pigs should always be supplied with shade and wallows)

The treatment is to inject antibiotics and NSAIDs and continue with water medication. Topical oily antibiotic creams should be applied. If the burns are too extensive, euthanasia should be considered.

Cuts

These are caused by:

- boar's tusks
- glass
- sharp metal

The treatment is to inject antibiotics and NSAIDs and continue with water medication. Topical antibiotic sprays should be applied. There should be no suturing unless the cuts are very large as pigs heal very well by second intention. If suturing is to be attempted, then a GA is recommended.

Haematomas

These normally occur in the ears of lop-eared breeds as a result of continuous shaking of the head caused by mange mites.

The underlying cause should be treated, i.e. treat the mange with injectable ivermectins. Antibiotics and NSAIDs should also be injected and water medication continued. Ear cleansers prepared for dogs should be applied. Draining the haematoma is not recommended as the haemorrhage will be profuse. Full aseptic surgery under GA could be attempted but is not recommended as healing will occur in time without surgery, leaving a not painful but 'cauliflower' ear.

Euthanasia

Euthanasia of piglets up to 10 kg

Euthanasia by trauma in baby pigs may be acceptable in a commercial situation but is not acceptable for pet pigs. Pet pigs up to 10 kg are best held on a sitting person's thighs with the head away from the handler. The handler holds the front legs firmly. The veterinary surgeon then stretches out the neck by pressure with one hand on the lower jaw and injects 5 ml 20% pentobarbitone sodium into the anterior vena cava just cranial to the thoracic inlet. The 3 cm 21 G needle that is used is directed slightly medially and caudally. This method is used because the ear vein is very difficult to inject in small piglets. A captive bolt may also be used at the point where the two lines from the ear to the opposite eye bisect on the head.

Euthanasia of larger pigs and adults using a gun

Larger and adult pigs should be shot by a licensed veterinary surgeon or slaughterman using a 0.32 humane killer at the point where the two lines from the ear to the opposite eye bisect on the head. If a veterinary surgeon does not possess a firearms licence it is permitted to use a 12 bore shotgun, with permission of the licensed owner, from 10–50 cm away and into the same spot as described above for piglets.

Chemical euthanasia

This creates a real problem. The ear vein is extremely difficult to inject in pot-bellied or kune kune pigs of any age although it can be managed in lop-eared adults of other breeds. The easiest protocol for adults is to give a GA im as described earlier, followed by an injection of 50 ml solution containing 400 mg/ml quinalbarbitone and 25 mg/ml cinchocaine hydrochloride, or 180 ml 20% pentobarbitone sodium into the heart with a 10 cm spinal needle. Growing pigs can be given less on a pro rata basis.

11

Domestic Poultry Medicine and Surgery

Introduction

This chapter starts with a discussion on animal husbandry of chickens, including a description of the healthy bird, its nutrition and nutritional deficiencies. Detailed information on the vaccines that are available for poultry in the UK is presented in a table, followed by brief comments on medication in general. Medical problems occurring in poultry are then described on a system by system basis, with sections on diseases of the gastroenteric system, the neurological system, the respiratory system, the circulatory system, the urinary system, the locomotory system and the integument. Two further sections follow on miscellaneous systemic diseases and notifiable diseases. The next two sections briefly describe analgesia, sedation and anaesthesia, before short accounts are given of various surgical conditions and procedures. The chapter concludes with advice on euthanasia. The focus throughout is predominantly on the UK.

Animal Husbandry of Chickens

Healthy chickens

They are lively, bright curious animals. Chicken are set apart from other birds by their combs and wattles. These are bright red and are secondary sex characteristics, which are usually larger in the male. Males develop spurs as a weapon for fighting which are occasionally prone to injury and it should be remembered that there is a large blood vessel in the spur so they should be filed, not cut.

The beak should be clean and dry. The legs should be smooth and covered with scales. The vent should be clean and surrounded by clean down feathers. The respiratory system is highly developed to enable gaseous exchange on both inspiration and expiration. Chickens have 13 air sacs for continuous gaseous exchange and short-term storage areas for each respiratory cycle. The respiratory rate should be 20–30 breaths/min but breathing should not be visible. Normal temperature is 40–42°C and heart rate is 250–300 beats/min. Life expectancy is 8–12 years.

Once food is ingested it is stored in the crop, a pouching out of the oesophagus by the thoracic inlet. From there, food is slowly taken into the proventriculus for chemical digestion. The next stage in the gastrointestinal (GI) tract is the strongly muscular gizzard which uses ingested insoluble grit to grind down seeds and grain. The food will reflux from the gizzard to the proventriculus several times before it continues into the duodenum. The ingesta then pass down the intestines for further digestion and absorption of nutrients.

Cellulose is broken down in the bilobed caecum by bacterial fermentation. Some 1 in 10 droppings will be much looser than the normal firm, black and white faeces; this is caecal voiding and completely normal. The whole process can take 3–25 h depending on how full the digestive tract is. The faeces are voided through the cloaca which is a common opening with the urinogenital tract.

Birds will start laying at about 20 weeks of age and depending on the breed will lay between 100 and 300 eggs a year. Birds lay in response to increasing day length so artificial light can be used – using sunset as the baseline and working back 6 min every day to give an optimum of 16 h a day. Chickens lay on a 25 h cycle, so will normally lay later and later every day until they miss a day and start again the next morning. Hens will usually return to the same place each day to lay again. This can be encouraged by using a clay egg that remains there, while any fresh eggs can be removed. It is important to remove eggs frequently because once a clutch has been laid it is very inviting for a hen to go broody and try to hatch them, regardless of whether there is a cockerel. Birds will stop laying once a year and moult. This takes 4 weeks as each feather and scale has to be replaced.

Birds should be handled frequently to check body condition and to look for ectoparasites. It is easiest to start off at night when birds are dozy. The bird should have both wings clamped to her body and her head tucked under the handler's arm. The legs can be held by one hand leaving the other free for examination. Never pick up a chicken by one leg as they can dislocate a hip very easily.

Wing clipping is necessary if hens need to be contained in a pen. They can be pinioned at 1 day old by sectioning the metacarpus and dipping the end into iodine. If this has not been done, the primary feathers on one wing can be cut. This has to be repeated after each moult.

Chicken have no external genitalia. The bottom of the cockerel's cloaca will form a groove of tissue to funnel the semen into the hen. The cockerel has two testes located near the kidneys, under the spine. He will ejaculate 0.5–1 ml of semen and this can be stored, viably, in the vagina for up to 14 days in chickens and 72 days in turkeys.

Once an egg has been laid it does not need to be incubated immediately; in fact it can cause problems if the eggs are too fresh, for they will hatch early. Equally, if they are too old then the chicks may have unhealed navels. Between 24 h and 10 days is about right for the age of egg before it is incubated. The broody hen will sit tight for 21 days, rarely venturing off to defaecate, eat and drink before scuttling back. It is possible to 'candle' lighter shelled eggs to see if they are growing a chick. This is done by shining a bright torch under one end of the egg after 7 days of incubation and looking for developing blood vessels. Incubation takes 21 days for chickens and 28 days for turkeys and guinea fowl.

A cockerel that is aggressive to humans will be made worse by fighting back. There is no treatment and they are best to be culled, particularly if children are at risk.

Nutrition

Nutrition for commercial poultry is very well researched and backyard poultry keepers would be well advised to feed specially prepared feed which will contain the correct nutrients and vitamins. If whole corn is being fed, keepers must realize that the diet will not be optimum, nor will any medication, e.g. coccidiostats be adequate. Household vegetables may be fed but no meat products.

Nutrient deficiencies

CALCIUM AND PHOSPHORUS   Chickens with calcium/phosphorus deficiency will show poor bone development and poor eggshell quality even if there are adequate levels of vitamin D. This deficiency is the cause of 'cage layer fatigue'. Pinpointing the difference between calcium/phosphorus deficiency and vitamin D deficiency is extremely difficult as both will result in rickets.

IODINE   Mature layers will become obese as a result of iodine deficiency and birds will show an enlarged thyroid gland.

IRON AND COPPER   Deficiencies of iron and copper are linked and cause marked anaemia. Turkeys will be found dead with aortic rupture.

MAGNESIUM   Magnesium deficiency is extremely rare but deficient baby chicks will be seen to pant.

MANGANESE   Deficiency of manganese in growing birds will cause perosis, and on maturity the birds will lay thin-shelled eggs. The deficiency is linked to that of calcium and phosphorus and will give similar signs to rickets.

SELENIUM   Selenium deficiency is seen as exudative diathesis in growing birds. It is linked with vitamin E deficiency.

SODIUM CHLORIDE   Deficiency of sodium chloride is seen as a deficiency of chloride which causes generalized muscle weakness and ataxia. Cannibalism will be noted in adult birds.

VITAMIN A   Vitamin A deficiency is very unlikely as birds would have to be on a deficient diet for a minimum of 2 months before egg laying ceases and emaciation is seen. White pustules will be seen in the mouth and there are secondary infections. Chicks, from eggs laid by mothers low in vitamin A will show signs of weakness, etc. after a week of life. Vitamin supplements for oral administration are available.

VITAMIN B
- Biotin deficiency results in dermatitis of the feet with perosis, and will cause a fatty liver and kidney syndrome.
- Choline deficiency is seen as perosis followed by twisted legs in growing birds.
- Folic acid deficiency is seen as poor growth and feathering, and anaemia in growing birds.
- Niacin is synthesized by embryos so deficiency should not occur unless there is an absence of the niacin precursor tryptophan. Chicks will show very inflamed oral mucosa at 2 weeks of age and adults will show a drop in egg production.
- Pantothenic acid deficiency will be manifest in hens as a severe drop in egg

production and hatchability of eggs. The eggs will show cutaneous haemorrhages.
- Pyridoxine deficiency results in poor growth and dermatitis with anaemia, which is particularly shown in growing ducks.
- Riboflavin deficiency affects the peripheral nerves so that growing birds show a curled toe paralysis.
- Thiamine deficiency is seen in growing birds as a polyneuritis with head tremors.
- Vitamin B_{12} deficiency is seen in growing chickens, which will show poor feathering and neurological signs.

VITAMIN D   Signs of osteoporosis and poor egg shell quality will be seen within 2 weeks of a diet deficient in vitamin D being fed. Beaks and claws become soft. Vitamin supplements for oral administration are available.

VITAMIN E   The three main disorders seen in vitamin E deficiency are encephalomalacia, exudative diathesis and muscular dystrophy. The deficiency is linked with selenium deficiency and deficiency of sulfur-containing amino acids. Signs will occur after 4 weeks of a deficient diet and can be reversed by 300 IU vitamin E/bird oral administered. Waterfowl are particularly prone to cardiac muscular dystrophy which will be manifest as 'capture myopathy'.

VITAMIN K   Deficiency of vitamin K causes a haemorrhagic syndrome and will be seen in chicks from deficient hens. Treatment is the inclusion of menadione in the diet.

ZINC   Zinc deficiency is extremely rare and will be shown as shortened leg bones in growing birds.

Vaccination

Vaccination is widely carried out in commercial flocks, with the smallest pack size available often being for a thousand birds. It can be carried out in small flocks if required, but large quantities of vaccine have to be wasted. Vaccines available in the UK are listed in Table 11.1, but are rarely required for small flocks.

Table 11.1. Licensed vaccines available for poultry in the UK.

Disease	Type of poultry	Notes
Avian cholera	Layers, ducks and turkeys	2 doses by injection, 1st injection at 6 weeks in chickens and turkeys, with the 2nd 4 weeks later; in ducks 1st injection at 3 weeks with the 2nd 3 weeks later
Avian encephalomyelitis	Layers and breeders	1 dose in drinking water from 10 weeks of age but not nearer than 4 weeks to point of lay
Avian infectious laryngotracheitis	Layers	1 dose by eye drop from 4 weeks before laying
Avian influenza	Chickens, ducks and other avian species	2 doses by injection from 8 days of age with an interval of 6 weeks
Chicken infectious anaemia	Broiler breeders	1 dose by injection from 6 weeks of age to within 6 weeks of laying
Coccidiosis	Broilers	Not for use in layers, to be given by spray or in the drinking water
Coccidiosis (2)	Chickens	To be given by spray or in feed at 1 day old or in drinking water from 3 days
Colibacillosis	Broiler breeders	2 doses by injection from 6 weeks of age with an interval of 6 weeks
Erysipelas	Turkeys	2 doses by injection from 6 weeks of age with an interval of 4 weeks
Gumboro disease	Layers	2 doses required by spray or drinking water
Gumboro disease	Broilers	1 dose in drinking water
Infectious bronchitis	Broilers and layers	Spray, intra-nasal/ocular from 3 weeks
Marek's disease	Chickens	1 dose by injection
Mycoplasma gallisepticum	Chickens	1 dose by spray from 6 weeks of age
Newcastle disease	Broilers and layers	Oral or ocular for individuals
Newcastle disease, infectious bronchitis, egg drop syndrome and avian rhinotracheitis (combined vaccine)	Layers	Inject after 18 weeks
Ornithobacterium rhinotracheale	Broiler breeders	2 doses by injection from 6 weeks of age with an interval of 6 weeks
Salmonellosis (*Salmonella enteritidis*)	Layers	1st injection at 6 weeks, 2nd injection 10 weeks later
Swollen head syndrome	Broilers and layers	1 dose in drinking water. May be repeated in laying birds
Turkey rhinotracheitis	Turkey breeders	1 dose by injection from 28 weeks
Turkey rhinotracheitis	Turkeys and broilers	1 dose by intra-nasal spray or eye drop from day old

Medication

There are several oral antibiotics licensed for chickens in the UK (see Chapter 2). These can be used in ducks and turkeys under the cascade principle. There are no injectable products in the UK but injectable antibiotics licensed for other species can be used under the cascade principle. When using off-licence products, a minimum of 28 days withhold period for meat and 7 days for eggs must be observed.

Diseases of the Gastroenteric System

Predominant signs

- Decreased egg production
- Diarrhoea
- General unthriftiness
- Poor growth and feed conversion of young birds

Intestinal viral diseases found in the UK

Coronaviral enteritis

This is restricted to young turkeys. Outbreaks will show a high morbidity but generally a low mortality. There is usually a growth check and transitory diarrhoea. There is no vaccine available but oral antibiotics seem to help.

Duck viral enteritis

This virus is restricted to waterfowl and causes 'duck plague'. It is caused by *Anatid herpesvirus 1* and is spread by inhalation and ingestion. There is a high mortality with bloody diarrhoea. Adult males may have a prolapsed penis. A diagnosis can be made on clinical signs and virus isolation. There is no treatment available.

Duck viral hepatitis

This disease is restricted to ducks and caused by a picornavirus. It is actually seen as a neurological disease with a high mortality in birds up to 6 weeks of age. Petechiae will be seen on the swollen spleen, liver and lungs. A diagnosis can be made by virus isolation or serology. There is no treatment available.

Fowlpox

This disease of chickens and turkeys is caused by an *Avipoxvirus* and occurs worldwide. There are also other poxviruses that occur in waterfowl. The common form shows as crusty lesions on the comb and in the mouth. There is a more acute form that affects the birds systemically and causes deaths. There is a vaccine available but it is not licensed in the UK.

Goose viral hepatitis

This disease is restricted to geese and Muscovy ducks. It is called 'goose plaque' or Derzy's disease and is caused by a *Parvovirus*. There is a very high mortality in young birds which show an ocular and nasal discharge and have a fibrinous membrane in the oral cavity. Diagnosis is by a PCR test. There is no treatment available.

Haemorrhagic nephritis enteritis of geese

This condition is restricted to geese and is caused by a *Polyomavirus*. There is a high mortality in 4–10 week old goslings which will often show neurological signs. They have enlarged kidneys on post-mortem (PM). The diagnosis is confirmed by a PCR test. There is no treatment available.

Newcastle disease

See below under 'Notifiable Diseases in the UK'.

Rotavirus

Rotavirus causes diarrhoea in young birds, with adults acting as carriers but not showing any disease signs. There is a high morbidity and a high mortality in game birds but a lower mortality in chickens and turkeys. Electron microscopy of faeces or intestinal contents, which tend to be frothy, will give a diagnosis. There is no vaccine available but good hygiene and broad-spectrum antibiotics will lower mortality.

Intestinal bacterial diseases found in the UK

Avian cholera

This disease is found in all species of poultry and is caused by *Pasteurella multocida*. The birds will show respiratory signs as well as enteric signs. There is a vaccine available for chickens but it is of doubtful efficiency in waterfowl. Treatment is with oxytetracyclines.

Campylobacter jejuni

The main importance of the disease caused by *C. jejuni* is its zoonotic implications, which are serious. There is rarely clinical disease in chicks, poults or ducklings but they pick up the disease in the litter and carry the organism. With a large exposure, young poultry species will die with acute haemorrhagic enteritis. Diagnosis is on culture and PM findings of enteritis and hepatic necrosis. Erythromycin is the antibiotic of choice.

Escherichia coli

This is the causative organism of colibacillosis, and will attack young chicks or ducklings, particularly if they are overcrowded or if the conditions are dirty. It is the normal organism isolated from hens suffering from egg peritonitis (see below under 'Miscellaneous Systemic Diseases'). Diarrhoea and lethargy will be seen, with a relatively high mortality. Treatment with antibiotics in the water may have to be changed depending on culture and sensitivity. There is a vaccine available.

Necrotic enteritis

This is an enterotoxaemia of young growing broilers and turkeys caused by *Clostridium (Cl.) perfringens*. It is found in the intestines of normal chickens as well as in the soil, and a trigger is required to spark off an outbreak. Affected animals will be depressed and have diarrhoea. Diagnosis can be confirmed by stained intestinal content smears. There is no vaccine available but treatment is normally successful using lincomycin in the water.

Salmonellosis

SALMONELLA ENTERITIDIS AND S. TYPHIMURIUM These organisms are very important in poultry as they are zoonotic, but rarely cause disease except in very young birds. Infection is likely from dirty eggs or vermin. Eggs should be washed in a Virkon disinfectant solution which is warmer than the eggs. Birds should be fed away from wild birds. There is a vaccine available against *S. enteritidis*.

SALMONELLA GALLINARUM This is specific to birds and causes the disease of fowl typhoid in all types of poultry. Signs are yellow diarrhoea and pale combs. The disease is seen in growers and layers but is now rare.

SALMONELLA PULLORUM This organism is specific to birds and causes the disease of bacillary white diarrhoea (BWD). It is now rare as carriers have been culled after showing positive to a compulsory blood test in the UK. It is spread in hatcheries and rearing units and so may be seen in backyard flocks.

Yersinia pseudotuberculosis

This organism is found in all species of poultry but most often in waterfowl. The disease caused is called pseudotuberculosis. There is no treatment available.

Intestinal protozoal diseases found in the UK

Coccidiosis

This is the most important enteric disease of poultry in the UK, and probably worldwide. Some of the most important causative species are *Eimeria acervulina*, *E. brunetti*, *E. maxima*, *E. mitis*, *E. necatrix*, *E. praecox* and *E. tenella*; these are the species contained in the chicken vaccine listed in Table 11.1 under Coccidiosis (2). There is also a broiler vaccine available. Most commercial food contains coccidiostats. The most common age for signs of enteritis – wet droppings or bloody droppings – is from 4 weeks old. All species of poultry are affected, with a prepatent period of less than 7 days. Diagnosis can be confirmed by oocyst counts on faeces samples. Treatment can be carried out with toltrazuril or amprolium in the drinking water. Sulfadimethoxine in the drinking water will provide effective treatment but it is only licensed in the UK for use in racing pigeons. See also 'Diseases of the Urinary System', '*Eimeria truncata*'.

Cryptosporidium *spp.*

This is mainly a disease of quail but may be rarely seen in turkeys. It is extremely rare in chickens. Diagnosis by finding the small oocysts in the intestines is difficult. There are no control measures available. Avian species of *Cryptosporidium* spp. are not zoonotic.

Hexamita

This is an opportunistic motile protozoan which can occur at times of stress and overcrowding, and causes listlessness and diarrhoea. Diagnosis is by seeing the motile protozoa in the gut contents of a fresh corpse (within 30 min of death). Treatment is nonspecific with oxytetracyclines.

Histomoniasis

After coccidiosis, this is the most important disease in turkeys, guinea fowl and peafowl in the UK. It is caused by *Histomonas meleagridis* and is commonly called 'blackhead'. Animals have yellow malodorous droppings or are found dead. Multiple necrotic circular lesions on the liver are pathognomic. There is no preventive or treatment available in the UK as dimetridazole is banned. As the life cycle involves earthworms and the caecal worm *Heterakis gallinarum* (see below under 'Intestinal nematode diseases found in the UK'), these should be controlled.

Trichomonas

In cases of infection by *Trichomonas*, a cheesy substance will be seen in the mouth and throat. The disease is called 'oral canker'. Treatment is with metronidizole.

Intestinal nematode diseases found in the UK

Amidostomum anseris (goose gizzard worm)

This is the most important intestinal worm in geese. It causes erosions which can result in death.

Ascaridia galli (roundworm)

This is the largest worm found in poultry and can be up to 12 cm long. It has a direct life cycle, with adults living in the small intestine. Larvae may do considerable damage to the mucosa. Adult worms may cause a total intestinal blockage resulting in death.

Capillaria *spp.*

Several species of *Capillaria* worms affect poultry. *C. anatis* is found in the caecum of ducks; the intermediate host unknown. *C. annulata* is found in the crop and oesophagus of turkeys; earthworms are the intermediate hosts. *C. bursata* is found in the small intestine of chickens; earthworms are the intermediate hosts. *C. caudinflata* is found in the small intestine of poultry generally; earthworms are the intermediate hosts. *C. contorta* is found in the crop and oesophagus of turkeys; earthworms are the intermediate hosts. *C. obsignata* is found in the small intestine in poultry generally; there is no intermediate host.

Echinuria uncinata

This worm is found in the proventriculus of waterfowl. It may cause ulceration and death.

Heterakis gallinarum (caecal worm)

This important worm is found in the caecum of turkeys, guinea fowl, peafowl and chickens. Earthworms are the intermediate host. It is 1–2 cm long and rarely causes clinical disease. The importance of *H. gallinarum* is that it carries the protozoan *Histomonas meleagridis*, which causes the fatal condition of 'blackhead' (see above under 'Intestinal protozoal diseases found in the UK', 'Histomoniasis').

Trichostrongylus tenuis (grouse worm)

This worm is found in the caecum of goslings and wild birds.

Treatment of intestinal nematodes with licenced products in the UK

- Medicated premixture containing 10 mg/g flubendazole for addition to a complete ration daily for 7 days. Dosages vary with type of poultry being treated. Will treat all poultry and game birds.

- Oral emulsion containing 100 mg/g flubendazole for addition to the water daily for 7 days. Can be used in laying hens and has a nil egg withdrawal, although a 4 day meat withdrawal.

Miscellaneous diseases of the enteric tract

Crop impaction

This is a common and potentially life-threatening condition which can be caused by gorging or, more often, by an impaction further down the enteric tract, e.g. gizzard impaction (see below). Treatment is traditionally carried out by gently massaging the crop but in the author's experience this can be very hazardous as the bird can inhale the vomit and die. A safer option is to carry out surgical emptying (see below under 'Surgical Conditions and Procedures').

Crossed beak

This likely to be an inherited condition and therefore euthanasia is indicated.

'Dropped tongue'

This occurs in Toulouse geese when the tongue gets trapped in the sagging fleshy part of the mandible and allows food, particularly grass in balls, to accumulate thus causing a local infection and a reduced appetite. These grass balls are easily removed using the fingers, but tend to recur as the muscles have been stretched. This can easily be cured by stitching the floor of the mouth together.

Gizzard impaction

This results from a shortage of insoluble grit or from gorging on long lush grass. It is rarely diagnosed but often suspected. There is no treatment and euthanasia should be carried out.

Pendulous crop

This will occur in single birds. They will not necessarily be ill but will have a pendulous crop. No action should be taken as they can live pain free for many months although the condition will deteriorate.

Peritonitis

This is a separate disease from egg peritonitis and is caused by sharp foreign bodies that have been swallowed and penetrate the gizzard. The condition is particularly common in waterfowl. In theory, a metal foreign body could be diagnosed in a pet bird by radiography and surgery could be undertaken. The likely course of events though is euthanasia after antibiotic therapy has been unsuccessful.

Sour crop

This is an infection with the yeast *Candida albicans* and can follow prolonged oral antibiotic therapy. There is a pungent sour odour. Treatment is with oral ketoconazole.

Starve out

This condition seen in young chicks in the first few days of life is very common in pheasants and partridges. Conditions of the incubator should be checked, i.e. that there are good lights, good temperature control, round pens, good drinkers, no wet spots and chick crumbs fed in multiple flat places. *E. coli* may be isolated. Normally antibiotics are not required, but oral vitamin supplements may be helpful.

Sudden death syndrome of broiler chickens

The cause of this disease is unknown but it is thought to be related to poor carbohydrates in the food. It is seen worldwide and the deaths are so acute that it is called the 'flip-over disease'.

Vent pecking

Birds are attracted to red colouring, so this tends to occur when birds are overcrowded, particularly in hot humid conditions. Birds may die and it is vital that any bird which is the victim of such attacks is isolated. Affected birds should be sprayed with oxytetracycline spray and, if badly pecked, be given an injection of long-acting oxytetracycline. Birds should not be returned to the same environment until fully healed. Debeaking of birds is no longer acceptable from a welfare stance.

Diseases of the Neurological System

Blue-green algal poisoning

Chickens, and particularly waterfowl, are both affected by blue-green algae and will show neurological signs. Drinkers and ponds should be kept clean as there is no antidote.

Botulism

This is caused by the ingestion of the toxin from the bacterium *Cl. botulinum*, which proliferates in carcasses; in hot weather this proliferation can be very rapid. Birds, and particularly waterfowl, will be found dead or suffering from flaccid paralysis. The normal route of infection seems to be the consumption of infected maggots. There is no treatment.

Chemical poisoning

Arsenic

Poisoning by arsenic is now rare as it is no longer used in pig food nor in rat bait. If such poisoning does occur, arsenic will cause neurological signs.

Copper

Copper fungicides will cause convulsions and rapid death.

Herbicides

Paraquat is very toxic to waterfowl when sprayed around ornamental ponds. It causes vomiting and rapid death.

Insecticides

Most insecticides will kill birds rapidly but organophosphorus compounds will also have a cumulative effect. Birds will become dull and start twitching before death. There is no effective antidote.

Lead

Lead poisoning is a condition of waterfowl which have consumed lead shot from the lines left by fishermen, and also of other poultry grazing on ground used for clay pigeon shooting. Birds will be ataxic and lethargic, and have bright green droppings. Treatment is with calcium edentate (EDTA).

Mercury

This is a common type of poisoning as mercury is used as a seed dressing. Poisoning is cumulative and animals will become listless and then go off their legs. There is no effective antidote.

Molluscicides

This is another common type of poisoning as metaldehyde is used in slug bait and is attractive to birds. Neurological signs are severe and there is no antidote.

Newcastle disease

See below under 'Notifiable Diseases in the UK'.

Phosphides

Poisoning is rare nowadays as phosphides are no longer used in rat bait. If phosphide poisoning does occur, there will be neurological signs. There is no antidote.

Diseases of the Respiratory System

Aspergillosis

All types of birds are susceptible to infection by *Aspergillus* spp. Mouldy bedding gives off the spores of the fungus, which are inhaled and cause respiratory distress and sudden death. The pathognomic finding on PM is grey plaques on the lungs. Treatment for individual birds is nebulization with the disinfectant F10 at a concentration of 1:250.

Avian chlamydiosis

This is not a problem in domestic poultry, but is very important in parrots, in which it causes psittacosis, a dangerous zoonotic disease. The causal bacterial organism is *Chlamydophila psittaci* (formerly *Chlamydia psittaci*), which causes respiratory signs. Diagnosis is by a PCR test on a swab from the choanae or the cloaca. Special precautions need to be taken before submitting possible infected birds for PM. Doxycycline is the antibiotic of choice.

Avian infectious laryngotracheitis

This is caused by a herpesvirus and affects large table birds and turkeys. There is a marked nasal discharge, and the disease has a high morbidity but a low mortality. There is normally a secondary bacterial infection which will respond to antibiotics. A vaccine is available.

Avian influenza

See below under 'Notifiable Diseases in the UK', 'Avian influenza'.

Avian tuberculosis (TB)

Avian TB (causative bacterium *Mycobacterium avium*) is a condition common in outdoor poultry as it is spread by wild birds. It causes rapid emaciation. Euthanasia is advised. The caseous lesions will be seen internally.

Gape worms

Syngamus trachea is the chicken gape worm, and *Cyathostoma bronchialis* is the waterfowl gape worm. The worms are aptly named as the pathognomic sign is gaping. Anthelmintic treatment is straightforward and is the same as for intestinal worms (see above under 'Diseases of the Gastroenteric System', 'Intestinal nematode diseases found in the UK').

Infectious bronchitis

This is a condition of young chicks, pheasants, partridges and guinea fowl that is caused by a coronavirus. There is a high mortality. Adult birds are carriers, with the virus causing poor-quality eggshells throughout life. There is a vaccine available.

Infectious coryza

This is a relatively common mild respiratory disease in small flocks and is caused by *Avibacterium paragallinarum*. Treatment is with oral antibiotics in the drinking water.

Leeches

Theromyzon spp. leeches are restricted to waterfowl. They are visible to the naked eye and cause head shaking, sneezing and conjunctivitis. Treatment is with ivermectins but waterfowl are very sensitive to these so strict attention should be paid to dosage.

Mycoplasmosis

This is caused by the two bacterial species *Mycoplasma gallisepticum* and *M. synoviae* in chickens and turkeys. The disease is characterized by foamy eyes, swollen sinuses and breathing difficulties. It is very contagious and is spread by wild birds. *M. synoviae* also causes infectious arthritis. The drug of choice is tylvalosin. There is a vaccine available.

Newcastle disease

See below under 'Notifiable Diseases in the UK'.

Ornithobacterium rhinotracheale

O. rhinotracheale causes respiratory disease of all ages of chickens, but mainly in growing broilers which will show respiratory signs. Antibiotics are helpful for treatment. There is a vaccine available.

Pasteurellosis

Pasteurellosis is a different syndrome from avian cholera (see above under 'Diseases of the Gastroenteric System', 'Intestinal bacterial diseases found in the UK'). It occurs in young ducklings and is caused by *Pasteurella anatipestifer*. Clinical signs include respiratory distress, blood in the mouth and sudden death. Significant lung consolidation is seen at PM. Treatment is with amoxicillin or lincomycin. There is no vaccine.

Swollen head syndrome

This often called avian pneumovirus infection as the primary causative agent is an avian pneumovirus. It is an acute, infectious respiratory disease. There is a vaccine available.

Turkey rhinotracheitis

This disease is caused by a *Metapneumovirus*. It is an acute highly contagious disease, mainly of young birds. It will cause an egg-drop syndrome in breeding birds. Antibiotics are helpful to treat the secondaries. There are vaccines available.

Diseases of the Circulatory System

Chicken infectious anaemia

This disease is caused by *Chicken anemia virus*, a *Gyrovirus* which kills 2 week old chicks. Symptoms are pallor and haemorrhages of the mucous membranes. The disease is contracted from the laying breeders via the egg. There is no treatment, but there is a vaccine available.

Fatal haemorrhage in turkeys

There are three syndromes recognized in fast-growing turkeys found dead with internal haemorrhage. These are: aortic rupture, perirenal haemorrhage syndrome and spontaneous cardiomyopathy. The cause of these atherosclerotic conditions in fast-growing turkeys is thought to be from the high level of circulatory fat, which could be controlled by dietary management.

Heart attack

This occurs in heavy breeds and may be anticipated by the appearance of a purple comb. The affected birds bruise very easily and will die if stressed.

Sodium toxicity

An excess of salt in the diet will lead to lesions in the heart muscle and sudden death.

Vitamin K deficiency

This is caused by the ingestion of rat poison. Animals will be found dead with bruising and abdominal haemorrhage.

Diseases of the Urinary System

Eimeria truncata

This coccidian parasite infects the kidneys of goslings, after it has been picked up from the environment and passed through the intestine. It can cause renal failure and death, or kidney swelling and lameness. Treatment with coccidiostats is often too late so prevention is important as sporulated oocysts are resistant to environmental extremes and can be infective for months.

Nephritis

This condition is caused by an astrovirus and affects newly hatched chicks in their first week of life. Diagnosis requires virus isolation. The virus is mainly spread by egg transmission so hygiene is vital as there is no treatment or vaccine available.

Nephrosis

This is a confusing condition as the cause is not known. Birds will go off their legs and be found on PM to have swollen kidneys. Antibiotics and dexamethazone do not appear to cure the condition.

Vent gleet

The vent will be moist, yellow, inflamed and malodorous. The condition is caused by a herpesvirus. Treatment is futile and euthanasia is indicated. In waterfowl, the condition is caused by bacteria (*Pseudomonas* spp.) and treatment can be attempted with enrofloxacin.

Visceral gout

The cause of this condition is not fully understood. Renal dysfunction decreases the clearance of uric acid from the blood and this is deposited in the joints, causing intense pain and lameness. Euthanasia is indicated.

Diseases of the Locomotory System

Angel wing

This is a disease of fast-growing geese. The rapid growth of the wing primary feathers puts a strain on the carpal joint which makes

the wing tip and the primary feathers twist out (Fig. 11.1). If caught early enough, the wing can be taped to itself for a week and the condition will resolve. The ultimate cure is amputation.

Avian encephalomyelitis

This is a viral disease of chickens, quail, turkeys and pheasants and is called epidemic tremor. The disease affects 7–10 day old birds. Muscular tremors can be seen on handling. There is normally a 5% mortality and morbidity. The virus is spread from laying birds. There is no treatment, but there is a vaccine available.

'Bumblefoot'

This occurs in all species of poultry and is essentially a staphylococcal infection of the foot pads (see Plate 17). It is predisposed by bruising, so owners must ensure that perches are rounded rather than square, are not too high and do not have bare concrete below them. Treatment is by debridement and strong iodine daily.

Deformities

Most deformities are inherited and so breeding stock should be selected carefully. Certain

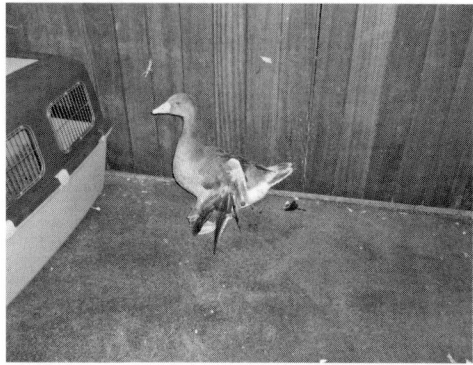

Fig. 11.1. Goose angel wing.

deformities, e.g. bent toes, do not cause a welfare problem but with most deformities euthanasia is indicated.

Fractures

Fractures of distal bones can be splinted, but if a joint is involved or the fracture is compound then euthanasia is indicated.

Marek's disease

This viral infection, which is caused by a herpesvirus, normally causes peripheral nerve paralysis and so the first sign may be lameness in growing birds. It can cause sudden death from lesions in the heart muscle and blood vessels. There is a vaccine available.

Rickets

This is caused by vitamin D deficiency or an imbalance of calcium and phosphorus in the diet. Birds will have poor growth and deformed legs.

Splay leg

This is seen in chickens and turkeys at birth and is likely to be a result of incorrect nutrition or incorrect incubation temperature. Given a good surface, many of these cases will correct themselves if the legs are tied like shackles with wool for 48 h.

Diseases of the Integument

Ectoparasites

Cnemidocoptes gallinae

This is the burrowing mite, which causes 'scaly leg', 'depluming itch' and 'scaly face or beak'. Treatment can be protracted but the best recommendation is daily dipping of

the legs into cypermethrin and weekly spraying of the bird with cypermethrin or fipronil. It should be remembered that the leg scales will only be replaced at the next moult.

Dermanyssus gallinae

This common blood sucking mite is termed the 'red mite', which lives in the cracks of wooden poultry houses and creeps out at night to suck blood from the birds. It causes anaemia, but deaths are rare as the mites retreat during the day. The birds should be sprayed with cypermethrin at night and the house should be sprayed during the day after the bedding has been removed and burnt.

Echidnophaga gallinacea

This is called the 'sticktight poultry flea' and is found in the subtropical and tropical parts of America. It causes anaemia and death. Control is with topical synthetic pyrethrums.

Holomenopon *spp.*

These are feather shaft lice which infest waterfowl and cause the 'wet feather syndrome'. The constant irritation leads to over-preening and loss of waterproofing. Treatment is with cypermethrin weekly for 3 weeks.

Menopon gallinae

This is the common fowl louse, which is about 2 mm long, flat and pale yellow in colour. The lice will move very quickly out of the light when the feathers are parted. They feed off skin debris, so are not life threatening to the bird but can be irritating. Infestations are controlled by louse powder.

Ornithonyssus sylvarum

This is the called the northern mite and is very similar to the red mite except that it spends its entire life on the bird and so anaemia and death are more common. The birds should be sprayed with cypermethrin or fipronil every 3 weeks.

Miscellaneous skin diseases

Breast blisters

These are caused by poor feathering, hard flooring and leg weakness. Antibiotics are helpful.

Feather pecking

This is a vice and results from stress, usually from overcrowding or competition for food and water.

Flank wounds

These are normally caused by the mounting of the male. There are back protectors available for turkeys.

Miscellaneous Systemic Diseases

Egg drop syndrome

The condition is caused by an adenovirus that is found in waterfowl and wild birds. It is characterized by the production of soft-shelled and shell-less eggs in apparently healthy birds. There is no treatment but there is a vaccine available.

Egg eating

This is not a disease but a vice and is often due to an inappropriate nesting box, or to eggs being laid in the wrong place. Once started, it is difficult to stop but several remedies are suggested:

1. Fill a 'blown egg' with strong mustard or curry powder in the hope of deterring the thief.
2. Scatter golfballs in the chicken house.
3. Collect the eggs several times a day.
4. Make the laying compartment dark.
5. If none of these remedies are successful, any bird caught egg eating must be culled.

Egg peritonitis

This is an infection with *E. coli*, either from an egg which does not drop into the oviduct or from an ascending infection from the vent. The condition is seen in ducks as well as hens. It mainly occurs in older birds, often in the spring or following a period of stress. Realistically it is untreatable, but morbidity can be reduced by oral antibiotics. Peritoneal flushing has been suggested for individual pet birds but this is outside the author's experience.

Erysipelas

Infection by *Erysipelothrix rhusiopathiae* has several manifestations in poultry. It mainly causes systemic illness in growing turkeys. Survivors may get endocarditis and then die suddenly. Treatment is with amoxicillin. There is a vaccine available.

Gumboro disease

This should be called 'infectious bursal disease' and is caused by an *Avibirnavirus* (*Infectious bursal disease virus*). The virus, which is spread in the faeces, is readily isolated from the bursa of Fabricius. Chickens show incoordination, watery diarrhoea and inflammation of the cloaca. There are vaccines available.

Haemorrhagic enteritis

This condition is caused by an adenovirus and is also called 'marble spleen disease'. It normally affects 6–12 week old chickens, which will be pale and have bloody droppings. Diagnosis is based on clinical and PM signs and can be confirmed by PCR. Antibiotics are helpful. There is a vaccine available for turkeys in Europe.

Notifiable Diseases in the UK

Avian influenza

This has been called 'Cathedral disease' owing to the silence in the turkey sheds when the workers went in in the morning. It was last seen in the UK in 2008. Clinical signs include; sudden egg drop, sudden death, respiratory distress, swelling around the head and diarrhoea. There is a vaccine available.

Newcastle disease

This viral disease, which is caused by a paramyxovirus, was last seen in the UK in 2006. It is seen in all species of poultry and can show respiratory, enteric and neurological signs. Diagnosis is by seeing haemorrhages in the proventriculus, or by virus isolation from lung and spleen, or serology. There is a vaccine available.

Further information on notifiable diseases in the UK is presented in Chapter 12.

Analgesia, Sedation and Anaesthesia

Analgesia

Buprenorphine can be used at 0.01–0.05 mg/kg im or ketoprofen at 5–10 mg/kg im.

Sedation

Ketamine can be used as a sedative either im or sub cut at a dose of 10 mg/kg for birds up to 1 kg, or 5 mg/kg for bigger birds.

Anaesthesia

Masking down using a mini Bain system and isoflurane is the method of choice. Ketamine can result in excessive wing flapping on recovery. Birds are extremely prone to hypothermia, so bubble wrap and heating devices should be used.

Surgical Conditions and Procedures

Cloacal prolapse

Birds will often be found dead with a prolapse, having been attacked by the others. The cause is likely to be stress, age or obesity. If the prolapse is fresh and undamaged it can be replaced and a purse string suture used to keep the prolapse in place. The bird should be given a deslorelin implant to stop her laying for a few weeks.

Crop evacuation

A small incision is made through the skin and into the crop after instilling 1 ml of local anaesthetic under the skin over the swollen crop. All the contents are removed with forceps. The crop is sutured with a single inverting horizontal mattress suture of catgut. The skin is sutured with a single everting horizontal mattress suture of monofilament nylon.

Egg-bound birds

Birds will look constipated, dull and depressed. Occasionally they will display tail pumping. Diagnosis can be confirmed with a radiograph. The egg binding is normally due to a calcium imbalance so the rest of the flock should be given ad lib oyster shell grit. The affected bird should be given 0.1 ml (1 IU) oxytocin in 0.5 ml of saline im together with calcium hypophosphite 4.84% w/v at 1 ml/kg im. The bird should be kept warm and its vent should be lubricated with warm obstetrical lubricant.

Orchidectomy

The main indication for this procedure in domestic poultry is male birds which are overly aggressive to other males. Birds which are aggressive to humans will not be affected by orchidectomy. The surgery and the anaesthesia are difficult and are outside the author's experience.

Penile prolapse

This is primarily a condition of waterfowl, and provided the prolapse is not long-standing it can be returned to its normal position with oily creams and secured with a temporary stitch, which should be removed in 48 h. If the prolapsed organ is damaged then euthanasia is indicated. The condition may be linked to duck viral enteritis (see above under 'Diseases of the Gastroenteric System', 'Intestinal viral diseases found in the UK'.

Salpingohysterectomy

The indications for this extremely difficult surgery are diverse. Clinicians should question the welfare implications. The surgical procedure is outside the author's experience.

Euthanasia

Neck dislocation

This is only suitable for an on-farm situation. It can be easily accomplished in chickens and smaller birds with two fingers around the neck and a sharp forwards pull. In large birds, e.g. geese, rest the bird on its chest on the ground and lay a broom stick on its neck. Tread on the broom stick and pull sharply up with the bird's legs.

Chemical euthanasia

There are various methods using triple-strength barbiturate injection:

1. Inject up under the breast bone with a 4 cm 19 G needle straight into the bird's liver. Death will be instantaneous.
2. Inject into the wing vein with a 1 cm 23 G needle while a competent handler holds the bird with the wing outstretched.
3. Inject into the breast muscles. Death will be slow but peaceful.

12

Notifiable Diseases

Introduction

The World Organisation for Animal Health, or OIE (formerly Office International des Epizooties), monitors specific epizootic diseases agreed by the member governments. Each member government has its own particular list of diseases. In the UK, the list is compiled by Defra (Department for Environment, Food and Rural Affairs). Certain diseases occur in several species and others are only found in single species. Both Defra and OIE lists are included below. All the lists include information on the species affected by the disease concerned, disease type (endemic, exotic or zoonotic and level of rarity). Note that Chapter 13 presents further information on zoonotic diseases.

Diseases Monitored in the UK

The main diseases monitored in the UK

Table 12.1 shows the main diseases of concern in farm livestock in the UK. These seven diseases are of real concern, not only to farmers, but also to the population as a whole, because a considerable amount of taxpayers' money is spent on their control.

Five of these diseases are considered to be exotic: avian influenza, bluetongue disease, foot-and-mouth disease (FMD), Newcastle disease and rabies. It is to be hoped that these do not return to the UK.

The two other diseases listed in Table 12.1 are bovine spongiform encephalopathy (BSE) and tuberculosis (TB). BSE has largely been controlled and it is hoped that it will no longer be considered endemic in the near future. However, the expensive extra safeguards that are in place at abattoirs are likely to remain so in the foreseeable future. At the time of writing, TB is still on the increase. Until a clear-cut programme for its control in cattle and badgers is agreed by all parties concerned, this unhappy state of affairs is likely to remain. It should be noted that Scotland is free of the disease. The increase in TB in South American camelids (SACs) is very alarming, especially as an owner has contracted the disease from her stock. Hope for the control of TB in SACs in the near future is unlikely as the skin test is not reliable in this species.

The above diseases are also described and discussed in earlier chapters of the book, where they can be found under the medicine of specific species (Chapters 3, 5, 7, 9 and 11).

©G.R. Duncanson 2013. *Farm Animal Medicine and Surgery: For Small Animal Veterinarians* (G.R. Duncanson)

Table 12.1. The seven main notifiable diseases of farm livestock in the UK.

Disease	Species affected	Disease type	Last occurred in UK
Avian influenza	Poultry	Exotic, zoonotic	2008
Bovine spongiform encephalopathy	Cattle	Zoonotic	Present
Bluetongue disease	Ruminants,[a] SACs[b]	Exotic	2008
Foot-and-mouth disease	Ruminants, SACs, pigs	Exotic	2007
Newcastle disease	Poultry	Exotic	2006
Rabies	Ruminants, SACs, pigs	Exotic, zoonotic	1970
Tuberculosis	Cattle, goats, SACs	Endemic, zoonotic	Present

[a]Cetruminantia.
[b]South American camelids.

Further diseases monitored in the UK

Table 12.2 shows a further 21 diseases that are monitored by Defra in the UK. These are of concern for the clinician who is carrying out farm animal practice not only in the UK, but also in Europe and North America. Brief comments on each disease are included below; the diseases are also discussed under the medicine of specific species (Chapters 3, 5, 7, 9 and 11).

African swine fever (ASF)

This viral disease, which occurs solely in pigs, was first recognized in Kenya in 1921 by R.E. Montgomery. He recognized the disease as an acute haemorrhagic fever infecting domestic pigs of European origin. The disease has never occurred in the UK but clinicians should always be vigilant as it occurs in Russia, Armenia and Sardinia, and throughout Africa south of the Sahara.

Aujeszky's disease

This viral disease was endemic in pig populations almost worldwide. It is also found in rodents, which spread the disease. It has very rarely been reported in cattle, sheep and humans. The disease has been eradicated from the UK, most of Europe and most of North America. It has never been seen in northern Africa or Australia.

Brucella abortus

This disease caused by this bacterium was originally called Bang's disease. It is an unpleasant zoonotic disease which has been eradicated from the UK and most of Europe and North America. Other areas have active eradication programmes based on vaccination and testing.

Brucella melitensis

The often fatal zoonotic disease caused by this bacterium was originally called Malta fever. It was first recorded in the Mediterranean area. It has never been recorded in the UK.

Brucella ovis

The rare disease of sheep caused by this bacterium has never been recorded in the UK.

Classical swine fever (CSF)

This is caused by a virus that solely affects pigs and is a totally separate disease from ASF. It is also called hog cholera. It has been eradicated from the UK and large areas of Europe and North America, by the use of vaccination in the 1960's. It still occurs in other areas of the world and has the ability to cause serious pandemics and so clinicians must be constantly vigilant and aware of the danger of the disease which could be spread by pig products.

Contagious agalactia

This rare disease caused by a mycoplasma has never been recorded in the UK.

Contagious bovine pleuropneumonia

This disease, which is caused by a mycoplasma, is now rare in the world and has not been recorded in the UK for over 100 years.

Table 12.2. Further notifiable diseases of farm livestock in the UK.

Disease	Species affected	Disease type	Last occurred in UK
African swine fever	Pigs	Exotic	Never
Anthrax	Ruminants,[a] SACs,[b] pigs	Zoonotic	2006
Aujeszky's disease	Pigs	Exotic	1989
Brucella abortus	Cattle	Exotic, zoonotic	2004
B. melitensis	Sheep, goats, SACs	Exotic, zoonotic	Never
B. ovis	Sheep, goats[c]	Exotic	Never
Classical swine fever	Pigs	Exotic	2000
Contagious agalactia	Sheep,[d] goats	Exotic	Never
Contagious bovine pleuropneumonia	Cattle	Exotic	1898
Enzootic bovine leucosis	Cattle	Exotic	1996
Goat pox	Goats	Exotic	Never
Lumpy skin disease	Cattle	Exotic	Never
Peste des petits ruminants	Sheep, goats	Exotic	Never
Rift Valley fever	Cattle, sheep, goats	Exotic, zoonotic	Never
Rinderpest	Cattle	Exotic	1877
Scrapie	Sheep, goats	Endemic	Present
Sheep pox	Sheep	Exotic	1866
Swine vesicular disease	Pigs	Exotic	1982
Teschen disease	Pigs	Exotic	Never
Vesicular stomatitis	Cattle, pigs	Exotic	Never
Warble fly	Cattle	Exotic	1990

[a]Cetruminantia.
[b]South American camelids.
[c]*B. ovis* affects only sheep, but historically legislators thought that it might affect goats as well, so the infection was made notifiable for both species.
[d]Contagious agalactia affects only goats, but historically legislators thought that it might affect sheep as well, so the infection was made notifiable for both species.

Practitioners should have the disease at the very back of their minds as bovine respiratory disease is extremely common worldwide, and causing a panic by diagnosing this disease by mistake could have serious consequences.

Enzootic bovine leucosis

This viral disease of adult cattle has to be distinguished from the condition called sporadic lymphosarcoma which is found in young cattle and has no relationship with enzootic bovine leucosis. Enzootic bovine leucosis is controlled in North America but is still widespread. It has been eradicated from the UK.

Goat pox

This viral disease can occur in sheep when it is called sheep pox. It has no connection with contagious pustular dermatitis. It has never been recorded in the UK or the New World. It is still seen rarely in Asia, Africa and the Middle East.

Lumpy skin disease

This viral disease of cattle is very similar to goat pox and sheep pox but it has never been recorded outside Africa.

Peste des petits ruminants (PPR)

This viral disease of sheep and goats is related to rinderpest but does not occur in cattle. It is showing a resurgence in tropical Africa and still occurs rarely in Asia. It has never been recorded in the UK or the New World.

Rift Valley fever

This zoonotic viral disease, which was first isolated in Kenya, is largely restricted to tropical

Table 12.3. Further diseases affecting farm livestock being monitored by the World Organisation for Animal Health (OIE) worldwide.

Disease	Species affected	Disease type	Last occurred in UK
Avian chlamydiosis	Poultry	Exotic, zoonotic	Present
Avian infectious bronchitis	Poultry	Endemic	Present
Avian infectious laryngotracheitis	Poultry	Endemic	Present
Avian mycoplasmosis (caused by *Mycoplasma gallisepticum*)	Poultry	Endemic	Present
Avian mycoplasmosis (caused by *M. synoviae*)	Poultry	Endemic	Present
Bovine anaplasmosis	Cattle	Extremely rare	Present
Bovine babesiosis	Cattle	Endemic in certain areas	Present
Bovine genital campylobacteriosis	Cattle	Extremely rare	Present
Bovine viral diarrhoea	Cattle	Endemic	Present (area eradication schemes in action)
Contagious caprine pleuropneumonia	Goats	Exotic	Never
Crimean-Congo haemorrhagic fever	Sheep, goats	Exotic, zoonotic	Never
Duck viral hepatitis	Ducks	Rare	Present
Echinococcosis	Cattle, sheep, goats, SACs[a]	Endemic, zoonotic	Present
Enzootic abortion of ewes	Sheep, goats, SACs	Endemic, zoonotic	Present
Epizootic haemorrhagic disease	Cattle	Exotic	Never
Fowl cholera	Poultry	Sporadic	Present
Fowl typhoid	Poultry	Sporadic	Present
Haemorrhagic septicaemia	Cattle	Exotic	Never
Heartwater	Cattle	Exotic	Never
Infectious bovine rhinotracheitis/ infectious pustular vulvovaginitis	Cattle	Endemic	Present
Infectious bursal disease	Poultry	Rare	Present
Japanese encephalitis	Pigs	Exotic, zoonotic	Never
Leptospirosis	Cattle, sheep, goats, SACs, pigs	Endemic, zoonotic	Present
Maedi-Visna	Sheep, goats	Endemic	Present
Marek's disease	Poultry	Endemic	Present
Nairobi sheep disease	Sheep	Exotic	Never
New world screw worm	Cattle, sheep, goats, SACs, pigs	Exotic	Never
Nipah virus encephalitis	Pigs	Exotic, zoonotic	Never
Old world screw worm	Cattle, sheep, goats, SACs, pigs	Exotic	Never
Paratuberculosis	Cattle, sheep, goats, SACs	Endemic	Present
Porcine cysticercosis	Pigs	Rare, zoonotic	Present
Porcine reproductive and respiratory syndrome	Pigs	Endemic	Present
Pullorum disease	Poultry	Endemic	Present
Q fever	Cattle, sheep, goats, SACs	Endemic, zoonotic	Present
Salmonella abortus ovis	Sheep, goats, SACs	Very rare, zoonotic	Present
Surra	Cattle, sheep, goats, SACs	Exotic	Never
Theileriosis	Cattle	Exotic	Never
Transmissible gastroenteritis	Pigs	Very rare	Present
Trichinellosis	Pigs	Exotic, zoonotic	Never
Trichomonosis	Cattle	Very rare	Present
Trypanosomiasis	Cattle	Exotic	Never
Turkey rhinotracheitis	Turkeys	Endemic	Present
Tularaemia	Sheep, pigs	Exotic, zoonotic	Never

[a]South American camelids.

Africa. It can affect sheep, cattle and goats. It has never been recorded in the UK or the New World.

Rinderpest

This has now been eradicated from the world.

Scrapie

This viral sheep disease is being rapidly controlled by the use of genetic blood testing. It is now rare in the UK and has been eradicated from Australia.

Sheep pox

This is the same disease as goat pox.

Swine vesicular disease (SVD)

The importance of this viral disease of pigs is its clinical similarity to FMD.

Teschen disease

This viral disease, which is thought to be the same as Talfan disease, causes neurological signs. It has never been recorded in the UK and was mainly a disease of Eastern Europe, where it was first recorded. It has largely been controlled by vaccination and herd management.

Vesicular stomatitis

This rare and relatively innocuous virus affects cattle, pigs, horses and deer and,
extremely rarely, humans. It was mainly seen on the eastern seaboard of the USA, and is vector spread. Its main importance is that it is clinically similar to FMD.

Warble fly

This parasite of cattle has been largely eradicated worldwide by the use of ivermectins. It has not been seen in the UK for over 20 years.

Diseases Monitored Worldwide

Table 12.3 shows further diseases – not already mentioned in Tables 12.1 and 12.2 – that are monitored by OIE worldwide. Clinicians should be aware that these diseases are monitored by both Defra and OIE. Many are endemic in the UK and are discussed under the medicine of specific species (Chapters 3, 5, 7, 9 and 11).

Concluding Comments

Disease patterns are constantly changing and practitioners are advised to consult their national regulatory authority regularly. Naturally, the world's press may be the first to highlight a serious disease situation, but practitioners should always seek clarification from reliable veterinary sources.

13

Zoonotic Diseases

_____

Introduction

Zoonotic diseases have always been important. However, they are now even more important as the number of emerging diseases with zoonotic implications is increasing rapidly. Veterinarians have a large role to play in controlling these diseases and in advising their medical colleagues on the real risks that animal diseases pose to humans. Zoonotic diseases can be viral, bacterial, fungal, protozoal or parasitic in origin. Veterinarians are uniquely qualified to advise on prevention of these diseases and reduce the chances of transmission to humans by proper education and management techniques. They have a duty of care to the general populace, the owners of the animals concerned, their own staff and themselves. One measure that can be taken is to wear washable protective clothing when possible.

There are other very simple measures that veterinarians can take to protect themselves, their families and their staff from zoonotic diseases. They can also advise their clients on how to protect themselves and their families, and any visitors to their farms:

- Never drink unpasteurized cow's or goat's milk.
- Never eat undercooked meat.
- Never cuddle newly born animals or give mouth-to mouth-resuscitation.

- Always wash your hands thoroughly after handling animals.
- Always wash hands before handling food.
- Always wash hands after handling fresh meat and milk before eating or handling cooked food.
- Remove dirty clothes before entering the kitchen.
- Pay particular attention to the hygiene of children.

Farmers, particularly if they are supplying milk or meat, or have an open farm, have an obligation to:

- Keep the farm clean.
- Keep animals, their feed and water clean.
- Handle dung, manure, slurry and sewage safely.
- Protect water supplies and watercourses.
- Practise 'clean milk production'.
- Reduce transport stress of animals.
- Keep transport vehicles clean.

This chapter presents information on the various types of zoonotic diseases that are common to farm animals categorized by their human medical names in the following order: viral (and prion) zoonotic diseases, bacterial zoonotic diseases, chlamydial and rickettsial zoonotic diseases, fungal zoonotic diseases, protozoal zoonotic diseases and parasitic zoonotic diseases.

©G.R. Duncanson 2013. *Farm Animal Medicine and Surgery: For Small Animal Veterinarians* (G.R. Duncanson)

Viral (and Prion) Zoonotic Diseases Categorized by their Human Medical Names

Bovine papular stomatitis

This is a skin disease caused by a *Parapoxvirus* called pseudocowpox or milker's nodules. It is found in cattle worldwide.

Bovine spongiform encephalopathy

This disease was first seen in the UK in 1986. It is caused by a prion and termed BSE but has now nearly been eradicated, and is only extremely rarely found in mainland Europe in cattle.

Contagious pustular dermatitis

This skin disease is caused by a *Parapoxvirus* and is called 'orf'. It is found in sheep, goats and South American camelids (SACs) worldwide.

Cowpox

This is a skin disease caused by an *Orthopoxvirus*. It is found in cattle worldwide.

Crimean-Congo haemorrhagic fever

This is a systemic disease affecting the blood vessels and caused by a *Nairovirus* which is spread by ticks. It is found in cattle, sheep, goats and pigs in Central Asia, Bulgaria and the Congo.

Encephalomyocarditis

This is a neurological and cardiac disease caused by a *Cardiovirus* and called three-day fever. It is found in cattle and pigs.

Foot-and-mouth disease

Foot-and-mouth disease (FMD) is a benign disease in humans and is caused by an *Aphthovirus*. It is found in cattle, sheep, goats, SACs and pigs.

Goat pox

This is a skin disease caused by a *Capripoxvirus*. It is found in goats in Africa, the Middle East, India and the Far East.

Influenza

Influenza is a generalized systemic disease caused by a variety of influenza viruses (*Influenzavirus*) and sometimes called grippe. It is found worldwide in pigs and poultry.

Japanese B encephalitis

This is a neurological disease caused by a *Flavivirus* which is spread by mosquitoes. It is found in pigs in India and the Far East.

Louping ill

This is another neurological disease caused by a *Flavivirus*. It is spread by the sheep tick *Ixodes ricinus* and is found in sheep worldwide, with a restricted occurrence in the UK.

Newcastle disease

This is a rare disease in humans in which it produces conjunctivitis. It is caused by a paramyxovirus. It is found in poultry on a restricted basis worldwide.

Rabies

This is a fatal neurological disease caused by a *Lyssavirus*. It is found in cattle, sheep, goats, SACs and pigs in most parts of the world except the UK, Scandinavia, Australia and New Zealand.

Rift Valley fever

This is a serious liver disease, often called enzootic hepatitis, and caused by a *Phlebovirus*. It is spread by mosquitoes and is found throughout Africa south of the Sahara and also in Egypt in cattle, sheep and goats.

Rotaviral gastroenteritis

This is a gastroenteric disease of children caused by a *Rotavirus*. It is found in calves, lambs, kids, crias and suckling pigs worldwide.

Russian and Central European spring–summer encephalitis

This is a neurological disease caused by a *Flavivirus* which is spread by ticks. It is found in cattle and goats in Eastern Europe and Asia.

Scrapie

This slow brain disease is caused by a prion. There is no direct link with Creutzfeldt–Jakob disease in humans. Scrapie is found in sheep and goats worldwide excepting Australia and New Zealand.

Swine vesicular disease

Swine vesicular disease (SVD) is a mild disease in humans which is caused by an *Enterovirus*. It is extremely rare in pigs worldwide and is important because it cannot be clinically differentiated from FMD.

Vesicular stomatitis

This disease, called 'sore mouth', is caused by a *Vesiculovirus*. It affects cattle and pigs in North and South America.

Wesselsbron disease

This mild disease is mosquito borne and caused by a *Flavivirus*. It affects cattle, sheep and goats in Africa.

West Nile fever

This is a serious disease in the elderly. It is mosquito borne and caused by a *Flavivirus*. The disease affects cattle, sheep, goats and poultry in Africa, southern Europe, Asia and northern America.

Bacterial Zoonotic Diseases Categorized by their Human Medical Names

Actinobacillosis

Actinobacillus ligniersii causes the condition called 'wooden tongue', and has been isolated in cattle, sheep, goats and SACs worldwide. The organism has been found in oral lesions in humans, but extremely rarely.

Actinomycosis

This granulomatous condition of the jaw in humans is normally caused by *Actinomyces israelii*. This bacterium is found in the normal flora of the human buccal cavity. It invades the soft tissue and bones when teeth are extracted. It also invades the genital tract of women using intrauterine contraceptive devices. The organism has never been isolated from animals. However, another *Actinomyces* sp., *A. bovis* is a common pathogen in cattle, in which it causes the condition of 'lumpy jaw'. It has been found in oral lesions in humans, but extremely rarely.

Animal erysipelas (human erysipeloid)

There is considerable confusion concerning this condition as a zoonosis. The disease is caused by the bacterium *Erysipelas rhusiopathiae*, an organism that is found in the soil all over the world. It commonly causes disease in pigs, and will also cause a joint infection in calves, lambs, kids, crias and poultry. The confusion arises because there is also a condition in humans termed erysipelas or 'fish sorters disease', which is not caused by *E. rhusiopathiae* but by a *Streptococcus* which is found in fish and in marine mammals.

Anthrax

This disease is caused by *Bacillus anthracis* which occurs in all mammals worldwide. It has three manifestations in humans. 'Woolsorters disease' is the invariably fatal pneumonic form caught from the skins of sheep and goats. Then there is an enteric form acquired by eating carcasses contaminated with *B. anthracis*. The third form, which is the most common, is the skin form.

Botulism

This disease is caused by the toxin produced by the anaerobic spore-forming bacterium, *Clostridium botulinum*. All warm-blooded animals are affected. Botulism is normally not an actual zoonosis as humans are poisoned by eating food in which the bacteria have produced toxin, e.g. in contaminated fish. Cases have been recorded worldwide. If farm animals and poultry carcasses contaminated by the toxin are consumed they will also cause death.

Brucellosis

This disease is caused by four bacteria:

1. *Brucella melitensis* is found in goats, and is common in the Mediterranean basin, the Middle East and Central Asia, but is not found in the UK.

2. *B. ovis* is found in both sheep and goats in tropical Africa and Latin America.
3. *B. abortus* is found in cattle worldwide but no longer occurs in the UK.
4. *B. suis* is found in pigs worldwide but not in the UK or northern Europe.

Campylobacteriosis

This disease is caused by *Campylobacter jejuni*. It is the main cause of acute bacterial enteritis in the UK. The most common animal host to be a danger to humans is the chicken. The disease is also found in cattle and sheep worldwide.

Clostridial food poisoning

Although the many *Clostridium* spp. are very important and prevalent in all farm animals, clostridial food poisoning is not an important zoonosis. The organism is found in soil and dust worldwide and so animals are not the main cause of infection. The clostridial species that occur in sheep and goats cause very mild enteritis in humans, which rarely lasts for more than 24 h, and is self-limiting. The important human pathogen is *Cl. difficile*, which is not pathogenic to or found in farm animals.

Clostridial wound infections

Tetanus is caused by *Cl. tetani*, which is found in soil worldwide. An animal is not required for the infection, which normally comes from a contaminated deep puncture wound. Other clostridial species will also infect wounds in humans or farm animals and cause serious gangrene and death, but humans cannot become infected from animals; the main organisms are *Cl. novyi*, *Cl. septicum* and *Cl. sordellii*.

Colibacillosis

This is a very important life-threatening zoonotic disease that is found worldwide and is caused by *Escherichia coli*. The most important highly pathogenic *E. coli* found in the UK is the verocytotoxigenic strain *E. coli* O157. In other countries, there are other verocytotoxigenic strains of *E. coli* (VTEC), e.g. O26. VTEC O157 is carried asymptomatically by animals, and owners of animals should be aware of the potential for zoonotic transmission of VTEC O157, even from healthy animals. The organism colonizes the rectal-anal junction, with certain individuals being super-shedders.

Corynebacteriosis

Corynebacterium diphtheria causes the very serious condition of diphtheria in humans but it does not occur in animals. *C. pseudotuberculosis* is a very important pathogen in sheep, goats and SACs worldwide. Cases of *C. pseudotuberculosis* reported in humans are extremely rare.

Dermatophilosis

This is an important skin condition in cattle, sheep, goats and SACs worldwide that is caused by *Dermatophilus congolensis*. It is not an important zoonosis.

Enterocolitic yersiniosis

This serious disease is caused by *Yersinia enterocolitica*. It occurs in pigs worldwide.

Leptospirosis

There is considerable confusion with this worldwide zoonotic disease. *Leptospira icterohaemorrhagiae* causes a very serious, often fatal, disease in humans that is called Weil's disease. This disease is passed to humans from rodents, which are normally symptomless carriers. Pigs can also get the disease and infect humans. Cattle will become infected with *Leptospira* serovar Hardjo, which does not cause a serious human disease.

Listeriosis

This disease, which occurs worldwide, is caused by *Listeria monocytogenes*. Infection is very serious in very young babies and will cause abortion in women. *L. monocytogenes* is found in cattle, sheep, goats, SACs and poultry.

Meliodosis

This disease is caused by *Pseudomonas pseudomallei* and is also called rodent glanders. It is mainly confined to sheep, goats and pigs in the tropics, particularly South-east Asia.

Necrobacillosis

This condition is caused by *Fusobacterium necrophorum*, which causes disease in cattle, sheep and goats. It is an extremely rare disease in humans.

Nocardiosis

This condition is caused by *Nocardia* spp. and starts as a pyogenic focus. It occurs worldwide in cattle, sheep and goats.

Pasteurellosis

There is confusion in the nomenclature of the two agents causing this disease, which both used to be *Pasteurella* spp. – *P. multocida* and *P. haemolytica*. *P. haemolytica* is now called *Mannheimia haemolytica*. These are both common pathogens worldwide in cattle sheep, goats, SACs, pigs and poultry. They cause severe pneumonia in mammals and fowl cholera in poultry.

Salmonellosis

Salmonella typhimurium is found in cattle, sheep, goats, SACs, pigs and (rarely) in poultry worldwide. It will cause enteritis in humans. *S. enteritidis* is mainly found in poultry worldwide and will also cause enteritis in humans. *S. dublin* is mainly found in cattle and rarely causes human enteritis. There are also other *Salmonella* species/subspecies/serovars causing salmonellosis which are ever present on farms, e.g. *S. enterica* subsp. *diarizonae* and *S.* Montevideo. Further, there are species-specific salmonellae, e.g. *S. pullorum* and *S. gallinarum*, both found in poultry, and *S. abortus ovis*, found in sheep. These species rarely cause human disease. Most human *Salmonella* infections are acquired as a result of eating contaminated food. Infection on farms is more commonly acquired by mouth from hands contaminated by infected animals, their bedding and surroundings. The following simple precautions will go a long way towards preventing people associated with livestock from becoming infected with salmonellosis:

1. Observe high standards of personal hygiene; wear rubber boots and protective overgarments when working with animals.
2. Change and launder overalls frequently and disinfect boots to avoid spreading the infection to other animals and people.
3. Wash hands using hot water and soap immediately after working with infected animals.
4. Wash hands before eating, drinking or smoking.
5. Ensure that anyone with diarrhoea, vomiting or flu-like illness consults a doctor, and informs the doctor if salmonellae have been isolated from livestock.
6. Don't take or wear dirty clothing and boots into the home.
7. Don't allow vulnerable people, including children, the elderly and pregnant women to come into contact with infected animals.
8. Don't drink raw milk or eat undercooked eggs from the herd/flock when salmonellae have been isolated – even healthy animals may excrete salmonellae.
9. Don't bring infected animals into any room where food is prepared or eaten.
10. Don't allow pets to come into contact with infected animals.

Tularaemia

This disease is caused by *Francisella tularensis*, which is spread by ticks. It is mainly seen in sheep in North America and Russia.

Yersiniosis

Yersinia pseudotuberculosis causes Parinaud's oculoglandular syndrome in humans. It causes a similar syndrome in goats.

Zoonotic tuberculosis

Tuberculosis (TB) in humans is normally caused by the human pathogen, *Mycobacterium tuberculosis*, although humans can also become infected by *M. bovis*. This is primarily a disease affecting cattle and badgers. It is a chronic condition eventually leading to severe caseous pneumonia and death in both cattle and badgers. Humans become infected by drinking unpasteurized contaminated milk. In sheep and pigs, *M. bovis* is extremely rare, but it is becoming quite common in the UK in goats and SACs. Avian TB does not cause disease in humans. TB occurs worldwide, excepting certain areas, e.g. Scotland.

Chlamydial and Rickettsial Zoonotic Diseases Categorized by their Human Medical Names

Avian chlamydiosis

This disease, which occurs worldwide, is caused by *Chlamydophila psittaci* (formerly *Chlamydia psittaci*). It causes a serious respiratory disease in humans. It is common in parrots but can also occur in ducks and turkeys. It is very rare in chickens.

Chlamydiosis

This is caused by *Chlamydophila abortus* (formerly *Chlamydia psittaci*), which is found in sheep and goats. It occurs worldwide.

Q fever

Q fever is caused by *Coxiella burnetti* and occurs worldwide. It can be spread between cattle, sheep and goats, and to humans through drinking water. It can also be spread by ticks. There has been a recent Q fever epidemic in the Netherlands which is the largest ever epidemic reported globally. The source of infection was aerosol transmission from a very high concentration of large, infected dairy goat units located close to the human population.

Fungal Zoonotic Diseases Categorized by their Human Medical Names

Dermatophytosis

Dermatophytosis, or ringworm, in sheep, goats, SACs and pigs is extremely rare compared with its occurrence in cattle. Sheep, goats, SACs and pigs will contract one of the causative organisms, *Trichophyton verrucosum*, from cattle. *Microsporum gypseum* has been recorded in lambs and kids. *Microsporum* spp. are not as contagious to humans as *Trichophyton* spp.; both are found worldwide.

Protozoal Zoonotic Diseases Categorized by their Human Medical Names

Babesiosis

Although this protozoan (*Babesia* spp.), which is spread by ticks, has a worldwide incidence, it is not an important zoonosis. This is because humans seem to be resistant to the disease, so that infections are extremely rare. The disease is also rare in sheep, goats and SACs, as it is primarily a cattle parasite.

Cryptosporidiosis

Cryptosporidiosis is caused by the protozoan *Cryptosporidium parvum*, which causes enteritis. It has a worldwide distribution. *C. parvum*

is mainly a parasite of cattle but is also seen in sheep, goats and SACs. Bottle-fed animals are often symptomless carriers and a danger to children visiting open, educational farms. The disease can be well contained by strict hygiene that involves/includes hand washing and not allowing eating and drinking near animals.

Sarcocystosis

In cattle, this disease is caused by *Sarcocystis hominis*. In pigs it is caused by *S. suihominis*. Humans are usually a symptomless carrier. The disease occurs worldwide.

Toxoplasmosis

The causal organism of toxoplasmosis is *Toxoplasma gondii*, which is pathogenic to humans. It causes abortion in cattle, sheep, goats and SACs worldwide. Cats and rodents are the main danger to humans.

Parasitic Zoonotic Diseases Categorized by their Human Medical Names

Acanthocephaliasis

Several species of acanthocephalan nematodes can cause this disease in humans. One of these, *Macracanthorhynchus hirudinaceous*, occurs in the small intestine of pigs (the definitive host) and humans (a secondary definitive host). The life cycle of the worm, which is known as the 'giant thorny-headed worm of swine' includes beetles of the genus *Melolontha* as intermediate hosts. *M. hirudinaceous* occurs worldwide but is most commonly found in Eastern Europe and Asia.

Ascariasis

There are two species of ascarid nematode that cause this disease, and they are very similar: *Ascaris lumbricoides* in humans and

A. suum in pigs. They can – but rarely – infect the heterologous host. They are found worldwide.

Clonorchiasis

This disease is caused by a fluke, *Clonorchis sinensis*, which affects humans and pigs. It has two intermediate hosts, a snail and a fish. It occurs in the Far East.

Coenurosis

This disease is caused by the larval stage of the tapeworm *Taenia multiceps*; this stage is known as *Coenurus cerebralis*. The normal life cycle occurs in the dog or wild canids, i.e. foxes, jackals and coyotes. These animals are definitive hosts of *T. multiceps* and harbour the tapeworm in their intestines. The normal intermediate host is the sheep or, rarely, the goat. Humans are not the normal intermediate host although rare cases have been recorded. The tapeworm is found worldwide in temperate areas.

Dicrocoeliasis

Dicrocoelium dendriticum is a lancet-shaped trematode (the lancet fluke) that lives in the bile ducts of cattle, sheep and goats, but can infect humans. It requires two intermediate hosts for its development, the first being a land snail and the second an ant. The parasite is found in North and South America, Europe, Asia and North Africa.

Echinostomiasis

Several species of *Echinostoma*, a trematode fluke, causes this disease, which is found in the Far East. It has two intermediate hosts, a snail and then another snail, a tadpole or a fish. Humans, pigs and poultry, particularly ducks and geese, are infected by eating the second intermediate host.

Fascioliasis

This is a very serious disease in cattle, sheep, goats and SACs. It is caused by the liver flukes *Fasciola hepatica* (found throughout the world) and *Fasciola gigantica* (found in Africa and Asia). The herbivores are the main hosts, with the amphibious snail *Lymnaea truncatula* as the intermediate host. Humans are a rare host and normally become infected by consuming contaminated watercress.

Gastrodiscoidiasis

Gastrodiscoidiasis is caused by the fluke, *Gastrodiscoides hominis*, which occurs in humans and pigs, and has a single intermediate host, an aquatic snail. This fluke occurs in Asia.

Hydatidosis

The main host for the tapeworm that causes this disease (*Echinococcus granulosus*) is found in the dog. The sheep, goat and, rarely, humans can become infected as secondary hosts. The disease is found worldwide, and used to be common in New Zealand until radical public hygiene measures were undertaken.

Linguatuliasis

This disease is caused by *Linguatula serrata*. The female of this linguiform parasite measures 10 cm long and the male 2 cm. It is found in the nasal passages and frontal sinuses of dogs and cats. Eggs are laid and pass to the environment by sneezing or spitting. They then need to be eaten by a secondary host – usually a small ruminant. This pentastomid worm is found in Europe, the Middle East and North Africa, and also throughout the New World. The larvae are asymptomatic in sheep and goats. Humans can become infected in two ways. The first is by ingesting eggs from vegetables or water. The larvae may then cause gastroenteric signs, while the nymphs may cause ocular infection by invading the anterior chamber of the eye. However the second type of infection is more common in humans, and results from ingesting contaminated offal. The infection is immediate as the nymphs invade the nasopharynx and cause pain in the throat and a runny nose.

Myiasis caused by larvae of *Oestrus ovis*

The adult of *Oestrus ovis*, a grey fly 12 mm in length, is larviparous, and deposits larvae in the nostrils of sheep, goats and, occasionally, humans. It is found throughout the world.

Taeniasis and cysticercosis

There are two cestodes, *Taenia solium* and *T. saginata*, which have humans as the definitive host. The secondary hosts are the pig and the ox, which carry the larval stages – which are known as *Cysticercus cellulosae* and *C. bovis*, respectively. They are now rare but occur worldwide.

Trichinosis

This disease is caused by a small filiform nematode, *Trichinella spiralis*. Humans are the end host. The pig can be both the intermediate and the main host. The disease occurs rarely in North and South America and

extremely rarely elsewhere. It is not found in the UK. The bush pig is the intermediate host in eastern and southern Africa.

Trichostrongyliasis

Trichostrongyliasis is caused by short slender nematodes of the species *Trichostrongylus*, which inhabit the small intestine and abomasums of sheep and goats. Humans are only very rarely infected by chance ingestion of the eggs. The disease that results should not be confused with that caused by the specific human parasite, *T. orientalis*, which is passed directly from human to human via the faeces. This nematode is found in Central Asia and the Far East. It is particularly prevalent in Central Iran.

Tungiasis

This condition, which occurs in pigs and humans, is caused by a small flea, *Tunga penetrans*. It occurs in tropical areas of Africa, the Caribbean, Central and South America.

Zoonotic scabies

Human scabies is caused by the mite *Sarcoptes scabiei*. A very similar mite, *Sarcoptes scabiei* var. *suis*, is found in pigs and can infect humans. It is found worldwide.

Glossary

_____

Abortion – the premature birth of young.

Annual – a plant which grows from seed, flowers and dies within a year.

Anthelmintics – drugs that expel parasitic worms from the body, generally by paralysing or starving them.

Antigen – a molecule or part of a molecule that is recognized by components of the host immune system.

Autosomal chromosome – a non-sex chromosome.

Awn – a bristle or hair-like appendage to a fruit or to a glume, as in barley and some other grasses.

Bacteraemia – bacteria in the blood.

Base pairs – in DNA, the four bases pair up to form the internal structure of DNA: adenine with guanine and thymine with cysteine.

Biennial – a plant which flowers and dies in the second year after growing from a seed.

Billy goat – a mature male goat.

Billy rag – a piece of cloth rubbed over a mature male goat, particularly its urine covered front legs, to stimulate a female goat to show signs of oestrus.

Bradycardia – a decrease in heart rate.

Bruxism – grinding of the teeth.

Buck – a mature male goat.

Calculi – stones formed in the urinary system.

Caprine – adjective applied to goats.

Cerebral – relating to the cerebrum, the largest part of the brain.

Cestodes – parasitic flatworms, commonly called tapeworms, which usually live in the digestive tract of vertebrates as adults and in the bodies of various intermediate hosts as juvenile stages.

Codon – sequences of three nucleotides that encode a specific single amino acid.

Colitis – inflammation of the colon: often used to describe an inflammation of the large intestine.

Coma – profound unconsciousness from which the patient cannot be roused.

Congestion – the presence of an abnormal amount of blood in an organ or part.

Contusions – bruises.

Convulsion – a violent involuntary contraction of muscles.

Corm – underground bulbous root.

Cria – a young South American camelid (SAC) in its first year.

Cryptorchid – see rig below.

Cull ewe – a ewe no longer suitable for breeding, and sold for meat.

Cystitis – inflammation of the bladder

Dag/s – clump/s of dung stuck to the wool of the rear and tail of a sheep, which may lead to fly strike.

Dagging – clipping off dags, or clipping the wool to prevent them forming.

Deciduous plants – those which shed all their leaves annually.

Detoxicate – to render a poison harmless.

Distension – the filling of a hollow organ to more than its usual capacity.

Diuresis – excessive urination.

DNA fingerprinting – much like the fingerprint used in human identification, but done with unique DNA characters for each individual animal. Utilizes the polymerase chain reaction (PCR, see below) to replicate small samples.

Doe – a mature female goat.

Draft ewe – a ewe too old for rough grazing, e.g. moorland or upland, and drafted on to better grazing on another farm.

Drenching – giving an anthelmintic dose by mouth.

Dysentery – an illness characterized by diarrhoea with blood in the faeces.

Dysphagia – difficulty in swallowing.

Dysphonia – hoarseness heard when vocalizing.

Dyspnoea – difficulty in breathing.

Dystocia – difficulty at parturition.

Egg reappearance period – the time taken (usually expressed in weeks) for eggs to reappear in the faeces after anthelmintic treatment. This is usually described for drug-sensitive worm populations at the time of product licensing.

ELISA (enzyme-linked immunosorbent assay) – a technique used primarily in immunology to detect the presence of an antibody or an antigen in a sample. Basically, an unknown amount of antigen is bound to the surface of a plastic well, then a specific antibody is added; if the antibody is specific to the test antigen it will bind that antigen. This antibody is linked to an enzyme or is detected by incubation with a second antibody that is linked to an enzyme. In the final step, a substance is added that the enzyme can convert to some detectable signal (usually a colour change which is detectable by a spectrophotometer).

Emaciation – excessive body wasting.

Emesis – vomiting.

Emetic – a substance that causes vomiting.

Emphysema – air or gas in the interstices of a tissue.

Enema – rectal injection.

Epidemiology – the study of factors affecting the health of populations and often of how diseases are transmitted.

Ewe – a female sheep which has had at least one lamb.

Exon – the coding part of a gene.

Faecal egg count reduction test (FECRT) – a test that measures the effect of anthelmintic treatment on faecal egg output. Generally, efficacy is assessed by comparing faecal egg counts (FECs) obtained on the day of treatment with those obtained 14 days after treatment. This is an important tool in detecting anthelmintic resistance in the field.

Flock – the collective word for a group of sheep.

Foetid – malodorous.

Fold – a pen in which flocks are kept overnight to keep them safe from predators.

Gelding – castrated South American camelid (SAC).

Gene mapping – mapping of a gene to/on a given chromosome.

Genetic engineering – the direct manipulation of genes to alter the physical appearance of an animal. Also used in recombinant vaccine technology.

Genome – an organism's entire hereditary information, encoded either in DNA or, for some types of virus, in RNA. The genome includes the genes that code the proteins and non-coding sequences of the DNA.

Genotype – the inherited instructions that an organism carries in its genetic code.

Gimmer – a female sheep which is mature enough to be served by a ram for the first time; also called a theave.

Glabrous –without hair of any kind.

Goatherd – a person who looks after a herd of goats.

Goatling – a young goat normally weaned.

Granules – small grains.

Gravid – the pregnant horn of a uterus.

Hembra – female South American camelid (SAC).

Haematuria – blood in the urine.

Haemoglobinuria – haemoglobin in the urine.

Haemolytic – a substance that causes breakdown of red blood corpuscles.

Hefting – the instinct in some breeds of keeping to a certain heft, or local area, throughout their lives. This allows farmers to graze sheep on different areas without fences. Lambs naturally stay on the area where they were born.

Helminths – a group of eukaryotic parasites that live inside their hosts. They are worm like and live and feed off animals.

Hepatitis – inflammation of the liver.

Herbaceous perennials – plants in which the greater part dies after flowering, leaving only the rootstock to produce next year's growth.

Heterozygous – a genotype consisting of two different alleles at a given locus.

Hogget – a one year old female sheep normally destined for meat (also hogg, hog or hoggat).

Homozygous – a genotype consisting two identical alleles at a given locus.

Herd – the collective word for a group of cattle, goats, pigs or South American camelids (SACs).

Iatrogenic – resulting from treatment.

Ileus – failure of peristalsis.

In cria – pregnant South American camelid (SAC).

In kid – pregnant goat.

In lamb – pregnant sheep.

In vitro – in the test tube.

In vivo – in the living body.

Indigenous – native of the country in which it was produced.

Intron – the non-coding part of a gene.

Jaundice – a disease in which bile pigments stain the mucous membranes.

Kid – a young goat in its first year.

Lamb – a young sheep in its first year.

Lambing – the process of giving birth in sheep.

Larvae – juvenile forms that many animals undergo before the mature adult stage. Larvae are frequently adapted to environments different to those that adult stages live in.

Leucocytosis – increase in white blood cells (WBCs) in the blood.

Leucopenia – decrease in white blood cells (WBCs) in the blood.

Linear leaves – those that are long and narrow.

Lumen – the inner space of a tubular structure, such as the intestine.

Macho – entire male South American camelid (SAC).

Markers – a short tandem repeat (STR) that may be used to aid in the identification of a trait.

Mediastinum – space in the chest between the lungs.

Melaena – dark tarry faeces indicating bleeding high in the intestinal tract.

Metritis – inflammation of the uterus.

Microsatellite – a stretch of DNA that is repeated several times in a row. These are located at random throughout a chromosome. The variation in these markers allows for parentage verification and other forensic activities.

Micturition – the passing of urine.

Mitochondrial DNA – DNA found only in the mitochondria. Only provided by the female and controls cellular metabolism.

Monoecious – when male and female flowers are separate, but on the same plant.

Mutations – alterations in DNA sequence in a genome that spontaneously occur during meiosis or DNA replication, or are caused by factors such as by radiation, viruses or chemicals. Mutations can have either no effect, or alter the product of a gene so that it does not function properly or at all.

Mutton – the meat of an older sheep.

Myiasis – fly strike.

Nanny goat – a mature female goat.

Narcosis – sleep induced by a drug or poison.

Nematodes – roundworms, one of the most diverse phyla of all animals.

Nodule – a small round lump.

Non-gravid – the non-pregnant horn of a uterus.

Nuclear DNA – DNA found in the nucleus of all cells of the body. A copy is provided by each parent. This DNA carries the code for phenotype (physical characteristics).

Nucleotide – the building blocks of DNA. Composed of deoxyribose sugars, a phosphate and one of four nitrogenous bases.

Old-season lamb – a lamb a year old or more.

Orchitis – inflammation of the testicle.

Ovine – adjective applied to sheep.

Ovoid – egg shaped.

Panacea – a cure all.

Paracentesis – the technique of puncturing a body cavity.

Pathogenicity – the ability of a pathogen to produce signs of disease in an organism.

Pathognomic – a single specific sign of a disease.

Pediculosis – lice infestation.

Phenotype – any observable characteristic or trait of an organism, such as its morphology, development, biochemical or physiological properties, or behavior. Phenotypes result from the expression of an organism's genes as well as the influence of environmental factors and possible interactions between the two.

Polled – inherited hornlessness.

Polydactyly – having an extra limb.

Polydipsia – abnormally intense thirst leading to the drinking of large quantities of fluid.

Polymerase chain reaction (PCR) – a technique to amplify a single or a few copies of a piece of DNA by several orders of magnitude that generates thousands to millions of copies of a particular sequence. PCR relies on cycles of repeated heating (DNA melting, to separate the two DNA strands), cooling (to allow annealing – the pairing of the DNA template so produced to a primer) and enzymatic replication of DNA. The primers (short DNA fragments), which contain sequences complementary to the target DNA region, along with a DNA polymerase (after which the method is named), are key components to enable selective and repeated amplification. As PCR progresses, the DNA generated is used as a further template for replication, setting in motion a chain reaction in which the original template is exponentially amplified.

Polyphagia – excessive eating.

Premix – medicine available in a concentrated form to be added to food.

Primer – several thousand copies of short sequences of DNA that are complementary to part of the DNA to be sequenced (see polymerase chain reaction).

Proctitis – inflammation of the rectum.

Ptyalism – excessive saliva production.

Purgative – a strong laxative.

Pyrexia – raised rectal temperature.

Raddle – a colour marker strapped to the chest of a ram to mark the backs of ewes he has mated with.

Ram – an uncastrated adult male sheep.

Recumbency – unable to get up.

Rhinitis – inflammation of the nose.

Rig – a male in which one or both testicles have not descended into the scrotum.

Ring womb – failure of the cervix to dilate.

Rostral – towards the nose.

Ryegrass – a commonly grown grass, *Lolium perenne*.

Schistosomus reflexus – a deformity of a fetus in which the spine is bent backwards.

Sclerosis – hardening of a tissue.

Septicaemia – pathogenic bacteria in the blood.

Shearling – a yearling sheep of either sex, also called a teg.

Shepherd – a person who looks after a flock of sheep.

Short tandem repeats (STR) – sections of DNA arranged in back-to-back repetition.

Slough – dead tissue that drops away from living tissue.

Spasm – involuntary contraction of a muscle.

Staggers – an erratic gait.

Stomatitis – inflammation of the mouth and gums.

Stricture – a narrowing of a tubular organ.

Subclinical – when the symptoms are not evident.

Syncope – fainting.

Syndrome – a group of symptoms.

Tachycardia – increased heart rate.

Tachypnoea – increased respiratory rate.

Teaser – a vasectomized ram.

Tenesmus – straining to pass urine or faeces.

Teratoma – a developmental embryological deformity.

Torpid – sluggish.

Tourniquet – an appliance for temporary stoppage of the circulation in a limb.

Trismus – locking of the jaw.

Tuis – 1 to 2 year-old South American camelid (SAC).

Tup – another term for a ram.

Tupping – another term for sheep mating.

Twin lamb disease – pregnancy toxaemia.

Tympanic – distended with gas.

Typhilitis – inflammation of the caecum.

Ubiquitous – everywhere.

Udder – mammary gland.

Ureter – the tube connecting the kidney to the bladder.

Urethra – the tube leading from the bladder to the outside.

Urethritis – inflammation of the urethra.

Urine scald – inflammation of the skin caused by persistent wetting with urine.

Urolithiasis – the formation of stones in the urinary system.

Urticaria – an acute inflammatory reaction of the skin.

Vaginitis – inflammation of the vagina.
Vagus – 10th cranial nerve.
Venereal disease – a disease spread by coitus.
Vesicle – a collection of fluid in the surface layers of the skin or of a mucous membrane.
Viraemia – virus particles in the blood.
Volatile – a substance that evaporates rapidly.
Wether – a castrated sheep, goat or South American camelid (SAC).
Zoonoses – diseases communicable between animals and man.

References

Agnello, S., Chetta, M., Vicari, D., Mancuso, R., Manno, C., Puleio, R., Console, A., Nicholas, R.A.J. and Loria, G.R. (2012) Severe outbreaks of polyarthritis in kids caused by *Mycoplasma mycoides* subspecies *capri* in Sicily. *Veterinary Record* 170, 416.

Angell, J. and Ross, T. (2011) Suspected bog asphodel (*Narthecium ossifragum*) toxicity in cattle in North Wales. *Veterinary Record* 169, 102.

Baird, G. (2003) Current perspectives on caseous lymphadenitis. *In Practice* 25, 62–68.

Baird, G. and Malone, F.E. (2010) Control of caseous lymphadenitis in six sheep flocks using clinical examination and regular ELISA testing. *Veterinary Record* 166, 358–362.

Ball, A.L. and Gregory, N.G. (2007) Prognostic indicators in cattle treated for uterine prolapse. *Journal of Commonwealth Veterinary Association* 23, 9–15.

Bell, C. (2011) Bleeding disorders in cattle. *In Practice* 33, 106–115.

Bravo, P.W., Bazan, P.J., Troedsson, M.H., Villalta, P.R. and Garnica, J.P. (1996) Induction of parturition in alpacas and subsequent survival of neonates. *Journal of the American Veterinary Medical Association* 209, 1760–1762.

Buxton, D. (1989) Toxoplasmosis in sheep and other farm animals. *In Practice* 11, 9–12.

D'Alterio, G.L., Callaghan, C., Just, C., Manner-Smith, A., Foster, A.P. and Knowles, T.G. (2005) Prevalence of *Chorioptes* sp. mite infestation in alpaca (*Lama pacos*) in the south-west of England: implications for skin health. *Small Ruminant Research* 57, 221–228.

Dawson, M., Moore, R.C. and Bishop, S.C. (2008) Progress and limits of PrP gene selection policy. *Veterinary Research* 39(4), 25.

Duncanson, G.R. (1984) Uterine torsion in cattle – a review of 18 severe cases. *Proceedings for 1984–85, British Cattle Veterinary Association*, pp. 133–135.

Fazili, M.R., Malik, H.U., Bhattacharyya, H.K., Buchoo, B.A., Moulvi, B.A. and Makhdoomi, D.M. (2010) Minimally invasive surgical tube cystotomy for treating obstructive urolithiasis in small ruminants with an intact urinary bladder. *Veterinary Record* 166, 528–532.

Foster, A. (2008) Skin diseases of South American camelids. *British Veterinary Zoological Society Proceedings, May 2008*, pp. 30–32.

Foster, G., Hunter, L., Baird, G., Koylass, M.S. and Whatmore, A.M. (2010) *Streptococcus pluranimalium* in ovine reproductive material. *Veterinary Record* 166, 246.

Goodchild, L.M., Dart, A.J., Collins, M.B., Dart, C.M., Hodgson, J.L. and Hodgson, D.R. (1996) Cryptococcal meningitis in an alpaca. *Australian Veterinary Journal* 74, 428–430.

Gregory, N. (2011) Problems associated with cattle welfare. *In Practice* 33, 328–333.

Grosche, A., Fürll, M. and Wittek, T. (2012) Peritoneal fluid analysis in dairy cows with left displaced abomasum and abomasal volvulus. *Veterinary Record* 170, 413.

Hoinville, L.J., Tongue, S.C. and Wilesmith, J.W. (2010) Evidence for maternal transmission of scrapie in naturally affected flocks. *Preventive Veterinary Medicine* 93, 121–128.

243

Ingoldby, L. and Jackson, P. (2001) Induction of parturition in sheep. *In Practice* 23, 228–231.

Jackson, P. (1986) Skin diseases in goats. *In Practice* 8, 5–10.

Jeffrey, M. (1993) Sarcocystosis in sheep. *In Practice* 15, 2–8.

Mason, C., Stevenson, H., Cox, A., Dick, I. and Rodger, C. (2012) Disease associated with immature paraphistome infection in sheep. *Veterinary Record* 170, 343–344.

Michell, S., Mearns, R., Richards, I., Donnan, A.A. and Bartley, D.J. (2011) Benzimidazole resistance in *Nematodirus battus*. *Veterinary Record* 168, 623.

Nodelijk, G., van Roermund, H.J.W., van Keulen, L.J.M., Engel, B., Vellema, P. and Hagenaars, T.J. (2011) Breeding with resistant rams leads to rapid control of classical scrapie in affected sheep flocks. *Veterinary Research* 42, 5, doi:10.1186/1297-9716-42-5.

Pearson, H. (1971) Uterine torsion in cattle: a review of 168 cases. *Veterinary Record* 89, 597–603.

Petridou, E.J., Gianniki, Z., Giadinis, N.D., Filioussis, G., Dovas, C.I. and Psychas, V. (2011) Outbreak of polyarthritis in lambs attributed to *Pasteurella multocida*. *Veterinary Record* 168, 50.

Quintas, H., Reis, J., Pires, I. and Alegria, N. (2010) Tuberculosis in goats. *Veterinary Record* 166, 437–438.

Rebhun, W.C., Jenkins, D.H., Riis, R.C., Dill, S.G., Dubovi, E.J. and Torres, A. (1988) An epizootic of blindness and encephalitis associated with a herpesvirus indistinguishable from equine herpesvirus 1 in a herd of alpacas and llamas. *Journal of the American Veterinary Medical Association* 192, 953–956.

Richey, M.J., Foster, A.P., Crawshaw, T.R. and Schock, A. (2011) *Mycobacterium bovis* mastitis in an alpaca and its implications. *Veterinary Record* 169, 214.

Rifatbegović, M., Maksimović, Z. and Hulaj, B. (2011) *Mycoplasma ovipneumoniae* associated with severe respiratory disease in goats. *Veterinary Record* 168, 565.

Rousseau, M., Anderson, D.E., Miesner, M.D., Schulz, K.L. and Whitehead, C.E. (2010) Scapulohumeral joint luxation in alpacas: 10 cases (2003–2009). *Journal of the American Veterinary Medical Association* 237, 1186–1192.

Sargison, N. and Edwards, G. (2009) Tick infestations in sheep in the UK. *In Practice* 31, 58–65.

Scott, P. (2000) Ultrasonography of the urinary tract in male sheep with urethral obstruction. *In Practice* 22, 329–333.

Scott, P. (2010) Intussusception in neonatal lambs. *Livestock* 15(2), 39–40.

Scott, P. (2011) Uterine torsion in the ewe. *Livestock* 16(2), 37–39.

Sharpe, A.E., Brady, C.P., Johnson, A., Byrne, W., Kenny, K. and Costello, E. (2010) Concurrent outbreak of tuberculosis and caseous lymphadenitis in a goat herd. *Veterinary Record* 166, 591–592.

Strugnell, B. and McAuliffe, L. (2012) *Mycoplasma wenyonii* infection in cattle. *In Practice* 34, 146–154.

Twomey, D.F., Allen, K., Bell, S., Evans, C. and Thomas, S. (2010) *Eimeria ivitaensis* in British alpacas. *Veterinary Record* 167, 797–798.

Uzal, F.J., Paulson, D., Eigenheer, A.L. and Walker, R.L. (2007) *Malassezia slooffiae*-associated dermatitis in a goat. *Veterinary Dermatology* 18, 348–352.

van der Burgt, G. (2010) *Mycobacterium bovis* causing clinical disease in adult sheep. *Veterinary Record* 166, 306.

Wessels, M.E., Payne, J., Willmington, J.A., Bell, S.J. and Davies, I.H. (2010) *Yersinia pseudotuberculosis* as a cause of ocular disease in goats. *Veterinary Record* 166, 699–670.

Wilsmore, A. (1989) Birth injury and perinatal loss in lambs. *In Practice* 11, 239–243.

Index

_____

Actinobacillosis 29, 230
Actinomycosis 29, 230
acute lameness
    arthrogryposis 204
    fractures 204
    infectious mycoplasma lameness 205
    Osteochondrosis 205
    slipped epiphysis, femoral head 205
    splay leg 205
African swine fever (ASF) 187, 224, 225
anaesthesia
    cattle 36, 53, 54–5, 61, 62, 69, 70, 73
    pigs 197, 198, 199
    poultry 207, 221
    SAC 165, 166, 167, 168, 170, 171, 175, 177
    sheep and goats 99, 121, 122, 123, 131, 133,
        134, 135, 139
    see also general anaesthesia
analgesia
    cattle 54
    pig 198
    poultry 207, 221
    SAC 166
    sheep and goat 122
Anaplasmosis 43
Animal erysipelas 231
anthrax 231
ASF, *see* African swine fever (ASF)
Aspergillosis 41, 215–16
Aujeszky's disease 224, 225
avian influenza 221–2, 223, 224
avian tuberculosis (TB) 216

Babesiosis 43–4
bacterial zoonotic diseases 230–3

BEF, *see* bovine ephemeral fever (BEF)
Besnoitosis 50
bluetongue disease 145–6, 223, 224
bluetongue virus (BTV) 83
BMC, *see* bovine malignant catarrh (BMC)
botulism 231
bovine ephemeral fever (BEF) 49
bovine malignant catarrh (BMC) 28
bovine papular stomatitis 49
bovine progressive degenerative
        myeloencephalopathy (BPDME) 71–2
bovine respiratory disease (BRD) 39–40
bovine spongiform encephalopathy (BSE) 35,
    223, 224
bovine viral diarrhoea virus (BVDV) 45
bovine viral diarrhoea (BVD) 29, 146, 159–60
BPDME, *see* bovine progressive degenerative
        myeloencephalopathy (BPDME)
BRD, *see* bovine respiratory disease (BRD)
Brucella abortus 224, 225
Brucella melitensis 224, 225
Brucella ovis 224, 225
Brucellosis 231
BSE, *see* bovine spongiform
        encephalopathy (BSE)
BTV, *see* bluetongue virus (BTV)
BVD, *see* bovine viral diarrhoea (BVD)
BVDV, *see* bovine viral diarrhoea virus (BVDV)

CAE, *see* Caprine arthritis encephalitis (CAE)
Campylobacter coli 30
Campylobacteriosis 231
Campylobacter jejuni 30
Caprine arthritis encephalitis (CAE) 97
caseous lymphadenitis (CLA) 113, 162

cattle medicines
    anti-inflammatory preparations 8–9
    antimicrobials
        bolus/tablet to calves, oral products 14
        injectables 10–14
        oral products, drinking water, milk or
            milk replacer 14–15
        topical products 15
    antiprotozoals 15
    cardiovascular and respiratory
        preparations 15
    circulatory system 42–4
    clinical examination 27–8
    common causes of cattle death 53
    dietary supplements and fluid
        metabolites 15–16
    diseases, gastroenteric system, *see*
        Gastroenteric diseases, cattle
    fat necrosis 33
    iatrogenic causes, sudden death 53
    liver diseases 33
    locomotory system 49–53
    metabolic diseases, *see* metabolic diseases, cattle
    mixed anti-inflammatory and antimicrobial
        preparations 9–10
    neurological system, *see* neurological diseases
    pathogenic causes, diarrhoea 33
    reproductive system, *see* reproductive
        system, cattle
    respiratory system, *see* respiratory diseases, cattle
    urinary system 44
cattle surgery
    anaesthesia 54–6
    analgesia 54
    euthanasia 80–1
    gastroenteric system, *see* gastroenteric system
    integument
        bull ring insertion 78
        dehorning, adults 78–9
        disbudding 79
        tail amputation 79–80
    locomotory system 72–8
    neurological system 62–3
    reproductive system, *see* reproductive system
    sedation 54
    urinary system, *see* urinary system
CCN, *see* cerebrocortical necrosis (CCN)
CCPP, *see* contagious caprine pleuropneumonia (CCPP)
cerebrocortical necrosis (CCN) 15, 34, 93, 97
chemical euthanasia
        cattle 80, 81
        pig 206
        poultry 222
        SAC 181
        sheep and goat 142
chemical poisoning
    arsenic 215

    copper 215
    herbicides 215
    insecticides 215
    lead 215
    mercury 215
    molluscicides 215
    Newcastle disease 215
    phosphides 215
chlamydial and rickettsial
    zoonotic diseases
    avian chlamydiosis 233
    chlamydiosis 233
    Q fever 234
Chorioptes caprae 116
Chorioptic mange 51
chronic lameness
    hoof abscess 205
    ligament damage 205
    septic arthritis 205
circulatory diseases
    cattle
        anthrax 42
        bleeding disorders 42
        bovine leucosis 42
        bovine petechial fever 42
        Cor pulmonale 42
        dilated cardiomyopathy 43
        endocarditis 43
        heartwater 43
        lightning strike 43
        lyme disease 43
        Mycoplasma wenyonii 43
        protozoa and treatment 43–4
    haemopoietic and lymphatic systems
        Babesiosis 106
        Theileriosis 106
        tick-borne fever 106
    heartwater 105
    poisonous plants 105
    rupture, aorta 105–6
    Schistosomiasis 106
    vegetative endocarditis 106
circulatory system
    cardiovascular system
        iliac arterial thrombosis 157
        vegetative endocarditis 158
        ventricular septal defects 158
        viral myocarditis 158
        white muscle disease 158
    chickens
        fatal haemorrhage, turkeys 217
        heart attack 217
        infectious anaemia 217
        sodium toxicity 217
        vitamin K deficiency 217
    haemopoietic and lymphatic systems
        Anaplasmosis 158

Babesiosis 158
Mycoplasma haemolamae 158
CLA, *see* caseous lymphadenitis (CLA)
classical swine fever (CSF) 187, 224, 225
clostridial diseases 30–1, 146–7
clostridial food poisoning 231
clostridial wound infections 231
CODD, *see* contagious ovine digital
    dermatitis (CODD)
Colibacillosis 231–2
contagious agalactia 224, 225
contagious bovine pleuropneumonia 224, 225
contagious caprine pleuropneumonia
    (CCPP) 103
contagious ovine digital dermatitis (CODD) 136
cornual block 55
coronavirus 29
Corynebacteriosis 232
CSF, *see* classical swine fever (CSF)

demodectic mange 51
Demodex caprae 116
Dermanyssus gallinae 51
Dermatophilosis 114, 232
Dermatophytosis 51
diseases, integument
    bacterial skin diseases
        actinobacillosis 113
        Actinomycetic mycetoma 113
        CLA 113
        Clostridial cellulitis 113–14
        Dermatophilosis 114
        fleece rot 114
        Morel's disease 114
        Nocardiosis 114
        Periorbital eczema 114
        scald 114
        Staphylococcal dermatitis 114–15
        Staphylococcal folliculitis 115
    fungal skin diseases
        Cryptococcosis 115
        Malassezia dermatitis 115
        Phaeohyphomycosis 115
        Pythiosis 115
        ringworm 115
    inherited skin diseases
        redfoot 111–12
        sticky goat syndrome 112
    neoplastic conditions 120
    parasitic skin diseases,
        sheep and goats
        flies and insects 117–18
        mites 116–17
    physical causes 119
    protozoal skin diseases
        Besnoitosis 115–16

Leishmaniasis 116
Sarcocystosis 116
skin, aetiology 120
toxic causes 119–20
viral skin diseases
    Caprine herpesvirus 112
    Caprine viral dermatitis 112
    Contagious pustular dermatitis 112
    goat pox 112
    Venereal orf 112–13
    Vesicular stomatitis 113
vitamin- and mineral-related skin 118–19
domestic poultry medicine and surgery
    anaesthesia 221
    analgesia 221
    animal husbandry, chickens
        healthy 207–8
        medication 210
        nutrition 208–9
        vaccination 209–10
    circulatory system, *see* circulatory
        system, chickens
    euthanasia 222
    gastroenteric system, *see* gastroenteric
        system, chickens
    integument, *see* integument, chickens
    locomotory system, *see* locomotory
        system, chickens
    miscellaneous systemic diseases 220
    neurological system, *see* neurological
        system, chickens
    notifiable diseases, *see* neurological
        system, chickens
    respiratory system, *see* respiratory
        system, chickens
    sedation 221
    surgical conditions and procedures
        cloacal prolapse 221
        crop evacuation 221
        egg-bound birds 221
        orchidectomy 221
        penile prolapse 221–2
        salpingohysterectomy 222
    urinary system, *see* urinary system, chickens

EAE, *see* enzootic abortion of ewes (EAE)
ectoparasites, chickens
    Cnemidocoptes gallinae 219
    Dermanyssus gallinae 219
    Echidnophaga gallinacea 219
    Holomenopon spp. 219
    Menopon gallinae 219
    Ornithonyssus sylvarum 219
egg drop syndrome 220
egg eating 220
egg peritonitis 220

EHV, *see* equine herpesvirus (EHV)
enteric diseases, cattle
    abomasal ulcers 32
    bacteria and treatment
        Actinobacillosis 29
        Actinomycosis 29
        calf diphtheria 30
        Campylobacter jejuni and *Campylobacter
            coli* 30
        clostridial disease 30–1
        E. coli 31
        Johne's disease 31
        Salmonellosis 31
    causes 28
    cleft palate 33
    congenital erythropoietic porphyria 33
    jejunal haemorrhagic syndrome 33
    parasites
        Fasciolisis 32
        PGE 32
    protozoa and treatment
        Candida albicans 31
        Coccidiosis 31–2
        Cryptosporidium parvum 32
    vagal indigestion 33
    viruses and treatment
        bluetongue disease 28
        BMC 28
        bovine papular stomatitis 28–9
        BVD 29
        coronavirus 29
        FMD 29
        rotavirus 29
enteric diseases, gastroenteric system
    bacteria
        clostridial diseases 146–7
        E.coli 147
        Johne's disease 147
    parasites
        intestinal cestodes 148–9
        nematodes 149
        trematodes 149
    protozoa
        Coccidiosis 147–8
        Cryptosporidiosis 148
        giardia 148
    viruses
        bluetongue disease 145–6
        BVD 146
        coronavirus 146
        FMD 146
        MCF 146
        rotavirus 146
enteric diseases, pig
    bacteria
        Campylobacter enteritis 184
        clostridial diarrhoea 184

        Escherichia coli diarrhoea 184–5
        Helicobacter pylori 185
        proliferative enteropathy 185
        Salmonellosis 185
        swine dysentery 185
        Yersinia 185
    causes 183
    endoparasites
        Ascaris suum 186
        control and resistance to
            anthelmintics 186
        Hyostrongylus rubidus 186
        Oesophagostomum dentatum and
            O. quadrispinulatum 186
        trichuris suis 186
    intestinal haemorrhagic syndrome 186
    poisons 186
    protozoa
        Coccidiosis 185–6
        Cryptosporidiosis 186
    viruses
        epidemic diarrhoea 183
        FMD 183–4
        rotavirus 184
        TGE 184
        vomiting wasting disease 184
enteric diseases, sheep and goat
    bacteria and treatment
        Bacillary haemoglobinuria 84
        blackleg 84
        Black's disease 84
        botulism 84
        braxy 84
        E.coli 85
        enterotoxaemia 85
        Johne's disease 85
        lamb dysentery 85
        malignant oedema 85
        Sordellii abomasitis 85–6
        struck 86
        tetanus 86
    BTV 83
    causes 82
    gastric disorders 89–90
    liver 90–1
    pancreas 91
    parasites and treatment
        intestinal cestodes 87
        intestinal nematodes 87–9
        trematodes 89
    protozoa and treatment
        coccidiosis 86
        cryptosporidiosis 86–7
        giardia 87
    viruses and treatment
        BTV 83
        FMD 83

MCF 83
NSD 83
PPR 84
rotavirus 84
Enterocolitic yersiniosis 232
entropion 126
enzootic abortion of ewes (EAE) 108
Enzootic bovine leucosis 225
epidural block 55
equine herpesvirus (EHV) 153, 160
Erysipelas 220
Escherichia coli (E. coli) 31
euthanasia
    cattle 33, 38, 40, 80
    captive bolt pistol 141–2
    chemical 142
    chickens
        neck dislocation 222
        triple-strength barbiturate injection 222
    firearm, free bullet 141
    pig 206
    poultry 222
    SAC 181
    sheep and goats 141
eye disorders 155

failure of passive transfer (FPT) 160
FMD, *see* foot-and-mouth disease (FMD)
foot-and-mouth disease (FMD)
    notifiable diseases 223, 224
    pig 183–4, 194
    zoonotic diseases 229
FPT, *see* failure of passive transfer (FPT)
fungal zoonotic diseases
    Dermatophytosis 234
    ringworm 234

GA, *see* general anaesthesia (GA)
gastric disorders
    acidosis 89–90
    bloat 90
    gastritis 90
    rumen atony 90
    rumen impaction 90
gastroenteric diseases
    cattle
        diagnosis 28
        enteric diseases, *see* enteric diseases, cattle
        predominant signs 28
    sheep and goat
        diagnosis 82
        enteric diseases, *see* enteric diseases
        predominant signs 82
gastroenteric system
    Actinobacillosis, oesophagus 57

bloat, choke 57–8
bloat without choke
    chronic bracken poisoning 58
    fore-stomach obstruction 58
    frothy bloat 58
    tetanus 58
    Traumatic reticulitis 58
chickens
    intestinal diseases, *see* intestinal
        diseases, chickens
    miscellaneous diseases,
        enteric tract 214–15
    predominant signs 211
congenital and hereditary conditions
    Atresia coli 145
    mega-oesophagus 145
enteric diseases, *see* enteric diseases,
    gastroenteric system
intestinal torsion 58–9
intussusception 59
LDA, *see* left-sided displacement
    of the abomasum (LDA)
left-sided volvulus, abomasum 60
liver abscess 60
mediastinum 57
pig
    diagnosis 183
    enteric diseases, *see* enteric diseases, pig
    infection mode 183
    predominant signs 182
    prevention 183
ptyalism and pseudoptyalism 145
RDA, *see* right-sided displacement of the
    abomasum (RDA)
rectal prolapse 61
SAC
    choanal atresia 168
    congenital and hereditary conditions 168
    fracture, mandible 168
    problems, teeth 169
    prolapsed rectum 169
    umbilical hernia 170
stomachs and intestines
    anatomy 149–50
    colic 150–1
    diagnosis 150
    gastric ulceration 151–2
    gastroliths 152
    grain overload 152
    liver 152
    spiral colon impaction 152
    surgical and medical cases 150
swellings, soft tissue 145
general anaesthesia (GA)
    cattle 53, 54 55
    hypothermia 123
    inhalation 122

general anaesthesia (GA) (*continued*)
    pigs 188, 197
    regurgitation, rumen contents 122
    SAC 166, 167, 168
    sheep and goats 121, 122
goat pox 225
gumboro disease 220

haemorrhagic enteritis 220
hepatic encephalopathy 155
hermaphroditism 110
herpes mammillitis 49
hypocalcaemia 155
hypoglycaemia 155
hypomagnesaemia 155

integument
    bacterial skin diseases 162
    cattle
        bacterial skin diseases 50
        frostbite 52
        fungal skin diseases 51
        mast cell tumour 52
        nutritional skin diseases 52
        parasitic skin diseases 51
        photosensitization 52
        protozoal skin diseases 50
        subcutaneous emphysema 52–3
        urticaria 53
        viral skin diseases 49–50
    chickens
        ectoparasites 219
        miscellaneous skin diseases 220
    fungal skin diseases 163
    neoplastic conditions 164–5
    parasitic skin diseases 163
    physical causes, skin disease 164
    pig
        causes 195
        skin diseases, *see* skin diseases, pig
        systemic diseases 195
    skin diseases, uncertain aetiology 165
    viral skin diseases 161–2
    vitamin and mineral related skin diseases 163–4
intestinal diseases, chickens
    bacteria
        avian cholera 211
        Campylobacter jejuni 212
        Escherichia coli 212
        necrotic enteritis 212
        Salmonellosis 212
        Yersinia pseudotuberculosis 212
    nematode
        amidostomum anseris 213
        ascaridia galli 213

Capillaria spp. 213
        echinuria uncinata 213
        heterakis gallinarum 213
        treatment 213–214
        Trichostrongylus tenuis 213
    protozoa
        coccidiosis 212
        Cryptosporidium spp. 212–13
        hexamita 213
        Histomoniasis 213
        trichomonas 213
    virus
        coronaviral enteritis 211
        duck viral enteritis 211
        fowlpox 211
        goose viral hepatitis 211
        haemorrhagic nephritis enteritis, geese 211
        hepatitis 211
        Newcastle disease 211
        rotavirus 211
intestinal nematodes
    anthelmintics 87
    grazing methods 88
    Haemonchus contortus infection 88, 89
intestinal obstruction, pig
    causes 199
    clinical signs 199–200
    foreign body, intussusception/volvulus 200
    inguinal hernia 200
    umbilical hernia 200
inverted L block 55

Johne's disease 31, 147

lameness
    adult sheep and goats
        CODD 136
        excess granulation tissue 136
        foot abscesses 136–7
        foot rot 137
        interdigital hyperplasia 137
        scald 137
        soil balling 137–8
        strawberry foot rot 138
        white line abscesses 138
    lambs and kids
        joint ill 138
        laminitis 137
        post-dipping septic arthritis 137
        swayback 137
        tetanus 137
        white muscle disease 137
LDA, *see* left-sided displacement
        of the abomasum (LDA)
left-sided displacement of the abomasum (LDA)
    description 59

double-flank surgical method 59
medical treatment 59
rolling 59–60
single-flank surgical method 59
toggling 60
ventral body wall stitching 60
leptospirosis 232
listeriosis 232
liver diseases, sheep and goat
abscesses 90
Black's disease 90
fascioliasis 90
plant toxicity 90
RVF 90–1
tumours 91
locomotory diseases, cattle
rickets 49
viral diseases 49
locomotory system
BPDME 72
carpal bursitis 72
chickens
angel wing 218
avian encephalomyelitis 218
bumblefoot 218
deformities 218–19
fractures 219
Marek's disease 219
rickets 219
splay leg 219
contracted tendons 72
digital dermatitis 72
digit removal 75–6
flying scapulas 72
'foul in the foot' 72
fracture, sacral/coccygeal vertebrae 73
hip dislocation 73
hock bursitis 73
interdigital hyperplasia 73–4
joint ill 74
lameness
adult sheep and goats 136–7
lambs and kids 137–8
laminitis 74
limbs
flying scapula 139
fractures 139
OCD 74
osteomyelitis 74
pedal bone, fracture 73
pig
acute lameness 204–5
chronic lameness 205
recumbency 205
progressive ataxia 74
progressive myelopathy 74–5
recumbent/downer cow 75

rupture, gastrocnemius muscle 76
SAC
angular limb deformity 178–9
bilateral luxating patellae 179
digital amputation 179
dropped pasterns 179
flying scapula 180
fractures 180
scapulo-humeral joint luxation 180
sequestrations 180
spondylosis 180
tendon contraction 180–1
sacroiliac luxation 76
sand cracks 76
septic pedal arthritis 76
shoulder bursitis 76
small ruminants 139–40
sole ulcer 77
spastic paresis 77
spastic syndrome 77
spinal muscular atrophy 77
stifle joint damage 77
stone, foot 77
'street nail operation' 77
super foul 77
white line infection 77–8
lower limb block 55
lumpy skin disease 49, 225

malignant catarrhal fever
(MCF) 83, 146, 161–2
Marek's disease 219
MCF, *see* malignant catarrhal fever (MCF)
meliodosis 232
metabolic diseases
cattle
acetonaemia 37
acidosis 37
hypocalcaemia 37–8
hypomagnesaemia 38
hypophosphataemia 38
predominant signs 37
trace element deficiencies 38–9
hepatic encephalopathy 155
hypocalcaemia 155
hypoglycaemia 155
hypomagnesaemia 155
pig
copper deficiency myelopathy 190
hypoglycaemi 190
osteomalacia 190
vitamin A deficiency 190
vitamin B deficiency 190
sheep and goat
diagnosis 100
hypocalcaemia 100

metabolic diseases (*continued*)
    hypomagnesaemia 100–101
    ketosis 101
    predominant signs 100
  uraemic encephalopathy 155
miscellaneous skin diseases, chickens
  breast blisters 220
  feather pecking 220
  flank wounds 220
miscellaneous systemic diseases, chickens
  egg drop syndrome 220
  egg eating 220
  egg peritonitis 220
  Erysipelas 220
  gumboro disease 220
  haemorrhagic enteritis 220
myiasis 51

Nairobi sheep disease (NSD) 83
nasal myiasis 156
necrobacillosis 232
neurological diseases
  adult cattle
    Aujeszky's disease 35
    BSE 35
    listeria monocytogenes 35
    nervous acetonaemia 35
    obturator nerve damage 35–6
    rabies 36
    sciatic nerve damage 36
  adult sheep
    botulism 95
    cervical injury 95
    fibronecrotizing pachymeningitis 95
    heartwater 95
    listeriosis 95
    Maedi-Visna (MV) 95–6
    scrapie 96
    spinal abscess 97
  by bacteria
    abscesses 188
    Actinobacillosis 188
    bowel oedema 188
    haemophilus parasuis meningitis 188
    Leptospirosis 188
    listeriosis 188
    middle ear infection 188
    Salmonellosis 188
    streptococcal meningitis 189
    tetanus 189
  Border disease 91
  calves
    bacterial meningitis 34
    brain abscess 34
    CCN 34
    femoral nerve damage 34

    lead poisoning 35
    middle ear infection 35
    radial paralysis 35
  cerebellar hypoplasia 91
  CNS, birth 92
  Dandy–Walker malformation 91
  eye conditions 99–100
  goats
    Border disease 97
    CAE 97
    CCN 97
    listeriosis 97–8
    scrapie 98
    spinal abscess 97
    swayback 98
  growing lambs
    CCN 93
    gid 93–4
    lead poisoning 94
    louping ill 94
    plant poisoning 94
    ryegrass staggers 94
    Sarcocystosis 94
    spinal abscess 94
    tetanus 95
  hereditary chondrodysplasia 91
  hypoglycaemia 91–2
  Myodystrophia foetalis deformans 92
  neonatal lambs and kids
    congenital cataracts 98
    microphthalmia 98
    split eyelid syndrome 98
    trauma 98–9
  ocular conditions
    Besnoitosis 36
    bovine iritis 36
    congenital cataracts 36
    foreign bodies 36
    Horner's syndrome 36
    infectious bovine
      keratoconjunctivitis 36–7
    squamous cell carcinoma,
      third eyelid 37
    Thelazia spp. 37
    vitamin A deficiency 37
  by poisoning
    arsenic 189
    congenital tremor 189
    iron toxicity 189
    metaldehyde 189
    nitrite/nitrate poisoning 189
    salt poisoning 189
    selenium poisoning 189
  swayback 92
  unweaned lambs
    delayed swayback 93
    Listeriosis 93

meningitis/encephalitis 93
spinal abscess 93
tetanus 93
tick pyaemia 93
by viruses
ASF 187
Aujeszky's disease 187
CSF 187
rabies 187
SVD 187
Talfan disease 187
Teschen disease 187–8
neurological system
chickens
blue-green algal poisoning 215
botulism 215
chemical poisoning 215
congenital conditions
atlanto-occipital malalignment 152
hydrocephalus 152
kyphosis 152
entropion 126
enucleation eye
antibiotics 127
disease recovering 126
local anaesthetic 126
eye disorders 155
infectious diseases
EHV 153
listeriosis 153
louping ill 153
meningeal worms 153
otitis media 153
protozoal meningitis 153
rabies 153
septic bacterial meningitis 153
WNV 153
miscellaneous conditions
facial paralysis 153
heat stroke 154
hypothermia 154
polioencephalomalacia 154
tumours, brain and spinal cord 154
musculoskeletal conditions 154
pig
bacteria 188–9
causes 187
Coccidiosis 189
diagnosis 187
heat stroke 189
poisoning 189
predominant signs 187
viruses 187–8
removal, eye 62–3
SAC
enucleation, eye 170
eye disorders 170

squamous-cell carcinoma 63
toxic conditions
botulism 154
ionophore toxicosis 154
ryegrass staggers 154
tetanus 154
traumatic conditions
cerebral hypoxia 154
fractured vertebrae 154–5
Newcastle disease 221, 223, 224
Nocardiosis 232
notifiable diseases
ASF 224, 225
Aujeszky's disease 224, 225
Brucella abortus 224, 225
Brucella melitensis 224, 225
Brucella ovis 224, 225
chickens
avian influenza 221–2
Newcastle disease 222
Contagious agalactia 224, 225
contagious bovine pleuropneumonia 224–5
CSF 224, 225
diseases monitored, UK
avian influenza 223, 224
bluetongue disease 223, 224
BSE 223
farm livestock 223, 224
FMD 223, 224
Newcastle disease 223, 224
rabies 223, 224
TB 223, 224
enzootic bovine leucosis 225
goat pox 225
lumpy skin disease 225
PPR 225
rift valley fever 225, 227
rinderpest 225, 227
scrapie 225, 227
sheep pox 225, 227
SVD 225, 227
Teschen disease 225, 227
vesicular stomatitis 225, 227
warble fly 225, 227
World Organisation for Animal
Health 226, 227
NSD, *see* Nairobi sheep disease (NSD)

OCD, *see* osteochondritis dissecans (OCD)
ocular disease, sheep and goat
infectious keratoconjunctivitis 99
Listeriosis 99–100
trauma 100
Yersiniosis 100
osteochondritis dissecans (OCD) 74
Ovine parainfluenza 3 (OPI3) 103

pancreatitis 91
parasitic gastroenteritis (PGE) 32
parasitic zoonotic diseases
    Acanthocephaliasis 234
    Ascariasis 234–5
    Clonorchiasis 235
    Coenurosis 235
    Dicrocoeliasis 235
    Echinostomiasis 235
    Fascioliasis 235
    Gastrodiscoidiasis 235
    Hydatidosis 235
    Linguatuliasis 235–6
    Myiasis 236
    Taeniasis and cysticercosis 236
    Trichinosis 236
    Trichostrongyliasis 236
    Tungiasis 236
    Zoonotic scabies 236
paravertebral block 55–6
Pasteurellosis 232
PDNS, *see* Porcine dermatitis and nephropathy
        syndrome (PDNS)
Pediculosis 51
peste des petits ruminants (PPR) 84, 225
PGE, *see* parasitic gastroenteritis (PGE)
pig medicines
    anti-inflammatory preparations 20–21
    antimicrobials
        injectables 21–3
        oral products, feed/drinking water 24
        oral products, mouth 24
        topical products 25
    cardiovascular and respiratory
            preparations 25
    clinical examination 182
    dietary supplements and fluid
            metabolites 25
    gastroenteric system, *see* gastroenteric
            system, pig
    iatrogenic causes, sudden death 196–7
    integument 195–6
    metabolic diseases 190
    neurological system, *see* neurological system, pig
    reproductive system, *see* reproductive
            system, pig
    respiratory system, *see* respiratory system, pig
    urinary system, *see* urinary system, pig
    vetrabutine 25
pig surgery
    anaesthesia
        epidural space 198
        GA, *see* general anaesthesia (GA), pig
    analgesia 198
    euthanasia 206
    sedation 198
    surgical conditions, *see* surgical conditions, pig

PMWS, *see* Post-weaning multi-systemic
        wasting syndrome (PMWS)
Porcine dermatitis and nephropathy
        syndrome (PDNS) 193, 195
Porcine reproductive and respiratory
        syndrome (PRRS) 191, 194
post-mortem (PM) 6
Post-weaning multi-systemic wasting
        syndrome (PMWS) 191
poultry medicines
    antimicrobials 26
    antiprotozoals 26
PPR, see Peste des petits ruminants (PPR)
protozoal zoonotic diseases
    Babesiosis 234
    Cryptosporidiosis 234
    Sarcocystosis 234
    Toxoplasmosis 234
PRRS, *see* Porcine reproductive and respiratory
        syndrome (PRRS)
pseudocowpox 50
Psoroptes Caprae 116
Psoroptes Ovis 116
psoroptic mange 51

rabies 223, 224
Raillietia Caprae 116
RDA, *see* right-sided displacement
        of the abomasum (RDA)
reproductive diseases
    female sheep
        caesarean section 131–2
        dystocia 129–31
        embryotomy 133–4
        induction, parturition 128–9
        lamb survival 132
        normal parturition 128
        prolapsed uterus 134
        prolapsed vagina 134
        reproductive ultrasonography 135
        retained placenta 132
        uterine torsion 132–3
    goats, females
        caesarean section 133
        dystocia 133
        embryotomy 133–4
        induction, parturition 133
        lamb survival 132
        normal parturition 133
        prolapsed uterus 134
        prolapsed vagina 134
        removal, supernumerary teats 134–5
        reproductive ultrasonography 135
    males
        castration (and tail docking) 135
        castration of animals, retained testicle 136

reproductive system
    abortion and causes
        Akabane 107
        Border disease 107
        Brucellosis 107
        Cache valley virus 107
        Campylobacteriosis 107–8
        Caprine herpesvirus 108
        concurrent disease 108
        EAE 108
        Leptospirosis 108
        Listeriosis 108
        Neosporosis 108
        nutritional causes 108
        Q fever 108–9
        rift Valley fever (RVF) 109
        Salmonellosis 109
        Sarcocystosis 109
        Schmallenburg virus (SBV) 109
        sporadic abortions 109
        Streptococcus pluranimalium 109
        stress 109–10
        Thogoto virus 110
        Tick-borne fever (TBF) 110
        Toxoplasmosis 110
    acquired infertility, females 161
    congenital and hereditary conditions in
            goats 110
    contagious agalactia 110–11
    disorders, goats
        clostridium septicum metritis 111
        false pregnancy 111
        maiden milkers 111
        oestrus 111
    embryonic death 160
    females
        antibiotics 65
        Caesarean section 65–6
        hung calf 66–7
        hydrops uteri 67
        post-partum arterial haemorrhage 68
        prolapsed cervix 67
        prolapsed uterus 67–8
        removal, supernumerary teats 69
        teat amputation 69
        teat lacerations 69
        teat obstructions 69
        transmissible viral
                fibropapillomatosis 69–70
        uterine abnormalities 70
        uterine torsion 68–9
    male infertility 161
    males
        castration 70–1
        corkscrew penis 71
        inguinal hernia 71
        persistent penile frenulum 71–2

    mammary gland 160
    mastitis 111
    nephritis 106
    tumours 111
reproductive system cattle
    abortion and causes
        akabane 44–5
        Arcanobacterium pyogenes 45
        Bacillus licheniformis 45
        Bovine herpesvirus 1 (BHV 1) 45
        Brucellosis 45
        BVDV 45
        Campylobacter foetus subsp.
                veneralis 45
        chlamydophila abortus 45
        Coxiella burnetii 45
        Leptospira icterohaemorrhagiae 45
        Leptospira serovar Hardjo 45–6
        Leptospira serovar pomona 46
        Listeria monocytogenes 46
        mycotic abortion 46
        Neospora caninum 46
        parachlamydia acanthamoeba 46
        Rift Valley fever 46
        Salmonellosis 46
        SBV 46
        ureaplasma diversum 47
        Wesselsbron disease 47
    endometritis 47
    mastitis
        contagious pathogens 47
        environmental pathogens 47–8
        summer mastitis 48
    mummified fetus 48
    pyometritis 48
    udder oedema 48–9
    udder rot 49
reproductive system pig
    Aujeszky's disease 193
    blue eye paramyxovirus 193
    Brucellosis 193
    carbon monoxide 193
    chronic mastitis 194–5
    erysipelas 193
    FMD 194
    Japanese B encephalitis virus 194
    Leptospirosis 194
    mycotoxins 194
    porcine circovirus 194
    porcine parvovirus 194
    PRRS 194
    Salmonella spp. 194
    SMEDI 194
    swine fever 194
    swine influenza 194
    Toxoplasmosis 194
    vitamin A deficiency 194

reproductive system SAC
    females
        dystocia 172–4
        fusion, vulval lips 174
        induction, parturition 172
        parturition 172
        persistent hymen and vaginal aplasia 174
        ultrasonography 175–7
        uterus 175
        vagina 175
    males
        castration 177
        inguinal hernia 178
        vasectomy 178
respiratory diseases, cattle
    anaphylaxis 41
    causes 39
    diagnosis 39
    fog fever 41
    fungi 41
    inhalation pneumonia 42
    lungworm (parasitic bronchitis) 41
    predominant signs 39
    viruses and bacteria and treatment
        bovine tuberculosis 40
        BRD 39–40
        CBPP 41
        shipping fever complex 41
respiratory diseases, sheep and goat
    bacteria, lower respiratory tract
        CCPP 103
        Histophilus somni 103
        Mannheimia haemolytica 103–4
        mycoplasmas 104
        Pasteurella multocida 104
        TB 104–5
    lower respiratory tract, non-infectious
        conditions
        aspiration pneumonia 102
        ruptured diaphragm 103
        squamous cell carcinoma 103
        thymomas 103
        winter cough 103
    non-infectious conditions, upper
        respiratory tract
        chondritis, larynx 101
        collar trauma 102
        nasal foreign bodies 102
        nasal tumours 102
    parasitic pneumonia 104–5
    upper respiratory tract, infectious conditions
        enzootic nasal adenocarcinoma 102
        nasal leeches 102
        nasal myiasis 102
        retropharyngeal lymph node abscesses 102
        rhinitis 102
    viruses, lower respiratory tract
        Jaagsiekte 103

OPI3 103
Ovine pulmonary adenomatosis 103
respiratory system
    chickens
        Aspergillosis 215–16
        Avian chlamydiosis 216
        avian infectious laryngotracheitis 216
        coryza 216
        infectious bronchitis 216
        influenza 216
        leeches 216
        Mycoplasmosis 216
        ornithobacterium rhinotracheale 217
        Pasteurellosis 217
        swollen head syndrome 217
        TB 216
        turkey rhinotracheitis 217
    infectious conditions, upper tract 156
    lower tract, infectious conditions
        lungworms 157
        pneumonia 157
        streptococcus equi 157
        TB 157
    non-infectious conditions, lower tract
        aspiration pneumonia 156
        diaphragmatic paralysis 156
        drowning 156
        pleural effusion 156
        trauma 156
    upper tract, non-infectious conditions
        hyperplasia, soft palate 155
        rhinitis 155–6
respiratory system, pig
    bacteria
        Actinobacillosis 191
        atrophic rhinitis 191–2
        enzootic pneumonia 192
        Glasser's disease 192
        Pasteurellosis 192
    causes 191
    diagnosis 190
    endoparasites
        Ascaris 192
        metastrongylus 192
    infection mode 191
    predominant signs 190
    prevention 191
    viruses
        inclusion body rhinitis 191
        PMWS 191
        PRRS 191
        swine influenza 191
    warfarin poisoning 192
retrobulbar block 56
Rift Valley fever (RVF) 90–1, 109, 225, 277
right-sided displacement of the
    abomasum (RDA)
    medical treatment, cows 61

rumenotomy 61
torsion, caecum 61–2
umbilical hernia 62
rinderpest 225, 277
rotavirus 29

SAC medicine, *see* South American Camelid (SAC)
    medicine
Salmonellosis 31, 232–3
Sarcoptes Scabiei 116–17
sarcoptic mange 51–2
SBV, *see* Schmallenburg virus (SBV)
Schmallenburg virus (SBV) 46, 109
scrapie 225, 277
sheep and goat medicines
    circulatory system, *see* circulatory diseases
    dead animals 121
    eye conditions 99–100
    gastroenteric system, *see* gastroenteric
        diseases, sheep and goat
    iatrogenic causes, sudden death 120–1
    metabolic diseases 100–1
    neurological system, *see* neurological diseases
sheep and goat surgery
    diseases, urinary system 127–8
    euthanasia 140–1
    GA 122–3
    gastroenteric tract
        atresia ani 123
        atresia recti 123
        cheek tooth removal 123–4
        colic 124
        fractured mandible 124
        incisor removal 124–5
        intussusception 125
        prolapsed rectum 125
        rumen cannularization 125
        rumenotomy 125–6
    integument
        animals, rudimentary horn stubs 140
        disbudding, kids 140
        removal, adult horns 140–1
        tail docking, adult sheep 141
    locomotory system 136–40
    neurological system 126–7
    regional anaesthesia
        epidural 123
        lower limb 123
    reproductive system, *see* reproductive diseases
sheep medicines
    anti-inflammatory preparations 17
    antimicrobials
        injectables 17–19
        oral products, mouth 19
        topical products 19
    clenbuterol 20
    dietary supplements and fluid metabolites 19–20

sheep pox 225, 277
skin diseases
    bacteria
        Actinobacillosis 162
        Actinomycosis 162
        CLA 162
        clostridial cellulitis 162
        Dermatophilosis 162
        necrotic dermatitis 162
        periorbital eczema 162
        staphylococcal folliculitis 162
    fungus 163
    neoplastic conditions 164–5
    parasite
        blowfly strike 163
        lice 163
        mites 163
    pemphigus foliaceus 165
    physical causes
        frostbite 164
        photosensitization 164
        sunburn 164
        trauma 164
    virus
        bluetongue disease 161
        contagious pustular dermatitis 161
        FMD 161
        MCF 161–2
    vitamin and mineral
        cobalt deficiency 163
        copper deficiency 163
        iodism 164
        sulfur deficiency 164
        vitamin A, C, E deficiency 164
        zinc deficiency 164
skin diseases, pig
    bacteria
        erysipelas 195
        greasy disease 195
        PDNS 195
    miscellaneous causes
        bite wounds 196
        dermatosis vegetans 196
        epitheliogenesis imperfecta 196
        frostbite 196
        pityriasis rosea 196
        pressure sores 196
        sunburn 196
        thrombocytopenic purpura 196
    nutritional problems
        biotin deficiency 196
        parakeratosis 196
    parasites
        flies 196
        lice 196
        sarcoptic mange 196
ringworm 195
swinepox 195

SMEDI, *see* stillbirths, mummification, embryonic
    deaths and infertility (SMEDI)
South American Camelid (SAC) medicine
    animal husbandry
        behavioural problems 144–5
        classification 143–4
        normal behaviour 144
    circulatory system, *see* circulatory system
    clinical examination 145
    description 143
    gastroenteric system, *see* gastroenteric system
    iatrogenic 165
    integument, *see* integument
    metabolic diseases, *see* metabolic diseases
    neurological system, *see* neurological system
    reproductive system, *see* reproductive system
    respiratory system, *see* respiratory system
    sudden deaths 165
    urinary system, *see* urinary system
South American Camelid (SAC) surgery
    analgesia 166
    antibiotic cover 166
    euthanasia 181
    GA, *see* general anaesthesia (GA), SAC
    regional anaesthesia 168
    sedation
        acepromazine 167
        diazepam 167
        xylazine 167
    surgical conditions, *see* surgical
        conditions, SAC
    tetanus cover 166
stillbirths, mummification, embryonic deaths and
    infertility (SMEDI) 194
surgical conditions, pig
    gastroenteric system
        atresia ani 198
        gastric torsion 198
        intestinal obstruction, *see* intestinal
            obstruction, pig
        prolapsed rectum 201, 202
        tooth problems 201, 202
        ulceration 198
    integument
        bites 205–6
        burns 206
        cuts 206
        haematomas 206
    locomotory system, *see* locomotory
        system, pig
    males reproductive system 204
    reproductive system, females
        after parturition 204
        parturition 203
    urinary system
        preputial damage 201–2
        retroversion, bladder 202

surgical conditions, SAC
    gastroenteric system 168–70
    locomotory system 179–81
    neurological system 171
    reproductive system 172–9
    urinary system 171–2
SVD, *see* swine vesicular disease (SVD)
swine vesicular disease (SVD) 187, 225, 230, 277
Swollen head syndrome 217

Talfan disease 187
TAT, *see* tetanus antitoxin (TAT)
TB, *see* tuberculosis (TB)
teat blocks 56
Teschen disease 187–8, 225, 277
tetanus antitoxin (TAT) 30–1
TGE, *see* transmissible gastroenteritis (TGE)
theileriosis 44
tick-borne fever (TBF) 110
tick infestation 52
trace element deficiencies
    cobalt deficiency 38
    copper deficiency 38–9
    iodine deficiency 39
    selenium deficiency 39
transmissible gastroenteritis (TGE) 183, 184
trematodes 89
Trombicula Autumnalis 117
trypanosomiasis 44
tuberculosis (TB)
    notifiable diseases 223, 224
    zoonotic 233
tularaemia 233

uraemic encephalopathy 155
urinary diseases
    nephritis 106
    nephrosis 106
    tumours 107
urinary system
    cattle
        post-parturient haemoglobinuria 44
        pyelonephritis 44
        renal amyloidosis 44
    chickens
        eimeria truncata 217–18
        nephritis 218
        nephrosis 218
        vent gleet 218
        visceral gout 218
    congenital and hereditary conditions 158
    infected urachus 63
    medical conditions
        nephritis 158
        prostatitis 159

pig
    bacteria 193
    diagnosis 192
    infection mode 192
    predominant sign 192
    urolithiasis 193
prolapsed prepuce 63–4
rupture, penis 64
SAC
    persistent patent urachus 171
    ruptured bladder 171–2
    urethral obstruction 172
urethrostomy 64
urethrotomy 64–5
urinary calculi 65

vesicular stomatitis 50, 225, 277
veterinary equipment
    dentistry
        dental elevators 4
        dental picks 4
        dental rasps 4
        drinkwater gag 4
        headlight 4
        molar extraction forceps 4
        molar spreaders 4
        mouthwashing syringe 4
        small ruminant gag 4
    diagnosis 1–2
    eyes
        fluorescein strips 4
        ophthalmoscope 4
    feet
        gutter tape 3
        hoof knife 3
        hoof trimmers 3
        small sheep-size hoof clippers 3
    handling 1
    limbs
        bandages and dressings 3
        oscillating saw 3
        splints 3
    reproductive system 6–7
    stitching
        artery forceps 5
        clippers 5
        drapes 5
        dressing forceps 5
        dressing scissors 5
        needle holders 5
        scalpel blades 5
        scalpel handle 5
        small ruminant gag 4
        stitch-cutting scissors 5
        suture material 5
        suture needles 5–6

        tissue forceps 6
        towel clips 6
    treatment 2–3
veterinary medicines
    cattle, *see* cattle medicines
    pig, *see* pig medicines
    poultry 26
    sheep 17–21
viral zoonotic diseases
    bovine popular stomatitis 229
    bovine spongiform encephalopathy 229
    contagious pustular dermatitis 229
    cowpox 229
    Crimean-Congo haemorrhagic
        fever 229
    encephalomyocarditis 229
    FMD 229
    goat pox 229
    influenza 229
    Japanese B encephalitis 229
    louping ill 229
    Newcastle disease 229
    rabies 229–30
    Rift Valley fever 230
    rotaviral gastroenteritis 230
    Russian and Central European spring-
        summer encephalitis 230
    scrapie 230
    SVD 230
    vesicular stomatitis 230
    Wesselsbron disease 230
    West Nile fever 230

warble fly 225, 277
warble fly infestation 52
Wesselsbron disease 47, 230
West Nile virus (WNV) 153, 230
white muscle disease 158
WNV, *see* West Nile virus (WNV)

Yersiniosis 233

zoonotic diseases
    bacterial, *see* bacterial zoonotic diseases
    chlamydial and rickettsial, *see* chlamydial
        and rickettsial zoonotic diseases
    description 228
    fungal, *see* fungal zoonotic diseases
    milk/meat, obligation 228
    parasitic, *see* parasitic zoonotic diseases
    protozoal, *see* protozoal zoonotic diseases
    veterinarians 228
    viral, *see* viral zoonotic diseases
zoonotic tuberculosis 233